Dietary Reference Intakes: Recommended Intakes for Individuals: Vitamins

Life Stage Group	Vitamin A (μg/day)[a]	Vitamin C (mg/day)	Vitamin D (μg/day)[b,c]	Vitamin E (mg/day)[d]	Vitamin K (μg/day)	Thiamin (mg/day)	Riboflavin (mg/day)	Niacin (mg/day)[e]	Vitamin B6 (mg/day)	Folate (μg/day)[f]	Vitamin B12 (μg/day)	Pantothenic Acid (mg/day)	Biotin (μg/day)	Choline[g] (mg/day)
Infants														
0–6 mo	400*	40*	5*	4*	2.0*	0.2*	0.3*	2*	0.1*	65*	0.4*	1.7*	5*	125*
7–12 mo	500*	50*	5*	5*	2.5*	0.3*	0.4*	4*	0.3*	80*	0.5*	1.8*	6*	150*
Children														
1–3 y	**300**	**15**	5*	**6**	30*	**0.5**	**0.5**	**6**	**0.5**	**150**	**0.9**	2*	8*	200*
4–8 y	**400**	**25**	5*	**7**	55*	**0.6**	**0.6**	**8**	**0.6**	**200**	**1.2**	3*	12*	250*
Males														
9–13 y	**600**	**45**	5*	**11**	60*	**0.9**	**0.9**	**12**	**1.0**	**300**	**1.8**	4*	20*	375*
14–18 y	**900**	**75**	5*	**15**	75*	**1.2**	**1.3**	**16**	**1.3**	**400**	**2.4**	5*	25*	550*
19–30 y	**900**	**90**	5*	**15**	120*	**1.2**	**1.3**	**16**	**1.3**	**400**	**2.4**	5*	30*	550*
31–50 y	**900**	**90**	5*	**15**	120*	**1.2**	**1.3**	**16**	**1.3**	**400**	**2.4**	5*	30*	550*
51–70 y	**900**	**90**	10*	**15**	120*	**1.2**	**1.3**	**16**	**1.7**	**400**	**2.4**[h]	5*	30*	550*
> 70 y	**900**	**90**	15*	**15**	120*	**1.2**	**1.3**	**16**	**1.7**	**400**	**2.4**[h]	5*	30*	550*
Females														
9–13 y	**600**	**45**	5*	**11**	60*	**0.9**	**0.9**	**12**	**1.0**	**300**	**1.8**	4*	20*	375*
14–18 y	**700**	**65**	5*	**15**	75*	**1.0**	**1.0**	**14**	**1.2**	**400**[i]	**2.4**	5*	25*	400*
19–30 y	**700**	**75**	5*	**15**	90*	**1.1**	**1.1**	**14**	**1.3**	**400**[i]	**2.4**	5*	30*	425*
31–50 y	**700**	**75**	5*	**15**	90*	**1.1**	**1.1**	**14**	**1.3**	**400**[i]	**2.4**	5*	30*	425*
51–70 y	**700**	**75**	10*	**15**	90*	**1.1**	**1.1**	**14**	**1.5**	**400**	**2.4**[h]	5*	30*	425*
> 70 y	**700**	**75**	15*	**15**	90*	**1.1**	**1.1**	**14**	**1.5**	**400**	**2.4**[h]	5*	30*	425*
Pregnancy														
≤ 18 y	**750**	**80**	5*	**15**	75*	**1.4**	**1.4**	**18**	**1.9**	**600**[j]	**2.6**	6*	30*	450*
19–30 y	**770**	**85**	5*	**15**	90*	**1.4**	**1.4**	**18**	**1.9**	**600**[j]	**2.6**	6*	30*	450*
31–50 y	**770**	**85**	5*	**15**	90*	**1.4**	**1.4**	**18**	**1.9**	**600**[j]	**2.6**	6*	30*	450*
Lactation														
≤ 18 y	**1200**	**115**	5*	**19**	75*	**1.4**	**1.6**	**17**	**2.0**	**500**	**2.8**	7*	35*	550*
19–30 y	**1300**	**120**	5*	**19**	90*	**1.4**	**1.6**	**17**	**2.0**	**500**	**2.8**	7*	35*	550*
31–50 y	**1300**	**120**	5*	**19**	90*	**1.4**	**1.6**	**17**	**2.0**	**500**	**2.8**	7*	35*	550*

Note: This table (taken from the DRI reports, see www.nap.edu) presents Recommended Dietary Allowances (RDAs) in **bold** type and Adequate Intakes (AIs) in ordinary type followed by an asterisk (*). RDAs and AIs may both be used as goals for individual intakes. RDAs are set to meet the needs of almost all (97 to 98 percent) individuals in a group. For healthy breastfed infants, the AI is the mean intake. The AI for all other life stage and gender groups is believed to cover needs of all individuals in a group, but lack of data or uncertainty in the data prevent being able to specify with confidence the percentage of individuals covered by this intake.

[a]As retinol activity equivalents (RAEs). 1 RAE = 1 μg retinol, 12 μg β-carotene, 24 μg β-carotene, or 24 μg β-cryptoxanthin in foods. To calculate RAEs from REs of provitamin A carotenoids in foods, divide REs by 2. For preformed vitamin A in foods or supplements and for provitamin A carotenoid in supplements 1 RE = 1 RAE.

[b]Cholecalciferol. 1 μg cholecalciferol = 40 IU vitamin D.

[c]In the absence of exposure to adequate sunlight.

[d]As α-tocopherol, which includes RRR-α-tocopherol, the only form of α-tocopherol that occurs naturally in foods, and the 2R-stereoisomeric forms of α-tocopherol (RRR-, RSR-, and RSS-α-tocopherol). Does not include the 2S-stereoisomeric forms of α-tocopherol (SRR-, SSR-, SRS-, and SSS- α-tocopherol), also found in food and supplements.

[e]As niacin equivalents (NEs). 1 mg niacin = 60 mg tryptophan; 0–6 months = preformed niacin (not NE).

[f]As dietary folate equivalents (DFE) 1 DFE = 1 μg food folate = 0.6 μg folic acid from fortified food or as a supplement consumed with food = 0.5 μg of a supplement taken on an empty stomach.

[g]Although AIs have been set for choline, there are few data to assess whether a dietary supply of choline is needed at all stages of the lifecycle, and it may be that the choline requirement can be met by endogenous synthesis at some of these stages.

[h]Because 10–30% of older people may malabsorb food-bound B12, it is advisable for those older than 50 years to meet their RDA mainly by consuming foods fortified with B12 or a supplement containing B12.

[i]In view of evidence linking folate intake with neural tube defects in the fetus, it is recommended that all women capable of becoming pregnant consume 400 μg from supplements or fortified foods in addition to intake of food folate from a varied diet.

[j]It is assumed that women will consume 400 μg from supplements or fortified foods until their pregnancy is confirmed and they enter prenatal care, which ordina occurs after the end of the periconceptional period—the critical time for neural tube formation.

Source: Dietary Reference Intake Tables: The Complete Set. Institute of Medicine, National Academy of Sciences available online at www.nap.edu.

Dietary Reference Intakes: Recommended Intakes for Individuals: Minerals

Life Stage Group	Calcium (mg/day)	Chromium (μg/day)	Copper (μg/day)	Fluoride (mg/day)	Iodine (μg/day)	Iron (mg/day)	Magnesium (mg/day)	Manganese (mg/day)	Molybdenum (μg/day)	Phosphorus (mg/day)	Selenium (μg/day)	Zinc (mg/day)	Sodium (g/day)	Chloride (g/day)	Potassium (g/day)
Infants															
0–6 mo	210*	0.2*	200*	0.01*	110*	0.27*	30*	0.003*	2*	100*	15*	2*	.12*	.18*	0.4*
7–12 mo	270*	5.5*	220*	0.5*	130*	11	75*	0.6*	3*	275*	20*	3	.37*	.57*	0.7*
Children															
1–3 y	500*	11*	340	0.7*	90	7	80	1.2*	17	460	20	3	1.0*	1.5*	3.0*
4–8 y	800*	15*	440	1*	90	10	130	1.5*	22	500	30	5	1.2*	1.9*	3.8*
Males															
9–13 y	1,300*	25*	700	2*	120	8	240	1.9*	34	1,250	40	8	1.5*	2.3*	4.5*
14–18 y	1,300*	35*	890	3*	150	11	410	2.2*	43	1,250	55	11	1.5*	2.3*	4.7*
19–30 y	1,000*	35*	900	4*	150	8	400	2.3*	45	700	55	11	1.5*	2.3*	4.7*
31–50 y	1,000*	35*	900	4*	150	8	420	2.3*	45	700	55	11	1.5*	2.3*	4.7*
51–70 y	1,200*	30*	900	4*	150	8	420	2.3*	45	700	55	11	1.3*	2.0*	4.7*
> 70 y	1,200*	30*	900	4*	150	8	420	2.3*	45	700	55	11	1.2*	1.8*	4.7*
Females															
9–13 y	1,300*	21*	700	2*	120	8	240	1.6*	34	1,250	40	8	1.5*	2.3*	4.5*
14–18 y	1,300*	24*	890	3*	150	15	360	1.6*	43	1,250	55	9	1.5*	2.3*	4.7*
19–30 y	1,000*	25*	900	3*	150	18	310	1.8*	45	700	55	8	1.5*	2.3*	4.7*
31–50 y	1,000*	25*	900	3*	150	18	320	1.8*	45	700	55	8	1.5*	2.3*	4.7*
51–70 y	1,200*	20*	900	3*	150	8	320	1.8*	45	700	55	8	1.3*	2.0*	4.7*
> 70 y	1,200*	20*	900	3*	150	8	320	1.8*	45	700	55	8	1.2*	1.8*	4.7*
Pregnancy															
≤ 18 y	1,300*	29*	1,000	3*	220	27	400	2.0*	50	1,250	60	13	1.5*	2.3*	4.7*
19–30 y	1,000*	30*	1,000	3*	220	27	350	2.0*	50	700	60	11	1.5*	2.3*	4.7*
31–50 y	1,000*	30*	1,000	3*	220	27	360	2.0*	50	700	60	11	1.5*	2.3*	4.7*
Lactation															
≤ 18 y	1,300*	44*	1,300	3*	290	10	360	2.6*	50	1,250	70	14	1.5*	2.3*	5.1*
19–30 y	1,000*	45*	1,300	3*	290	9	310	2.6*	50	700	70	12	1.5*	2.3*	5.1*
31–50 y	1,000*	45*	1,300	3*	290	9	320	2.6*	50	700	70	12	1.5*	2.3*	5.1*

Note: This table (taken from the DRI reports, see www.nap.edu) presents Recommended Dietary Allowances (RDAs) in **bold** type and Adequate Intakes (AIs) in ordinary type followed by an asterisk (*). RDAs and AIs may both be used as goals for individual intakes. RDAs are set up to meet the needs of almost all (97–98%) individuals in a group. For healthy breastfed infants, the AI is the mean intake. The AI for all other life stage and gender groups is believed to cover needs of all individuals in the group, but lack of data or uncertainty in the data prevent being able to specify with confidence the percentage of individuals covered by this intake.

Source: Dietary Reference Intake Tables: The Complete Set. Institute of Medicine, National Academy of Sciences. Available online at www.nap.edu.

Acceptable Macronutrient Distribution Ranges (AMDR) for Healthy Diets as a Percent of Energy

Age	Carbohydrate	Added Sugars	Total Fat	Linoleic Acid	α-Linolenic Acid	Protein
1–3 y	45–65	≤ 25	30–40	5–10	0.6–1.2	5–20
4–18 y	45–65	≤ 25	25–35	5–10	0.6–1.2	10–30
≥ 19 y	45–65	≤ 25	20–35	5–10	0.6–1.2	10–35

Source: Institute of Medicine, Food and Nutrition Board. "Dietary Reference Intakes for Energy, Carbohydrates, Fiber, Fat, Protein, and Amino Acids." Washington, D.C.: National Academy Press, 2002.

Dietary Reference Intakes: Recommended Intakes for Individuals: Carbohydrates, Fiber, Fat, Fatty Acids, Protein, and Water

Life Stage Group	Carbohydrate (g/day)	Fiber (g/day)	Fat (g/day)	Linoleic Acid (g/day)	α-Linolenic Acid (g/day)	Protein (g/kg/day)	Protein (g/day)	Water (liters)
Infants								
0–6 mo	60*	ND	31*	4.4*†	0.5*‡	1.52*	9.1*	0.7*
7–12 mo	95*	ND	30*	4.6*†	0.5*‡	1.5	13.5	0.8*
Children								
1–3 y	130	19*	ND	7*	0.7*	1.10	13	1.3*
4–8 y	130	25*	ND	10*	0.9*	0.95	19	1.7*
Males								
9–13 y	130	31*	ND	12*	1.2*	0.95	34	2.4*
14–18 y	130	38*	ND	16*	1.6*	0.85	52	3.3*
19–30 y	130	38*	ND	17*	1.6*	0.80	56	3.7*
31–50 y	130	38*	ND	17*	1.6*	0.80	56	3.7*
51–70 y	130	30*	ND	14*	1.6*	0.80	56	3.7*
> 70 y	130	30*	ND	14*	1.6*	0.80	56	3.7*
Females								
9–13 y	130	26*	ND	10*	1.0*	0.95	34	
14–18 y	130	26*	ND	11*	1.1*	0.85	46	2.1*
19–30 y	130	25*	ND	12*	1.1*	0.80	46	2.3*
31–50 y	130	25*	ND	12*	1.1*	0.80	46	2.7*
51–70 y	130	21*	ND	11*	1.1*	0.80	46	2.7*
> 70 y	130	21*	ND	11*	1.1*	0.80	46	2.7*
Pregnancy	175	28*	ND	13*	1.4*	1.1	RDA + 25g	3.0*
Lactation	210	29*	ND	13*	1.3*	1.1	RDA + 25g	3.8*

ND = not determined   *Values are AI (Adequate Intakes)   † Refers to all n-6 polyunsaturated fatty acids   ‡ Refers to all n-3 polyunsaturated fatty acids

Source: Institute of Medicine, Food and Nutrition Board. "Dietary Reference Intakes for Energy, Carbohydrates, Fiber, Fat, Fatty Acids, and Protein." Washington, D.C.: National Academy Press, 2002.

eGrade Plus

www.wiley.com/college/grosvenor
Based on the Activities You Do Every Day

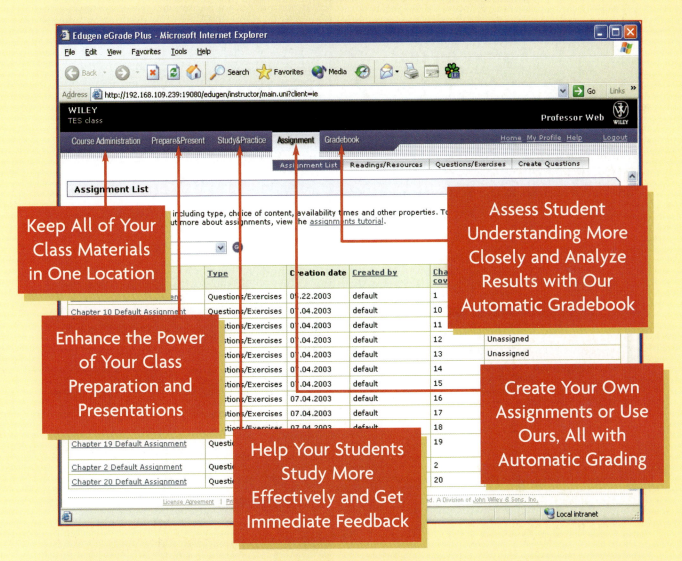

All the content and tools you need, all in one location, in an easy-to-use browser format.

Choose the resources you need, or rely on the arrangement supplied by us.

Now, many of Wiley's textbooks are available with eGrade Plus, a powerful online tool that provides a completely integrated suite of teaching and learning resources in one easy-to-use website. eGrade Plus integrates Wiley's world-renowned content with media, including a multimedia version of the text, PowerPoint slides, and more. Upon adoption of eGrade Plus, you can begin to customize your course with the resources shown here.

See for yourself!

Go to **www.wiley.com/college/egradeplus** for an online demonstration of this powerful new software.

Students,
eGrade Plus Allows You to:

Study More Effectively

Get Immediate Feedback When You Practice on Your Own

eGrade Plus problems link directly to relevant sections of the **electronic book content,** so that you can review the text while you study and complete homework online. Additional resources include **interactive simulations, interactive case studies,** and **integrated answers to end of chapter questions.**

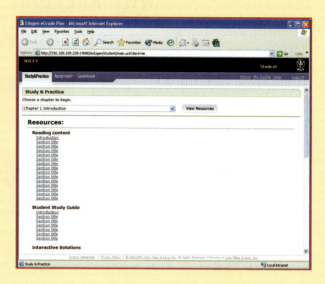

Complete Assignments / Get Context-Sensitive Help

An **Assignment** area keeps all your assigned work in one location, making it easy for you to stay "on task." In addition, many homework problems contain a **link** to the relevant section of the **multimedia book,** providing you with a text explanation to help you review the text as you complete assignments. You will have access to a variety of **interactive animations and case studies,** as well as other resources for building your confidence and understanding.

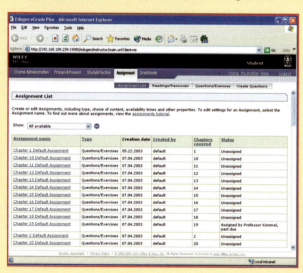

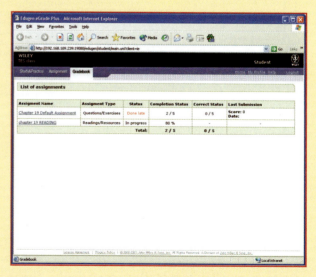

Keep Track of How You're Doing

A **Personal Gradebook** allows you to view your results from past assignments at any time.

NUTRITION
Everyday Choices

For information on the 2005 Dietary Guidelines and the USDA's new food guidance system, MyPyramid: Steps to a Healthier You, go to the Grosvenor, Smolin: Nutrition: Everyday Choices web site at www.wiley.com/college/grosvenor. Here you will find the author's summaries of these new recommendations as well as links to the respective government web sites, www.healthierus.gov/dietaryguidelines/ and www.mypyramid.gov/.

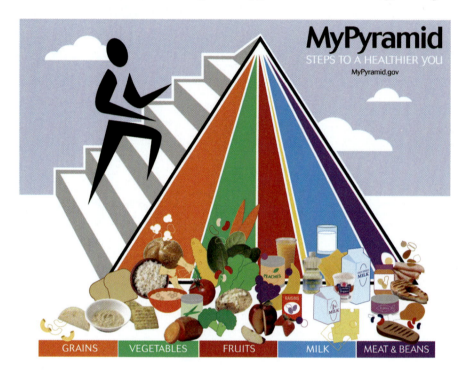

NUTRITION
Everyday Choices

Mary B. Grosvenor, M.S., R.D.

Lori A. Smolin, Ph.D.
University of Connecticut

WILEY

John Wiley & Sons, Inc.

EXECUTIVE EDITOR	Bonnie Roesch
PROJECT EDITOR	Mary O'Sullivan
SENIOR PRODUCTION EDITOR	Elizabeth Swain
EXECUTIVE MARKETING MANAGER	Clay Stone
DESIGN DIRECTOR	Harry Nolan
COVER DESIGN	Howard Grossman
INTERIOR DESIGN	Brian Salisbury
ILLUSTRATION EDITOR	Anna Melhorn
PHOTO EDITOR	Hilary Newman
PHOTO RESEARCHER	Bridget Small
SENIOR MEDIA EDITOR	Linda Muriello
COVER PHOTO	Front cover © Lew Robertson/Foodpix/PictureArts Corp.
	Back cover: © David McGlynn/Taxi/Getty Images
CONTENTS PHOTOS	© PhotoDisc, Inc./Getty Images

This book was set in 10.5/12 Adobe Garamond Regular by GGS Book Services, Atlantic Highlands and printed and bound by Von Hoffmann Press. The cover was printed by Von Hoffmann Press.

This book is printed on acid free paper.

To order books or for customer service please, call 1-800-CALL WILEY (225-5945).

Library of Congress Cataloging-in-Publication Data
Grosvenor, Mary B.
    Nutrition: everyday choices / Mary B. Grosvenor, Lori A. Smolin. – 1st ed.
       p.   cm.
    Includes index.
    ISBN 0-471-66876-1 (pbk.: alk. paper)
    1. Nutrition. I. Smolin, Lori A. II. Title.

QP141.G766 2006
613.2–dc22

                                                2004062039

Printed in the United States of America

10 9 8 7 6 5 4 3 2

To Peter, David, and John for your patience and forbearance through the many hours, days, and weeks spent researching, writing, and editing this book. Thank you for reminding me that there is more to life than work.

MBG

To my husband David for his patience and support, and for providing the technical expertise required to keep my computers up and running. To my sons Zachary and Max for dragging me away from my writing often enough to stay in touch with the world.

LAS

Mary B. Grosvenor, M.S., R.D. Mary Grosvenor received her B.A. degree in English from Georgetown University and her M.S. in Nutrition Sciences from the University of California at Davis. She is a registered dietitian with experience in public health, clinical nutrition, and nutrition research. She has published in peer-reviewed journals in the areas of nutrition and cancer and methods of assessing dietary intake. She has taught introductory nutrition at the community college level and currently lives with her family in a small town in Colorado. She is continuing her teaching and writing career and is still involved in nutrition research via the electronic superhighway.

Lori A. Smolin, Ph.D. Lori Smolin received her B.S. degree from Cornell University, where she studied human nutrition and food science. She received her doctorate from the University of Wisconsin at Madison. Her doctoral research focused on B vitamins, homocysteine accumulation, and genetic defects in homocysteine metabolism. She completed postdoctoral training both at the Harbor–UCLA Medical Center, where she studied human obesity, and at the University of California at San Diego, where she studied genetic defects in amino acid metabolism. She has published in these areas in peer-reviewed journals. Dr. Smolin is currently at the University of Connecticut, where she teaches both in the Department of Nutritional Sciences and in the Department of Molecular and Cell Biology. Courses she has taught include introductory nutrition, lifecycle nutrition, food preparation, nutritional biochemistry, general biochemistry, and introductory biology.

WE all make choices everyday that involve our nutrition and health. What should I have for breakfast? Should I have one scoop of ice cream or two? Should I walk up the stairs or take the elevator? Each of these decisions is small, but small choices add up. When taken together these daily choices can affect your health today and in the future. The goal of this text is to teach students how to make wise nutrition choices—both about the foods they eat and the nutrition information they encounter.

To make wise choices, students need to understand the basics of the science of nutrition. *Nutrition: Everyday Choices* teaches basic nutrition science in a style that is easily accessible to non-science majors. From this base, it guides students through the critical thinking processes needed to apply this information to their everyday choices. As they progress through the text, students grow in their nutrition knowledge and become savvy consumers. They develop the decision-making skills they need to navigate the scores of choices they face when deciding what to eat and what to believe.

Students enroll in nutrition classes for many reasons. They want to know if and how what they eat will affect their health, their weight, or their physical performance. To continuously feed this hunger for knowledge about how nutrition affects their lives, *Nutrition: Everyday Choices* has integrated the information students find most interesting throughout the text. Including information in each chapter about the relationship between diet and health, the importance of exercise, and which foods offer which benefit engages students early on and holds their interest. This approach also makes the more difficult concepts such as metabolism and digestion more palatable. Rather than thinking, "Why do I need to know this?" students can see, for example, that a nutrient's function in metabolism determines its role in health and disease. Students are then more motivated to learn the basics and are prepared to apply them to their personal health and nutrition.

In addition to capturing student interest by tapping into what students want to know, this text entices them with its writing style and visual impact. The writing is friendly, engaging, and personal while at the same time concise and consistent. The layout of the book is colorful and fun, and the carefully developed art program taps into the visual aspects of learning. Consistent colors and shapes are used to create appealing artwork that supports and visually enhances the written information.

To keep abreast of this ever-changing field, *Nutrition: Everyday Choices* provides up-to-date coverage of the most recent advances in nutrition science. The latest DRIs and recent changes in recommendations regarding healthy blood cholesterol levels and blood pressure are included. Although this text went to press before the newest release of the Dietary Guidelines for Americans and the Food Guide Pyramid were available, the latest information is available on our web site.

Choosing to use *Nutrition: Everyday Choices* for your nutrition course is one small choice that can make a big difference in how your students understand and apply nutrition principles every day for the rest of their lives.

FEATURES

This text includes features that both spark student interest and help educate them about nutrition.

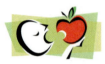

86   Chapter 4

germ is
dosper
tamins
germ a
clude
from j
the
fined
ents lo
remove
min B₆

When deciding whether whole wheat bread is healthier than white bread, consider that white bread is enriched with certain B vitamins and iron, but is lower in other vitamins, and minerals, as well as fiber because they are lost in milling and not added back in enrichment.

Add
in n

Refine

JUST A TASTE

Each chapter begins with a taste of what's to come. Just a Taste is a set of three or four intriguing questions that introduce information covered in the chapter. Students can use them to check their current understanding or misconceptions of the material that will be covered in the chapter. For example, Chapter 7 asks "Can obesity be prevented?" To follow through with these questions the Just a Taste icon then appears in the text where this information is discussed and a brief answer to the question is provided in the margin.

CHAPTER CONCEPTS

This bulleted list at the start of each chapter highlights the important concepts that will be discussed in the chapter.

CHAPTER INTRODUCTION

Nutrition is always in the headlines. We take advantage of this by opening each chapter with a clip from a recent news article relevant to the information in the chapter. For example, Chapter 4 begins with a story about how bakery profits are falling due to the low-carb diet craze; Chapter 5 starts with a clip about McDonald's removing *trans* fat from their french fries; and Chapter 8 begins with an article about the growing problem of vitamin D deficiency. What better way to spark student interest than to illustrate how the nutrition topics in the text relate to the news and issues that affect students every day? This gets students thinking about one of the nutrition topics discussed in the chapter.

chapter introduction

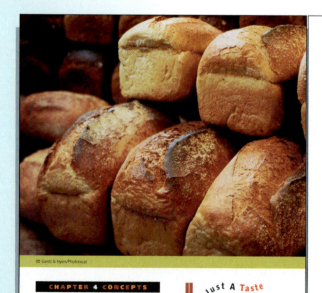

Chapter Concepts

OFF THE LABEL

"Off the Label" boxes included in each chapter present a discussion about the specifics of food labels. This material is designed as a supplement to the information included in the body of the chapter and to show students how to use food labels to make wise food choices. For example, an Off the Label box in Chapter 4 tells students how food labels can be used to avoid foods that are high in added sugars. Chapter 6 has an Off the Label box that discusses how to use food labels to avoid foods they are allergic to, and the Off the Label box in Chapter 15 discusses differences in food labels around the world.

YOUR CHOICE

"Your Choice" boxes included in each chapter provide a critical review of products or issues that are the focus of individual consumer choices. This feature has been developed to show students how to make decisions regarding foods and supplements. Each box addresses a choice to which consumers might be exposed, such as whether to include soy products in their diet or whether sports bars are a good choice during a workout. For example, the Your Choice box in Chapter 10 discusses the risks and benefits of choosing fortified foods and the box in Chapter 13 discusses the nutritional impact of choosing carbonated soda versus milk.

PIECE IT TOGETHER

These unique exercises use a critical thinking approach to walk students through the thought processes needed to make decisions and solve problems related to nutrition. One or two of these exercises appears in each chapter throughout the book. They help students learn to apply their nutrition knowledge to every-day situations by presenting a nutrition-related issue and then showing the student the logical progression of thought needed to collect information and solve the problem. Some of these exercises will take the student by the hand and lead them step by step through all the thought processes, while others show the student the way and then expect them to follow the path by solving some of the problems themselves. Many of these exercises focus on optimizing a diet to reduce disease risk or maintain health and thus also integrate health promotion and disease prevention issues that concern students the most. For example, one of the exercises in Chapter 5 takes the student through the process of evaluating the risk of developing heart disease. In addition, the use of case histories and diets that span many cultures helps increase ethnic diversity. For example, Chapter 6 shows the students how to use complimentary protein sources in a vegetarian diet that is based on traditional Indian cuisine. To provide the feedback needed to enhance learning, answers to these are included in Appendix M.

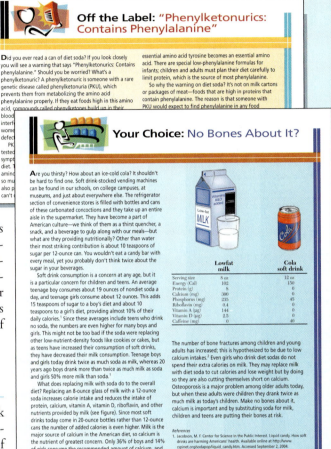

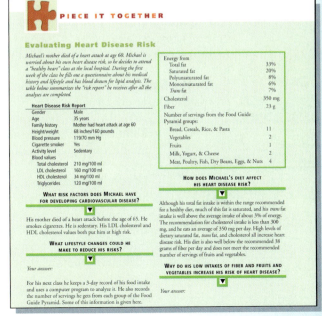

SO, WHAT SHOULD I EAT?

This feature provides simple, doable tips on what to eat to follow the recommendations included in the chapter. Students often complain that although they understand the technical concepts of nutrition, they still can't easily use this information when making food choices. This section will help the student translate nutrition recommendations into healthy food choices.

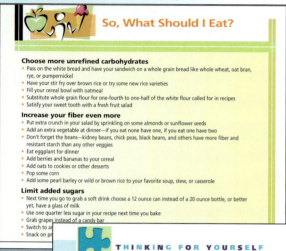

THINKING FOR YOURSELF

This feature, which appears at the end of each chapter, is a variation of the "Piece it Together" exercises. Instead of presenting a case history, these exercises ask students to consider their own dietary and health choices. The feature uses a critical thinking approach to help students apply the chapter material to their own diet.

MARGINAL FEATURES

In addition to the Just a Taste answers, the text includes a number of other margin features that aid student comprehension and enhance interest.

A running glossary of key terms These provide easy access to new terms as they appear in the text. These and other terms are included in an extensive Glossary at the end of the text.

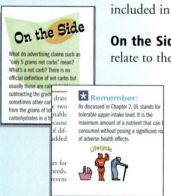

On the Side These feature interesting tidbits of information that relate to the text discussion.

Remember These remind students about relevant information that has been covered in an earlier chapter.

Lifecycle icons These highlight places in the text that feature discussions of how life stage affects nutritional requirements and concerns.

On the Web This feature, which appears throughout each chapter, provides websites where additional information relevant to the chapter can be found.

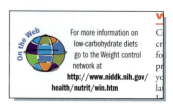

MAIN CONCEPTS AS SECTION TITLES

The section heads used in *Nutrition: Everyday Choices* allow students and instructors to find out at a glance the main concept covered in each section of the text. For example, a section head in Chapter 1 tells you that "Your nutrient intake affects your current and future health." A head in Chapter 4 explains that "Added refined sugars are low in nutrient density," and a Chapter 5 head informs that "Just cutting fat doesn't make your diet healthy." Including the main concept in the headings provides an excellent and easily accessible study tool because the title of each section tells the student in a few words the basic concept presented.

REVIEW QUESTIONS

This set of questions appears at the end of each chapter to test students' understanding of the key points covered. It can be used as a study tool.

CHAPTER SUMMARY

Each chapter ends with a summary that highlights important concepts addressed in the chapter.

CHAPTER BY CHAPTER OVERVIEW

Chapter 1 begins the journey by emphasizing that what you eat affects your current and future health. It also defines the basic principles of balance, variety, and moderation that are key to a healthy diet and introduces the process of science and the steps students need to follow to sort accurate from inaccurate nutrition information.

Chapter 2 takes the science out of the laboratory and shows how advances in nutrition knowledge have been used to develop the Dietary Reference Intakes (DRIs) and tools for diet planning, including the Food Guide Pyramid, Exchange Lists, food labels, and the Dietary Guidelines for Americans.

Chapter 3 presents digestion and absorption by showing how a specific meal is digested, its nutrients absorbed into the body and transported to the cells where metabolism occurs, and finally how wastes are removed.

Chapters 4, 5, and 6 focus on the energy-yielding nutrients; carbohydrates, lipids, and proteins. In addition to covering the functions of these, emphasis is placed on the types and proportions of each that are optimal for health. Chapter 4 discusses carbohydrates and emphasizes that despite the low-carb diet craze, high-carbohydrate foods are an important part of the diet. What should be limited are refined grains and foods high in added sugar, not fiber-rich whole grains. Chapter 5 covers lipids. It points out that Americans are not eating too much fat, but are typically choosing the wrong types of fat for optimum health. Chapter 6 discusses animal and plant sources of protein and points out that either can meet protein needs, but that different protein sources bring with them different combinations of nutrients. This chapter also provides information on how to plan a healthy vegetarian diet.

Chapter 7 introduces energy balance and the role of excess body fat in disease risk. This chapter discusses the obesity epidemic and shows how small changes in diet and behavior can alter long-term energy balance. This chapter also includes a comprehensive section on eating disorders and body image.

Chapters 8 and 9 cover vitamins, minerals, and water. Study of these nutrients is often tedious for students, but to enhance interest each discussion begins with a point that both captures interest and is one of the critical points to remember about that nutrient.

Chapter 10 discusses the role of foods, fortified foods, and supplements in meeting our nutrient needs. Many people can get all they need from unfortified foods, but fortified foods help prevent deficiencies in the population, and supplements are recommended to some groups.

Chapter 11 discusses the relationships among physical activity, nutrition, and health. The chapter emphasizes the connection between exercise and disease as well as the impact a healthy diet can have on exercise performance.

Chapters 12 and 13 focus on the importance of nutrition and changing needs throughout the lifecycle.

Chapter 14 discusses the risks and benefits associated with the U.S. food supply and includes information on the impact of microbial hazards, chemical toxins, food additives, irradiation, and genetically modified foods.

Finally, Chapter 15 discusses the problems of hunger and undernutrition as well as obesity both at home and globally.

TO THE STUDENT

In today's world of mad cow disease, low-carb diets, and biotech foods, even a non-science student is faced with a need to understand the process of science. We wrote *Nutrition: Everyday Choices* not only to provide you with the science base you need to understand issues in the world around you, but also to allow you to apply this knowledge to choices you make. Most of you have questions about nutrition: Is this food good for me or bad for me? Should I be eating a low-fat diet? Should I take a protein supplement to improve my athletic performance? Is a low-carbohydrate diet really the healthiest way to lose weight? The answers to these questions are in the pages of this text along with the tools you need to make our own nutrition decisions. Our goal is not to tell you to stop eating candy bars, to give up fast food, or to always eat your vegetables. Instead, it is to provide you with the tools you need to conclude for yourselves that fresh fruit may be a better everyday choice while candy bars can be an occasional treat; that fast food is something to indulge in every now and then; and that although not everyone always eats their vegetables, they should find ways to include them often. We hope that you are able to take this knowledge out of the classroom and apply the nutrition you have learned to your everyday lives.

ANCILLARIES

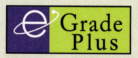

Helping Teachers Teach and Students Learn
ww.wiley.com/college/grosvenor

This title is available with eGrade Plus, a powerful online tool that provides instructors and students with an integrated suite of teaching and learning resources in one easy-to-use website. eGrade Plus is organized around the essential activities you and your students perform in class.

For Instructors

- **Prepare & Present:** Create class presentations using a wealth of Wiley-provided resources—such as an online version of the textbook, PowerPoint slides, Lecture Launchers, images from the Nutrition Visual Library, and interactive animations—making your preparation time more efficient. You may easily adapt, customize, and add to this content to meet the needs of your course.

- **Create Assignments:** Automate the assigning and grading of homework or quizzes by using Wiley-provided question banks, or by writing your own. Student results will be automatically graded and recorded in your gradebook eGrade Plus can link the pre-lecture quizzes and test bank questions to the relevant section of the online text, providing students with context-sensitive help.
- **Track Student Progress:** Keep track of your students' progress via an instructor's gradebook, which allows you to analyze individual and overall class results to determine their progress and level of understanding.
- **Administer Your Course:** eGrade Plus can easily be integrated with another course management system, gradebook, or other resources you are using in your class, providing you with the flexibility to build your course, your way.

For Students

Wiley's eGrade Plus provides immediate feedback on student assignments and a wealth of support materials. This powerful study tool will help your students develop their conceptual understanding of the class material and increase their ability to answer questions.

- **A "Study and Practice"** area links directly to text content, allowing students to review the text while they study and answer questions. Additional resources can include interactive animations, pre-lecture quizzes, clinical case studies, and other problem-solving resources.
- **An "Assignment"** area keeps all the work you want your students to complete in one location, making it easy for them to stay "on task." Students will have access to a variety of interactive self-assessment tools, as well as other resources for building their confidence and understanding. In addition, all of the pre-lecture quizzes contain a link to the relevant section of the multimedia book, providing students with context-sensitive help that allows them to conquer problem-solving obstacles as they arise.
- **A Personal Gradebook** for each student will allow students to view their results from past assignments at any time.

Please view our online demo at www.wiley.com/college/egradeplus. Here you will find additional information about the features and benefits of eGrade Plus, how to request a "test drive" of eGrade Plus for this title, and how to adopt it for class use.

MATERIALS AVAILABLE FOR STUDENTS

DIET ANALYSIS SOFTWARE
0-471-69994-2 (Web) 0-471-69992-6 (CD-ROM)

Now offered in two formats, online or CD-ROM, this user-friendly, visually appealing dietary assessment software will enhance the study of the nutritional components of food and how to meet dietary needs.

NUTRIENT COMPOSITION OF FOOD
SUPPLEMENT (0-471-71309-0)

Bundled with every copy of the textbook, this printed version of the food table found in the *Diet Analysis Software* has been packaged as a separate supplement from the textbook for easy reference. This table will also appear in pdf format on the Study Companion Web Site.

STUDY GUIDE (0-471-69983-7)

Written by Christine Graber of Ohio University, Chillicothe, this includes chapter outlines, multiple-choice questions, matching exercises, short-answer review questions, and a variety of learning activities designed for use by individual students and by groups in the classroom.

ENERGY ACQUISITION: THE DIGESTIVE SYSTEM AND METABOLISM (0-471-26524-X)

This CD-ROM from the popular series, *Interactions: Exploring the Functions of the Human Body*, uses animations, interactivity, and clinical correlations to enhance student understanding of the difficult concepts of metabolism and the structures and functions of the digestive system.

STUDENT COMPANION WEB SITE (www.wiley.com/college/grosvenor)

This dynamic website rich with many activities for review and exploration includes Chapter Overview and Objectives, Practice Quizzes for each chapter, Clinical Case Studies, Web Links linked to chapter content, Nutrition Update Newsletters, and study tools and tips.

MATERIALS AVAILABLE FOR INSTRUCTORS

INSTRUCTOR'S MANUAL

Written by Sally Weerts of the University of North Florida, the manual is available online from the Instructor Companion web site (www.wiley.com/college/grosvenor) and provides many resources for preparing and presenting lectures. Included are key concepts, chapter outlines, new Critical Thinking Exercises, key terms, student self-assessment forms, and sources for other teaching materials, including useful web sites that are in addition to those listed in the text.

WILEY'S VISUAL LIBRARY FOR NUTRITION CD-ROM (0-471-69995-0)

This all-new cross-platform CD-ROM includes all of the illustrations from the textbook in labeled, unlabeled, and unlabeled with leader line formats. In addition, illustrations and photographs not included in the text, but which could easily be added to enhance lecture or lab, are included. Search for images by chapter, or by using key words.

TEST BANK (0-471-69984-5)

The Test Bank, written by Neil Shay of Notre Dame University, includes multiple-choice and short-answer questions as well as short case studies for each chapter of the text.

COMPUTERIZED TEST BANK CD-ROM (0-471-69982-9)

This electronic version of the printed Test Bank provides a user-friendly interface allowing users to easily view, edit, and add questions. This CD makes preparing clear, concise tests quick and easy.

OVERHEAD TRANSPARENCIES (0-471-69981-0)

This set of full-color overheads helps instructors show the book's concepts in the classroom. This set can be supplemented by using the image bank from Wiley's Visual Library for Nutrition CD-ROM to create additional overheads for classroom use.

WEBCT/BLACKBOARD

Available online with content correlated to the textbook, this is available for both course management packages. Written by Roger McDonald of University of California, Davis.

INSTRUCTOR'S COMPANION WEB SITE (www.wiley.com/college/grosvenor)

This dedicated companion website for instructors provides many resources for preparing and presenting lectures, including Lecture Launchers—videos from the Discovery Channel plus web links directly correlated to each chapter, PowerPoint Lecture Slides integrating text and images, and all text tables and images in pdfs and jpegs for easy download.

CLASSROOM RESPONSE SYSTEMS

The Classroom Response System content to support this course contains 5–10 multiple choice questions per chapter. Some of the questions are tied to the Just A Taste teasers at the beginning of each chapter. The questions cover current topics that help stimulate in-class discussion and promote critical thinking.

ACKNOWLEDGMENTS

The authors wish to thank the many professors and students who helped in the development of this text. Their endless hours of careful reading and their many thoughtful suggestions from diverse viewpoints have helped to make this text the best available on today's market. The reviewers, who offered comments and suggestions on both the presentation and the accuracy of this information, include the following:

Helen Anderson-Lee, *California State University, Long Beach*
Wayne Askew, *University of Utah*
Nancy Berkoff, *Los Angeles Trade Technical College*
Gregory Biren, *Rowan University*
Amy Brown, *University of Hawaii*
Thomas Castonguay, *University of Maryland*
Erin Caudill, Southeast *Community College, Lincoln*
Melissa Chabot, *SUNY Buffalo*
Dorothy Chen-Maynard, *California State University, San Bernardino*
Wendy Cunningham, *California State University, Sacramento*
Earlene Davis, *Bakersfield College*
Marci DeWitt, *Liberty University*
Carol Eady, *University of Memphis*
Marjorie Fitch-Hilgenberg, *University of Arkansas*
Tanya Fitschen, *Western Wyoming Community College*
Allison Ford, *Florida Atlantic University*
Victoria Getty, *Indiana University – Bloomington*
Christine Graber, *Ohio University, Chillicothe*
Carolyn Gunther, *Purdue University*
Lauren Haldeman, *University of North Carolina at Greensboro*
Nancy Harris, *Eastern Carolina University*
Cindy Heiss, *California State University, Northridge*
Candace Hines-Tinsley, *Saddleback College*
Jasminka Ilich-Ernst, *University of Connecticut*
Caryl Johnson, *Eastern New Mexico University*
Laura Kruskall, *UNLV*
Alice Lindeman, *Indiana University, Bloomington*
Mohey Mowafy, *Northern Michigan University*
Linda Rankin, *Idaho State University, Pocatello*
Tonia Reinhard, *Wayne State University*
Shridhar Sathe, *Florida State University*
Terry Shaw, *Austin Community College*
Ingrid Skoog, *University of Oregon*
Mollie Smith, *California State University, Fresno*
LuAnn Soliah, *Baylor University*
Stasinos Stavrianes, *Willamette University*
Wendy Stuhldreher, *Slippery Rock University of Pennsylvania*

Norman Temple, *Athabasca University*
Kathy Timmons, *Murray State University*
Josephine Umoren, *Northern Illinois University*
Jennifer Weddig, *Metropolitan State College, Denver*
Donna Winham, *Arizona State University East*

We are grateful to the editorial, marketing, production, and design staff at John Wiley & Sons for their help and support. We thank our Executive Editor, Bonnie Roesch, for her enthusiasm and excitement about publishing in the field of nutrition, our Project Editor, Mary O'Sullivan, for managing the day-to-day and minute-to-minute problems that occur during the course of writing a book, and who also carefully developed all the ancillaries, and our Executive Marketing Manager, Clay Stone, for coordinating the advertising, marketing, and sales efforts for the book and its supplements. We also thank our Photo Editor, Hilary Newman, for ensuring the outstanding quality of the photos in this text, our Illustration Editor, Anna Melhorn, for assuring high-quality artwork, even when last minute corrections were needed, our Design Director, Harry Nolan, for delivering an attractively designed text, and our Senior Production Editor, Elizabeth Swain, for her patience and efficiency in guiding this project through production.

BRIEF CONTENTS

CONTENTS

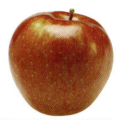

Chapter 8

The Vitamins   235

Chapter 11
Nutrition, Fitness, and Physical Activity 363

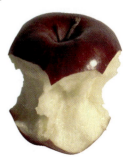

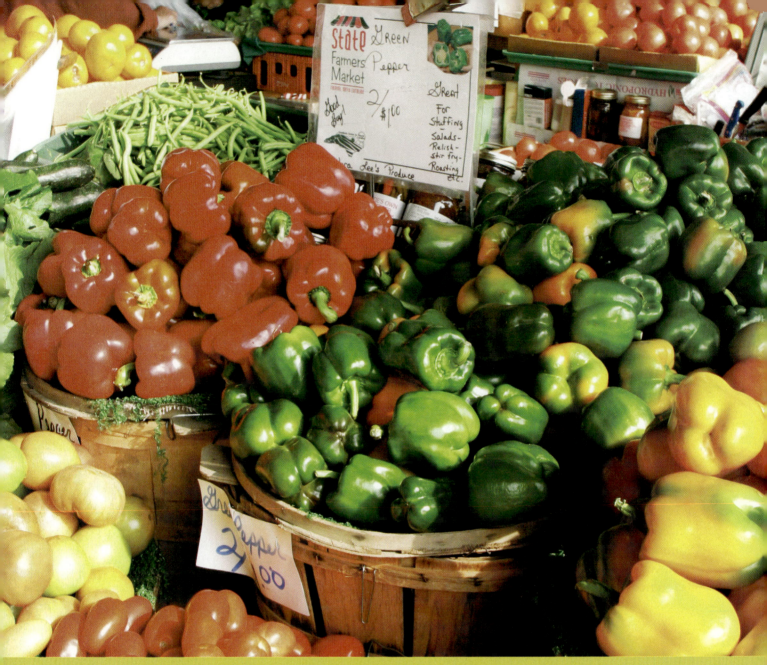

(Jeff Greenberg/Age Fotostock America, Inc.)

CHAPTER 1 CONCEPTS

- The foods you choose determine which nutrients you consume. Nutrient-dense foods provide more essential nutrients in fewer calories.
- Your nutrient intake affects your health in the short and long terms.
- Nutrients fuel our bodies, provide structure, and regulate body processes.
- A healthy diet is based on variety, balance, and moderation.
- We choose foods for many reasons other than their nutrient content.
- Advances in nutrition knowledge are made by using the scientific method.
- Nutrition information should be critically examined before it is accepted as true.

Just A Taste

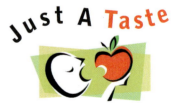

Can your food choices today affect your health later in life?

Do people naturally choose a healthy diet?

Are there foods you should never eat?

Nutrition: Choices for Health

INTRODUCTION

NBC's Today Show

Foods that Put the 'Super' in Supermarket

By *Phil Lempert, Food Editor*

(Updated 11:47 A.M. Eastern time, Apr. 22, 2004)—As an increasing number of Americans realize that they are overweight—and therefore more liable to fall victim to heart disease and diabetes—they are taking extra time to read those nutrition labels and seek out the most healthful foods.

But with more than 40,000 products in the typical supermarket, this can be a tough task. And while many food marketers claim that their products are the best for your health, only a few can really make that claim.

For more information on this article, go to www.msnbc.msn.com/id/4787822/.

Are you concerned about your diet and how it affects your health? You are not alone. More Americans than ever before are seeking information about nutrition and how to improve their diets.[1] But there is so much information that it is often hard to know what foods to choose and which reports to believe. Should you be cutting down on carbs, supplementing with soy, or drinking calcium-fortified orange juice? Should you believe the story you saw on the news about vitamin E and heart disease? Filtering out the worthless and understanding the worthwhile can be a mind-boggling task. To make healthy nutrition choices you need to know what nutrients you require, what roles they play in health and disease, and what foods contain them (Figure 1.1). You must also be able to know whether you can trust the nutrition information you encounter.

1

Your Food Choices Affect Your Health

Did you ever hear the saying "you are what you eat"? Well, it isn't literally true, but what you eat has an enormous impact on how much you weigh, how healthy you are now, and how likely you are to develop a chronic disease like heart disease or diabetes in the future. The foods you choose determine the **nutrients** you consume. There are over 40 different **essential nutrients** that we need to stay healthy. Because the foods we eat vary from day to day, so do the amounts and types of nutrients we consume.

✴ **Nutrients** Substances in food that provide us with energy and structure and regulate body processes.

✴ **Essential nutrients** Nutrients that must be consumed in the diet to maintain health.

✴ **Nutrient density** A measure of the nutrients provided by a food relative to its calorie content.

What you eat determines your nutrient intake

Some days you may feel like you're eating constantly and others hardly at all. One day you may go out for a fast food lunch and on the next just have a salad. Some days you may snack on the run while other days you sit down to three healthy meals. All of this is part of normal eating. And it can add up to a healthy diet as long as your average intake over a period of days or weeks provides all of the nutrients you need. Unfortunately, many Americans do not choose the healthiest of diets (Table 1.1).

To make your diet healthy, it is important to choose nutrient-dense foods. **Nutrient density** is a measure of the nutrients a food provides in comparison with its calorie content. More nutrient-dense foods contain more nutrients per calorie than do less-nutrient-dense foods (Figure 1.2). For example, a slice of whole wheat toast is a more

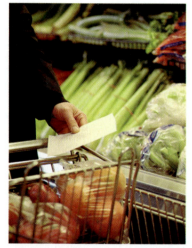

FIGURE 1.1

Modern grocery stores offer enormous variety. People try to choose foods they like and that keep them healthy. (Rob Melnychuk/Photo Disc, Inc./Getty Images)

TABLE 1.1
How Healthy Is the Typical American Diet?

Food Group	Daily Recommendation	Typical Diet
Grains	6–11 servings—most should be whole grains	50% do not eat even 6 servings; most people eat only one serving of whole grains
Vegetables	3–5 servings—include legumes, leafy greens, and yellow-orange vegetables	59% do not meet recommendations; 33% of vegetable servings are white potatoes, only 3% are leafy greens, and 6% are legumes
Fruits	2–4 servings	76% do not meet recommendations—48% do not eat any at all
Dairy	2–3 servings	77% do not meet recommendations; over 80% of women do not meet recommendations
Meats	2–3 servings or a total of 5–7 ounces	52% of men and 25% of women consume more servings than recommended
Fats and sweets	less than 30% fat; limit added sugars to less than 12 teaspoons per day	The typical diet contains 33% fat and includes 19 teaspoons of added sugars per day

From: Cleveland, L. E., Cook, A. J., Wilson, J. E., et al. Pyramid servings data, ARS Food Survey Research Group. Available online at www.barc.usda.gov/bhnrc/foodsurvey/home.htm.

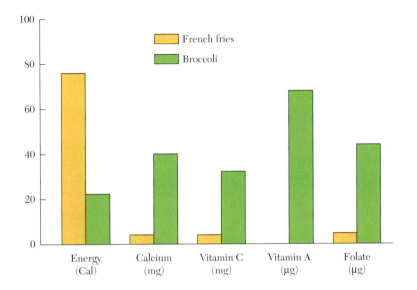

FIGURE 1.2

What vegetable you choose to have with dinner affects the number of calories and the essential nutrients you consume. Choosing a half cup of broccoli will provide more calcium, vitamin C, vitamin A, and folate and fewer calories than would be provided by a half cup of french fries.

nutrient-dense breakfast choice than a doughnut. The whole wheat bread has about 80 Calories and is a good source of B vitamins and fiber. The doughnut has about 240 Calories. It is still a good source of B vitamins but has little fiber, and the extra calories come from added sugar and fat, which bring few essential nutrients with them. This doesn't mean you always need to skip the doughnut and have whole grain toast for breakfast. But it does mean that if many of your choices throughout the day are soft drinks, snack foods, and baked goods that are low in nutrient density, it will be hard to meet your nutrient needs. On the other hand, if you know how to choose nutrient-dense foods, you can meet all your nutrient needs and have calories left over for occasional treats, like doughnuts, that are low in nutrients and high in calories.

Your nutrient intake affects your current and future health

To stay healthy, the foods you eat must provide the right proportions of all the nutrients. An optimal mix of nutrients will prevent **malnutrition**, which can be caused by either too much or too little energy or nutrients. Malnutrition can affect your health today and can impact on your health 20, 30, or 40 years from now.

Malnutrition Any condition resulting from an energy or nutrient intake either above or below that which is optimal.

Too little or too much can cause serious symptoms When your intake is less than your needs, you will suffer from **undernutrition**. The symptoms of undernutrition vary, depending on which nutrient is lacking. For example, vitamin A is needed for vision, so a deficiency affects your vision. Vitamin D is needed for healthy bones, so a deficiency will affect your bones. The degree of the deficiency also determines the symptoms. A mild deficiency may cause nonspecific symptoms, such as fatigue or a decreased ability to fight infection. A severe deficiency may cause more dramatic symptoms such as blindness and bone deformities and can be life-threatening.

Some nutrient deficiencies cause symptoms quickly. In only a matter of hours an athlete exercising in hot weather may become dehydrated because of a deficiency of water. Drinking water relieves the headache, fatigue, and dizziness caused by dehydration almost as rapidly as they appeared. Other nutritional deficiencies may take much longer to become visible. The symptoms of starvation, the most obvious form of undernutrition, may take weeks to become obvious (Figure 1.3a). The symptoms of the vitamin C deficiency disease scurvy do not occur until the diet has been deficient in vitamin C for months. Too little calcium in your teens causes no immediate symptoms but can cause your bones to be weak and break too easily when you reach your 50s or 60s.[2]

Undernutrition A condition resulting from an intake of calories or nutrients below that which meets nutritional needs.

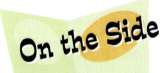

On the Side

Scurvy was common among sailors of old because fresh fruits and vegetables, which are the source of vitamin C in the diet, could not be stored for long aboard ships. More than half of Vasco da Gama's crew died from scurvy on his first trip (1497-1499) around the Cape of Good Hope.

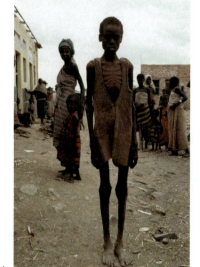

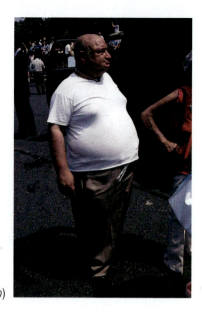

FIGURE 1.3

(*a*) Starvation is an obvious form of malnutrition. (*b*) Obesity is also a form of malnutrition that increases the risk of other chronic diseases. (*a*: Peter Turnley/Corbis Images. *b*: Van Bucher/Photo Researchers)

(*a*)   (*b*)

⚠️ **Overnutrition** Poor nutritional status resulting from a dietary intake in excess of that which is optimal for health.

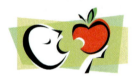

What you eat today affects how healthy you will be tomorrow. Too much saturated fat can increase your risk of heart disease. Too little calcium can increase your risk of osteoporosis, too much salt can raise your blood pressure, and too many calories can lead to obesity.

Excessive amounts of some nutrients can also cause severe symptoms. For example, an overdose of iron can cause liver failure, and too much vitamin B_6 can cause nerve damage. Because foods generally do not contain high enough concentrations of nutrients to be toxic, most nutrient toxicities result from taking large doses of vitamin and mineral supplements.

Too much contributes to chronic disease in the long term

The kind of malnutrition that is common in the United States today is not undernutrition but rather **overnutrition** (Figure 1.3*b*). Excessive intakes of calories and certain nutrients are associated with the development of heart disease, diabetes, and cancer, which are the major causes of illness and death in the U.S. population. Adults in their 50s and 60s are not the only ones affected by these chronic diseases. Heart disease and diabetes are now appearing in younger and younger groups. The genes you inherit from your parents contribute to your risk of developing these diseases, but they are not the only factor. An unhealthy diet and lack of physical activity also play a role. These two factors contribute to over 400,000 deaths annually in the United States, only tobacco use causes more preventable deaths.[3]

Six Classes of Nutrients Keep Us Alive and Well

⚠️ **Macronutrients** Nutrients needed by the body in relatively large amounts. These include water, carbohydrates, lipids, and proteins.

⚠️ **Micronutrients** Nutrients needed by the body in relatively small amounts. These include vitamins and minerals.

⚠️ **Carbohydrates** The class of nutrients that includes sugars, starches, and fibers. Chemically they all contain carbon, hydrogen, and oxygen in the same proportions as water.

⚠️ **Fiber** Substances in food that are not broken down by the digestive processes in the human stomach and small intestine.

There are six classes of nutrients that we need to stay alive and healthy, to grow, and to reproduce: carbohydrates, lipids, proteins, water, vitamins, and minerals. The amount of each we need varies. Water, carbohydrates, lipids, and proteins are needed in large amounts. These are considered **macronutrients**. Macronutrient requirements are measured in grams (g) or liters (L). Vitamins and minerals are needed only in milligram (mg) or microgram (μg) amounts. They are considered **micronutrients**.

Although we tend to think of carbohydrates, lipids, and proteins as single nutrients, there are actually many different types of molecules in each of these classes. **Carbohydrates** include starches, sugars, and **fiber**. Some high-carbohydrate foods like potatoes, pasta, and white bread contain mostly starch; some, like oatmeal, berries, kidney beans, and broccoli are high in fiber; and others like cookies, cakes, and carbonated beverages are high in added sugars (Figure 1.4). Foods that are high in fiber and low in added sugar tend to be higher in nutrient density, containing more vitamins and minerals per calorie than low-fiber, high-sugar foods. There are

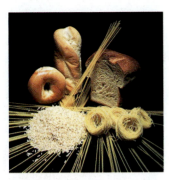

FIGURE 1.4

The carbohydrate in these foods is primarily starch. (Charles D. Winters)

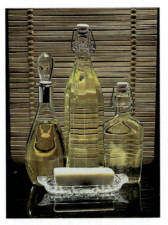

FIGURE 1.5

Not all fats are the same. Butter is high in saturated fat, and vegetable oils are higher in unsaturated fat. (Charles D. Winters)

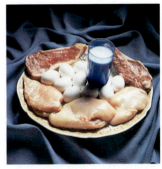

FIGURE 1.6

These animal products provide proteins that easily meet our need for amino acids. The right combination of plant proteins can also meet our protein needs. (Charles D. Winters)

several types of **lipids** that are important in nutrition. The ones we hear most about are cholesterol and saturated and unsaturated fats. Consuming a diet high in cholesterol and saturated fats, from foods like butter, meat, and milk, increases your risk of developing heart disease. Consuming a diet high in unsaturated fats from foods like vegetable oils, olives, and avocados lowers your risk (Figure 1.5). **Protein** is also not a single substance. There are thousands of different proteins in your body and your diet. All of these are made up of units called amino acids. Different combinations of amino acids are linked together to form different types of proteins. The amino acids we eat in animal products better match our needs than do the amino acids from plant proteins such as those in grains and legumes. However, both plant and animal proteins can provide all the amino acids we need if the diet is chosen wisely (Figure 1.6).

Water, unlike the other nutrient classes, has only one member. Water makes up about 60% of an adult's body weight. We can't store water so body losses must constantly be replaced by water in the diet. In the body water acts as a lubricant, a transport fluid, and a regulator of body temperature.

Vitamins are small **organic** molecules that must be consumed in the diet to maintain health. There are 13 different vitamins. Each provides a unique function in the body, from maintaining vision to helping blood to clot. **Minerals** are inorganic **elements**. Like vitamins, they are needed for a variety of diverse functions such as keeping our bones strong and transporting oxygen in our blood. We consume vitamins and minerals in almost all of the foods we eat. Some foods are natural sources of vitamins and minerals: oranges contain vitamin C, milk provides calcium, and carrots give us vitamin A. Other foods have vitamins and minerals added to them; breakfast cereals often have almost 100% of the recommended intake of many vitamins added to them. Dietary supplements are also a source of vitamins and minerals for some people.

The nutrients in food provide energy, structure, and regulation

Together the macronutrients and micronutrients in our diet provide us with energy, contribute to the structure of our bodies, and regulate the biological processes that go on inside us. Each nutrient provides one or more of these functions, but all nutrients together are needed to provide for growth, to maintain and repair the body, and to allow reproduction.

Lipids The class of nutrients that we commonly call fats. Chemically they are organic molecules, most of which do not dissolve in water.

Proteins The class of nutrients that is made up of one or more intertwining chains of amino acids.

Vitamins Organic molecules needed in the diet in small amounts to promote and regulate the chemical reactions and processes needed for growth, reproduction, and the maintenance of health.

Organic Molecules containing two or more carbon atoms.

Minerals Inorganic elements needed by the body in small amounts for structure and to regulate chemical reactions and body processes.

Elements Substances that cannot be broken down into products with different properties.

On the Side

Over 50% of Americans take a vitamin supplement on a regular basis. Supplements can help meet needs but they also increase the risk of consuming toxic amounts.

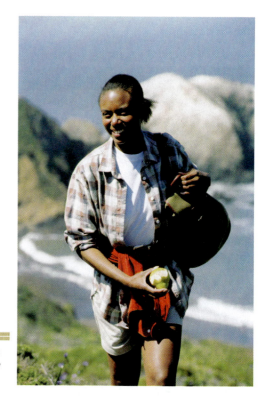

FIGURE 1.7

The calories provided by the nutrients in food fuels our activities. (Doug Menuez/PhotoDisc, Inc./Getty Images)

Calorie A unit of heat that is used to express the amount of energy provided by foods.

Kilocalorie 1000 calories. Can be expressed by spelling Calorie with a capital C.

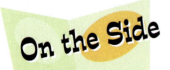

In Europe, the Joule rather than the Calorie is the standard measure of energy in food and the body. It takes 4.18 Joules to equal 1 Calorie.

Energy is measured in calories The term **calorie** is familiar to most people. Many of us think of calories as something to avoid, but we need calories to keep us alive and moving. Calories are the units we use to quantify the amount of energy a food provides when eaten. So, technically we don't eat calories; we eat food that provides energy measured in calories. Food and the energy it provides are essential to maintain life. Energy is used to do body work, whether it is breathing, walking to the mailbox, or running a marathon (Figure 1.7). When our diets provide the same number of calories as we use each day to stay alive and active, our body weight remains the same. If we consume more calories than we need, the extra energy is stored in our bodies, mostly as fat, and we gain weight. If we consume fewer calories than we need, our bodies use their stored energy and we lose weight.

The calories people talk about and you see listed on food labels are actually **kilocalories**, units of 1000 calories (abbreviated as kcalorie or kcal). When it is spelled with a capital "C," Calorie means kilocalorie.

Carbohydrates, lipids, and proteins are the nutrients that provide energy. They are often referred to as the energy-yielding nutrients. Carbohydrates provide 4 Calories per gram; they are the most immediate source of energy for the body. Lipids also help fuel our activities and are an important storage form of energy in the body. One gram of fat provides 9 Calories. Protein can supply 4 Calories per gram but is not the body's first choice for meeting energy needs, because protein has other more important roles. Alcohol, although it is not a nutrient because it is not needed for life, provides about 7 Calories per gram. Water, vitamins, and minerals do not provide any calories.

Nutrients provide structure Most of our body weight is due to water, protein, and fat. These nutrients, along with the minerals, are needed to form and maintain the shape and structure of the body. For instance, the muscles that help define our body contours are made up of water and protein. Proteins form the ligaments and tendons that hold our bones together and attach our muscles to our bones. Protein is also important in the structure of bones and teeth because it forms the framework that is hardened by mineral deposits. Fat also has an effect on the size and shape of our bodies. Someone with more fat is rounder and softer than someone with less fat and more muscle. On a smaller scale, lipids, proteins, and water form the structure of cells. Lipid and protein make up the membranes that surround each cell, and water fills the cells and the spaces around them.

Nutrients help regulate body processes In order to keep your body functioning, thousands of chemical reactions and physiological processes are going on all the time. Despite all this activity, your body temperature, blood pressure, blood sugar level, and hundreds of other parameters remain relatively constant. This state in which conditions inside the body are maintained in a healthy range is called **homeostasis**. Nutrients help regulate body processes to maintain homeostasis. All six classes of nutrients have important regulatory roles. Water helps to regulate body temperature; when your body temperature increases, you sweat to help keep you cool. Lipids and proteins are needed to make regulatory molecules called hormones that turn on or turn off various body processes, and proteins, vitamins, and minerals are needed to help regulate how quickly chemical reactions take place throughout the body.

Homeostasis A physiological state in which a stable internal body environment is maintained.

Food provides other substances that have health benefits

In addition to nutrients, food also contains substances that although not essential to life, can be beneficial for your health. Substances found in plant foods that have health-promoting properties are called **phytochemicals**. They are one of the many reasons you should eat your vegetables. A phytochemical found in broccoli called sulforaphane may reduce the risk of cancer, phytochemicals in soybeans help lower blood cholesterol, and some of the phytochemicals in dark green, leafy vegetables such as spinach and collard greens help prevent eye disorders (see Chapter 10). Animal foods also contain substances that have health-promoting properties. These are called **zoo-chemicals**. An example of a zoochemical is a type of fat found in dairy products; it is reported to have anticancer properties. Likewise, a type of fat in fish can help protect you from heart disease.

Phytochemical A substance found in plant foods that is not an essential nutrient but may have health-promoting properties.

Zoochemical A substance found in animal foods that is not an essential nutrient but may have health-promoting properties.

We Choose Foods for Reasons Other than Their Nutrients

Do you eat strawberries because they are a good source of vitamin C? Do you stop for an ice cream cone to add a little calcium to your diet? Probably not. Most of us choose these foods because we enjoy them. We need nutrients such as vitamin C and calcium to survive—but we choose foods, not individual nutrients (Figure 1.8). There are hundreds of food choices to make and almost as many reasons for making them. Sometimes we choose a food simply because that is what is put in front of us; often our decisions also depend on what suits our personal preferences, what we have learned to eat, what is socially acceptable, and sometimes what we think is a healthy choice. All of these factors are involved because food does more than meet our physiological requirements. It provides sensory pleasure and helps to meet our social and emotional needs. We eat chocolate to cheer us up. We eat cookies or cinnamon rolls while walking through the mall because the smell entices us to buy them. We eat lunch at noon out of social convention, not necessarily because we are hungry.

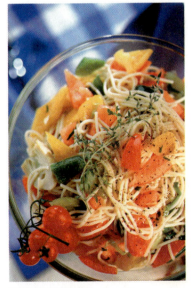

FIGURE 1.8

We don't eat nutrients; we eat foods that we choose for a variety of reasons, including taste, color, and texture. (© Image State)

We choose foods that help meet our emotional and psychological needs

Food is associated with comfort, love, and security. We develop this association as infants suckling while cradled in our mother's arms. As children and as adults, comfort foods such as hot tea and chicken soup help us to feel better when we are sick. We use food as a reward when we are good: a good report card is celebrated with an ice cream cone. We sometimes take away food as punishment: a child who misbehaves is sent to

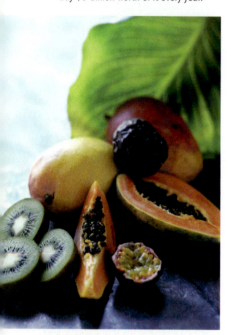

FIGURE 1.9

In the United States we enjoy year-round access to foods from around the world. (Alison Miksch/Foodpix/PictureArts Corp.)

bed without dinner. We consider ourselves good when we eat healthy foods and bad when we order a decadent dessert. We celebrate milestones and reward life's accomplishments with food. Food may also be an expression and a moderator of mood and emotional states. When upset, some of us turn to chocolate, while others stop eating altogether.

We choose from foods that are available to us

In February in Minnesota, fresh strawberries are hard to come by. The season, along with geography, socioeconomics, and health status, all affect the foods available to us as individuals and populations. In many parts of the world, food choices are limited to foods produced locally. Nutrients that are lacking in local foods will be lacking in the population's diet. In more developed parts of the world, the ability to store, transport, and process food allows year-round access to many seasonal foods and foods grown and produced at distant locations (Figure 1.9).

Even if foods are available in the store, it doesn't mean that they are available to everyone. Socioeconomic factors such as income level, living conditions, and lifestyle as well as education affect the types and amounts of foods available to us. Individuals with limited incomes can choose only the foods that they can afford. Individuals who don't own cars can purchase only what they can carry home. Those without refrigerators are limited to foods that are eaten right away or can be stored without refrigeration. And those who can't or don't have time to cook are limited to prepared foods and restaurant meals.

Health status also affects the availability of food. People who cannot carry heavy packages are limited in what they can purchase. People with food allergies, digestive problems, and dental disease are limited in the foods that are safe and comfortable for them to eat. People consuming special diets to manage disease conditions are limited to foods that meet their dietary prescriptions.

We choose foods we have learned to eat

Have you ever eaten grasshoppers or silkworms? If you grew up in Asia or Africa, the answer would likely be yes (Figure 1.10). In many parts of the world certain insects are considered a delicacy and can make an important nutritional contribution, but in American culture insects are considered food contaminants. If you didn't grow up in a culture that eats insects you may be unwilling to try them now. Food preferences and

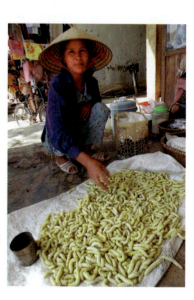

FIGURE 1.10

A plate of silkworms such as these being sold in a market in Vietnam may not be very appealing to you, but insects are a part of the diet in many parts of the world. (AFP/Getty Images)

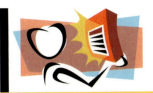

Off the Label: Read the Whole Label to Know What You Are Choosing

Healthy! Fresh! Light! The first thing that may catch your eye when shopping is a large-print banner describing some nutritious feature of a product. Food labels with eye-catching banners and names sell better. Although food labels must conform to federal guidelines and use standard definitions for most terms, they can still be misleading. Understanding what these terms mean on food labels will help you know what you are choosing and how it fits into your diet.

Many food labels highlight individual nutrients, and just as no single food determines the healthiness of a diet, no single nutrient makes a food good or bad for you. Look beyond the banner and see what other contribution the food makes to your diet. For example, chocolate cookies labeled "fat free" may not be your best choice if you are trying to reduce your sugar intake or increase the amount of fiber in your diet. A food labeled "fresh" may sound appealing, but the term "fresh" doesn't provide any information about the nutrient content of the product or how long it took for this food to travel from the farm to the grocery store shelf. Any raw food that has not been frozen, heat processed, or otherwise preserved can be labeled fresh. "Healthy" is another attractive byline that applies to more than a single nutrient. It implies that the product is wholesome and nutritious. In fact, to be described as "healthy," a food must be low in fat and saturated fat, contain limited amounts of sodium and cholesterol, and be a good source of one or more important nutrients. Since vegetables, fruits, and grain products are an important part of a healthy diet, fresh fruits and vegetables and some canned and frozen ones as well as enriched grain products may be labeled healthy even if they are not a good source of one or more of the specified nutrients. While all of the qualities specified by the term "healthy" are part of a healthy diet, foods that fit this definition are not necessarily the basis for a healthy diet. For instance, many fruit drinks fit the labeling definition of healthy. They are low in fat, saturated fat, cholesterol, and sodium and supply at least 10% of the recommended intake for vitamin C. But they are a good choice only in limited quantities because they are high in added refined sugar and contain few other nutrients. Likewise, a food that doesn't meet the labeling definition of healthy is not necessarily a poor choice. Vegetable soup, for example, contains more sodium than the definition of healthy will allow, but if the rest of the diet is not high in sodium, the soup can be a healthy choice.

Product names can also be misleading and unless you have memorized the labeling regulations, you may not be able to tell exactly what you are buying. These regulations determine how much beef is in a beef enchilada, how much chicken is in chicken soup, and how much fruit is in a Fruit Roll-Up. Product names must comply with legal definitions, but they don't have to make sense to consumers. For example, "lasagna with meat sauce" must be 6% meat, but "lasagna with meat and sauce" must be 12% meat.

To get the whole picture, you need to look beyond the healthy-sounding banner and the name of the product. Since the nutrient content of foods must be listed, along with information on how a food fits into the diet as a whole, reading the label thoroughly will provide you with the information you need to make wise choices. The discussion of labeling regulations in Chapter 2 and Off the Label boxes throughout this book provide more information on how to read food labels.

---

eating habits are learned as part of each individual's family, cultural, national, and social background. They are among the oldest and most entrenched features of every culture. In Japan rice is the focus of the meal, whereas in Italy pasta is always included. Curries characterize Indian cuisine, and we expect refried beans and tortillas when we go out for Mexican food. The foods we are exposed to as children influence what foods we buy and cook as adults.

What would a birthday be without a cake, or Thanksgiving without a turkey (Figure 1.11)? Each of us associates holidays such as Christmas, Easter, Passover, New Year's, and Kwanza with specific foods that are traditional in our family, religion, and culture. Seventh-Day Adventists are vegetarians; Jews and Muslims do not eat pork, Sikhs and Hindus do not eat beef. Even for those who choose not to observe religious dietary rules, habit may dictate many mealtime decisions. Jewish kosher laws prohibit the consumption of meat and milk in the same meal. Often Jews who do not follow kosher law may choose not to serve milk at dinner because they never had it as children.

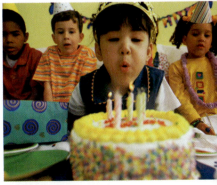

FIGURE 1.11

We expect to have a cake at a birthday party because it is a tradition. (Ryan McVay/PhotoDisc, Inc./Getty Images)

PIECE IT TOGETHER

How to Build a Healthy Diet

Courtney's class project is to interview four of her classmates and evaluate their diets to see if they follow the principles of variety, balance, and moderation. She starts by interviewing her friend Amy and then talks with other students in her dorm.

Amy says she likes the variety of foods offered at the cafeteria. She often has two different fruits at breakfast, several different greens in her salads, and two or three different vegetables at dinner. Despite these healthy choices, she has gained 10 pounds since she started college. By asking a few more questions, Courtney finds that Amy keeps a supply of cookies, candy, and chips in her room to snack on while studying.

DOES AMY'S DIET FOLLOW THE PRINCIPLES OF VARIETY, BALANCE, AND MODERATION

Amy's diet was varied, but she is short on moderation. While studying she tends to eat without paying attention to how much she is having. Apparently, despite her healthy meals, her high-calorie snacks are not balanced with enough exercise so they are adding the extra pounds.

Amad loves fast food. He often has breakfast at the doughnut shop, has burgers and fries for lunch, and goes out for tacos or pizza at dinner time.

HOW DOES AMAD'S DIET STACK UP?

His diet includes a variety of fast foods, but eating these foods every day adds up to a diet that is high in calories and fat and low in some vitamins and minerals. He doesn't have to give up fast food if he can balance his fast food choices that are low in nutrient density with ones that are higher in nutrient density. For example, if he plans on burgers for

dinner, he can have a sandwich on whole grain bread with lots of vegetables and a glass of milk for lunch. If his meals are high in calories, he can snack on low-calorie, nutrient-dense fresh fruits and vegetables.

Eric says he eats lots of fruits and vegetables, but when Courtney reviews his diet it turns out the only vegetables he ever eats are carrots and potatoes, and the only fruits he eats are oranges and apples.

WHAT IS MISSING FROM ERIC'S DIET?

Eric is getting enough servings of fruits and vegetables but he is missing out on variety. By limiting his choices to carrots, potatoes, oranges, and apples, he is missing nutrients and phytochemicals as well as tastes and textures that other fruits and vegetables provide.

Helen likes routine. She has cereal with milk for breakfast every day, a peanut butter sandwich for lunch, and meat with rice and a salad for dinner.

HOW COULD HELEN IMPROVE HER DIET?

Your Answer:

Emma loves sweets. She eats ice cream and cookies every day for a snack, and her meals are not complete unless they include a sweet dessert.

HOW COULD EMMA IMPROVE HER DIET?

Your Answer:

We choose foods that are socially acceptable

In addition to being part of our cultural heritage, food is the centerpiece of our everyday social interactions. We get together with friends for dinner or for a cup of coffee and dessert. The family dinner table is often the focal point for communication—a place where experiences of the day are shared. Social events dictate our food choices for a number of reasons. For example, when invited to a friend's house for dinner, we may eat foods we don't like out of politeness to our hosts. We may alter our food choices because of peer pressure. An adolescent may feel that stopping for a cheeseburger or taco after school is an important part of being accepted by his or her peers.

We choose foods that appeal to us

Tradition, religion, and social values may dictate what foods we consider appropriate, but personal preferences for taste, smell, appearance, and texture affect which foods we actually consume. Think of three of your favorite foods. How would you feel about giving them up? Probably not too good, and you are not alone. Even though most Americans understand that nutrition is important to their health, many do not choose a healthy diet because they don't want to give up their favorite foods and they don't want to eat foods they don't like.[1] Personal convictions also affect food choices; a vegetarian would not choose a meal that contains meat, and an environmentalist may not buy a food packaged in a non-recyclable container.

We choose foods that we think are healthy

Often a person's attitudes about what foods they think are good for them affect what they choose. For example, you may choose a low-carb diet because you think it helps you lose weight, organic produce because you are concerned about exposure to pesticides, or green tea to increase your intake of cancer-fighting antioxidants. Some healthy choices are easy. It is pretty obvious that having a salad and sandwich for lunch is a more nutritious choice than just a candy bar, but these decisions are not always clear. Is whole wheat bread healthier than white? Does honey provide more nutrients than table sugar? Will high-protein foods help you lose weight? People often base their food choices on what they think is healthiest, but they may not always have all the facts. Knowing how to use nutrition information is important in choosing nutritious foods.

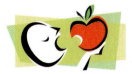

Choosing a healthy diet might come naturally if you had only nutrient-dense foods from which to choose. But grocery stores are packed with foods designed more to appeal to your senses than to supply your nutrient needs. Because of this, you should consider health and nutrition as well as taste when you choose which foods to include in your diet.

Variety, Balance, and Moderation Are Key to Choosing a Healthy Diet

A healthy diet is one that provides the right number of calories to keep your weight in the desirable range; the proper balance of carbohydrates, proteins, and fats; plenty of water; and sufficient but not excessive amounts of essential vitamins and minerals. It is rich in whole grains, fruits, and vegetables; high in fiber; moderate in fat, sugar, and sodium; and low in saturated fat, cholesterol, and *trans* fat. Choosing this healthy diet doesn't mean giving up your favorite foods. None of the foods we choose are good or bad in and of themselves, but together they make up a healthy or not-so-healthy diet. You also don't need a nutrient score card at every meal; what is important is your overall intake over the course of days, weeks, and months. A healthy diet is based on variety, balance, and moderation. Using these principles you can develop a personal strategy for making better choices and maintain your health for the long term (Figure 1.12).

On the Web
For more information on food intake patterns in the United States, go to the USDA Economic Research Service at **www.ers.usda.gov**.

Variety is important because no single food has it all

Variety is the spice of life. This is especially true when it comes to foods and nutrients. No single food can provide all the nutrients the body needs for optimal health. Eating a variety of foods helps ensure an adequate nutrient intake. Variety means choosing

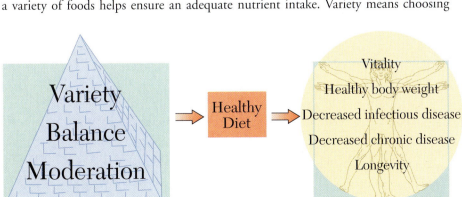

Variety
Balance
Moderation → Healthy Diet → Vitality
Healthy body weight
Decreased infectious disease
Decreased chronic disease
Longevity

FIGURE 1.12

A diet that follows the principles of variety, balance, and moderation will help you to live a longer, healthier life.

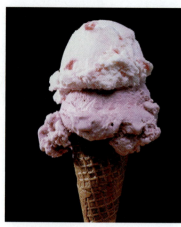

FIGURE 1.13

Ice cream cones and other favorite foods can be part of a healthy diet if they are balanced with choices that are lower in calories, fat, and sugar. (PhotoDisc, Inc./Getty Images)

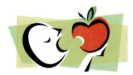

You shouldn't eat cake at every meal or guzzle soft drinks throughout the day, but if you limit foods that are low in nutrient density, any food can fit.

foods from different food groups—meats, dairy products, vegetables, grains, and fruits. Some of these are rich in protein and minerals, and others in vitamins and phytochemicals, but all are important. Variety also means choosing diverse foods from within each food group. Even similar types of foods provide different nutrients and different tastes. For instance, if you choose three vegetables a day and they are all potatoes, it is unlikely that you will meet your nutrient needs. Potatoes provide vitamin C but are lacking in vitamin A. If instead you have a salad, potatoes, and broccoli, you will be getting vitamin C along with more vitamin A and K than just potatoes could provide. If you always choose red meat to supply your protein, you will be missing out on the fiber in beans and the healthy fats in nuts. Variety comes from choosing different foods not only each day, but also each week and throughout the year. If you had apples and grapes today, have blueberries and cantaloupe tomorrow. If you can't find tomatoes in the winter, replace them with a winter vegetable like squash.

Balance allows you to include all foods in your healthy diet

Do you like fast food? Are you someone who can't live without chocolate? Whatever foods you love can be included in your diet if you balance your choices. There is no such thing as a good food or a bad food—only healthy diets and unhealthy diets. Any food can be part of a healthy diet as long as your total diet throughout the day or week provides enough of all of the nutrients you need without excesses of any. When you choose a food that is lacking in fiber, for example, balance this choice with one that provides lots of fiber. When you choose a food that is very high in fat, then balance that choice with a low-fat one. Balance involves mixing and matching foods so you get enough of the nutrients you need and not too much of ones that might harm your health. A balanced diet provides enough but not too much of each of the vitamins and minerals, as well as protein, carbohydrate, fat, and water. It also balances the calories you take in with the calories you use up in your daily activities so your body weight stays in the healthy range (Table 1.2; Appendix B). Balancing your choices allows foods that would not usually be considered healthy choices to fit into an overall healthy diet (Figure 1.13). For example, cookies, chips, and sodas should be balanced with nutrient-dense choices such as salads, fresh

TABLE 1.2
Balance Bigger Portions with Extra Exercise

If You Choose . . .	You Have Increased Your Calories By	To Balance Your Calories, You Need to Add
A 20-oz bottle of soda instead of a 12-oz can	100	2000 extra steps
A super-size fries instead of a small order	390	An hour of fast biking
A bagel from the bagel shop instead of two slices of toast	150	Half an hour at aerobics class
A Big Mac instead of a plain burger	260	An hour of golf, carrying your clubs
A grande mocha frappuccino instead of regular iced coffee	370	An hour of jogging
Three cups of pasta instead of one	400	An hour of hiking
A cup of spaghetti with cream sauce instead of marinara sauce	200	An hour of gardening
Fried chicken with skin instead of barbequed chicken with no skin	280	An hour of bowling

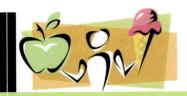

So, What Should I Eat?

Eat a variety of foods
- Snack on dried cranberries
- Put almonds on your salad
- Tired of carrots? Try jicama
- Try a new vegetable or fruit every week
- Vary your meats by having fish one day and pork, poultry, or beef on others
- Skip the meat and have beans with dinner

Balance your low-nutrient-density choices with higher ones
- Going out to dinner? Have a salad for lunch
- Add a veggie instead of pepperoni to your pizza
- When you have cookies for a snack, have fruit for dessert
- Had soda with lunch? Have milk with dinner
- If today's breakfast was a pastry, have oatmeal tomorrow

Everything in moderation
- Push back from the table before your are stuffed, and go for a walk
- Reduce your ice cream serving by scooping it into a smaller bowl
- Skip the seconds
- Have dessert every other day
- If you eat some extra fries, take some extra steps
- Split your restaurant meal with a friend

fruit, and low-fat dairy products. If your favorite meal is a burger, french fries, and a milkshake, enjoy it but balance it with asparagus, brown rice, and baked chicken at the next meal.

Moderation means having enough but not too much

Everything in moderation. Moderation means everything is OK, as long as you don't overdo it. It means watching your portions and passing up the super sizes. Have you ever sat down in front of the TV with a bag of chips and before you knew it, half the bag was gone? If you have, then you know how easy it is to let portion sizes get out of control. Moderation means not having too many calories, too much fat, too much sugar, too much salt, or too much alcohol. Choosing moderately will help you maintain a healthy weight and help prevent some of the chronic diseases like heart disease and cancer that are on the rise in our population. The fact that more than 60% of adult Americans are obese demonstrates that we have not been practicing moderation when it comes to calorie intake.[4] Moderation will make it easier to balance your diet and will allow you to enjoy a greater variety of foods.

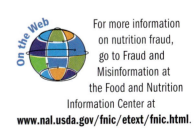

For more information on nutrition fraud, go to Fraud and Misinformation at the Food and Nutrition Information Center at www.nal.usda.gov/fnic/etext/fnic.html.

You Can't Believe All the Nutrition Advice You Hear

To choose a healthy diet you need to have the right information. We certainly get enough nutrition information. We are literally bombarded with it in our everyday lives. The evening news, the morning newspaper, and the Web all give us tidbits of nutrition advice. Food and nutrition information that would take physicians and dietitians years to disseminate now travels via the media, reaching millions in a matter of hours or days. Much of this information is reliable, but some can be misleading. It may be exaggerated to sell products or to make news headlines more enticing: carbohydrates make you fat, vitamin C cures the common cold, vitamin E slows aging. The motivation for news stories is often to sell subscriptions or improve ratings, not to promote the nutritional health of the population. Sifting through this information and distinguishing the useful from the useless may seem overwhelming. An understanding of how nutrition information is determined by using the methods of science will allow you to develop the nutrition savvy you need to judge the validity of nutrition headlines.

Nutrition discoveries are made by using the scientific method

⭐ **Scientific method** The general approach of science that is used to explain observations about the world around us.

⭐ **Hypothesis** An educated guess made to explain an observation or to answer a question.

⭐ **Theory** An explanation based on scientific study and reasoning.

Advances in our understanding of nutrition are made by using a systematic, unbiased approach called the **scientific method**. This process begins by making an observation and asking questions about that observation. For example, someone might observe that people who are overweight tend to skip breakfast. The next step is to propose an explanation for this observation. This explanation is called a **hypothesis**. In this example the hypothesis might be that people who skip breakfast eat more high-calorie foods later in the day, leading to weight gain. Once a hypothesis has been proposed, experiments can be designed to test it. In this example, the experiment might compare the total calorie intake of breakfast-skippers with that of breakfast-eaters. If the results from repeated studies support the hypothesis and do not prove it to be wrong, a scientific explanation or **theory** can be established (Figure 1.14). A single experiment is not enough to develop a theory; rather, repeated experiments showing the same conclusion are needed to develop a sound theory. A theory is not a fact. As new information becomes available, even a theory that has been accepted by the scientific community for years can be proved wrong. To generate reliable theories, the experiments done to test hypotheses must produce reliable results and be interpreted accurately.

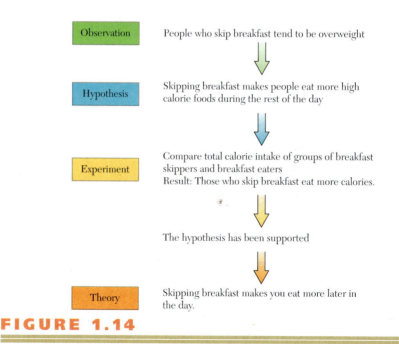

FIGURE 1.14

This example illustrates how the scientific method can be used to formulate hypotheses based on observations, design experiments to test these hypotheses, and interpret the results to support or disprove the hypotheses, helping establish a theory.

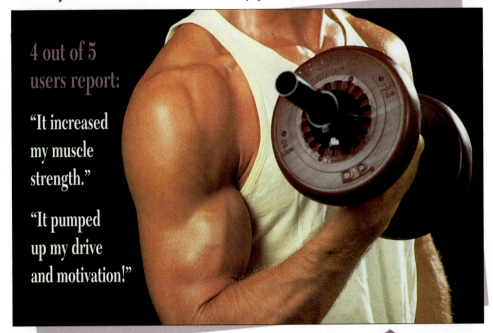

POWER BOOST
BOOST your STRENGTH • POWER up your DRIVE • MAXIMIZE your MASS

4 out of 5 users report:

"It increased my muscle strength."

"It pumped up my drive and motivation!"

Years of research have developed this special nutritional formulation. Just mix with water and stack one shake with every meal or snack.

University Study Shows: 25 experienced weight lifters added one POWER BOOST shake at meals and snacks 5 times a day for 4 weeks.
Body muscle mass and fat mass were measured by underwater weighing before POWER BOOST was added and after 4 weeks of training with POWER BOOST.

RESULTS
The weight lifters gained an average of 5.2 pounds of lean muscle and lost 4.5 pounds of unwanted fat.

FIGURE 1.15

This hypothetical advertisement illustrates the types of nutrition claims that consumers must be prepared to evaluate. (Lawrence Migdale/ Photo Researchers)

A good experiment provides quantifiable data Scientific experiments should provide data that can be quantified and repeated. Data that can be quantified include measures like body weight and blood pressure; they can be measured reliably and repeatedly. Feelings are more difficult to assess. They can be quantified with standardized questionnaires, but individual testimonies or opinions are not objective measures. The advertisement for Power Boost illustrated in Figure 1.15 describes a study that supports its claim to increase muscle mass and decrease body fat. The study used measures that provide quantifiable, repeatable data on the amount of body muscle and fat. In contrast, this ad also quotes users who report increased muscle strength and pumped-up motivation. This information it not quantifiable; it is merely the feelings and impressions of individual users.

A good experiment uses proper controls In order to know if what you are testing has an effect, you need to be able to compare it with something. A **control group** acts as a standard of comparison for each factor or **variable** being studied. A control group is treated in the same way as the **experimental group** except no experimental treatment is given. For example, in the experiment described in the

Control group A group of participants in an experiment that are used as a basis of comparison. They are identical to the experimental group but do not receive the experimental treatment.

Variable A factor or condition that is changed in an experimental setting.

Experimental group A group of participants in an experiment who undergo an experimental treatment.

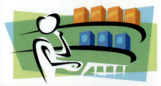

Your Choice: Would YOU Want to Be a Guinea Pig?

Being called a guinea pig usually means you are the first to try something. If you volunteer to be a subject in a research study you are doing just that. Sound adventurous? Or just scary? Oftentimes the only way to increase our understanding of human nutrition is to study humans. But this doesn't mean people need to risk their lives or safety for these studies. The government has strict regulations on what kinds of human research studies can be done and how the risks and benefits need to be presented to the subjects.

Before anyone becomes a human guinea pig, the researchers doing the study must explain the purpose of the research, the procedures used, and the possible risks and benefits. In addition to talking with the researchers, each subject must be given a written description of the study and its risks and benefits. Those who choose to participate must then sign a consent form stating exactly what they have agreed to do. And just because a person has consented doesn't mean he or she must stay in the study; if it turns out to be more than they bargained for, subjects can leave a study at any time. This informed consent process is part of the strict safety and ethical guidelines that must be followed when research involves human subjects. This system ensures that studies are conducted ethically, without undue risk to participants. Before a researcher can even look for study subjects, the study must be reviewed by a committee of scientists and nonscientists to ensure that the rights of the subjects are respected and that the risk of physical, social, and psychological injury is balanced against the potential benefit of the research. This committee can request that

changes be made in the study and can even stop a study if the researcher is not following the rules or if the trial appears to be causing unexpected harm to the participants. Studies can also be stopped if they demonstrate a strong benefit, so that the treatment can be made widely available.

Studies involving animals must follow similar rules. Although animals do not sign consent forms, the federal government mandates that panels of scientists review experiments in which the investigators propose to use animals. These panels consider whether the need for animals is justified and whether all precautions will be taken to avoid pain and suffering. Animal housing and handling are strictly regulated, and a violation of these guidelines can close a research facility.

Even research that uses only cells or genes from humans or animals is carefully reviewed and regulated. These newer types of studies have given rise to ethical issues regarding the manipulation of genes and the sources of genes and cells. For instance, stem cells obtained from embryos may be useful for treating diseases in adults, but many question the ethics of using these cells. As a result, funds for doing stem cell research are limited. Guidelines for the manipulation of genes and cells are constantly being revised to stay abreast of advances in this field.

So would you want to be a guinea pig? Some people do it to help contribute to medical breakthroughs. Others do it just because they get free medical care or other compensation. Whatever the reason, human guinea pigs can rest assured that there are safeguards at every step along the way to protect their physical and mental health.

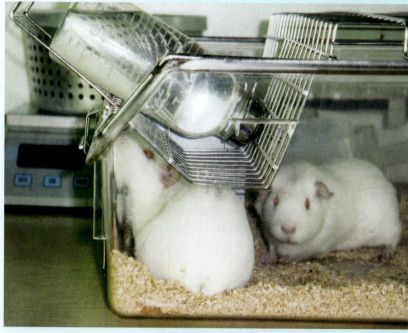

(Courtesy Lori Smolin)

Power Boost ad, the experimental group includes athletes consuming the Power Boost drink for 4 weeks. An appropriate control group would consist of athletes of similar age, gender, and ability eating similar diets and following similar workout regimens but not consuming Power Boost. The amount of body fat and muscle mass would be measured in both groups before and after the 4-week period.

In order to make the control and experimental groups indistinguishable, a **placebo** is sometimes used. A placebo, often a sugar pill, is identical in appearance to the actual treatment but has no therapeutic value. In the Power Boost example, the experimental group is consuming a protein drink. An appropriate placebo for the control group would be a drink that looks and tastes just like Power Boost but doesn't contribute any nutrients. Using a placebo prevents participants in the experiment from knowing if they are receiving the actual supplement. When the subjects do not know which treatment they are receiving, the study is called a **single-blind study**. Using a placebo in a single-blind study helps to prevent the expectations of subjects from biasing the results. For example, if the athletes think they are taking Power Boost, they may be convinced that they are getting stronger, and as a result they may work harder in their training and develop bigger muscles even without the supplement. Errors can also occur if investigators allow their own desire for a specific result to affect the interpretation of the data. This type of error can be avoided by designing a **double-blind study** in which neither the subjects nor the investigators know who is in which group until after the results have been analyzed.

A good experiment uses the right experimental population
For an experiment to produce reliable results, it must study the right group of people. For example, if Power Boost claims to improve performance in trained athletes, it should be tested in trained athletes. If a supplement claims to increase bone strength in older women, it must be tested in older women.

The number of subjects included in a study is also important. To be successful, an experiment must show that the treatment being tested causes a result to occur more frequently than it would by chance. The number of subjects needed depends on what is being studied. Fewer subjects are needed to demonstrate an effect that rarely occurs by chance. For example, if only one person in a million can increase the size of their muscles by weight training for 4 weeks, then the experiment to see if Power Boost increases muscles in 4 weeks would require only a few subjects to demonstrate an effect. However, if one out of four athletes can increase his or her muscle size by weight training for 4 weeks, then many more subjects are needed. A well-designed study considers how many subjects are needed to demonstrate an effect of the experimental treatment before a study is begun.

Experimental results must be interpreted correctly
Many different types of experiments are used to enhance our nutrition knowledge. Some study entire human populations, some study just a few people, some use animals, and some use just cells or molecules (Table 1.3). Regardless of the type of study, interpreting the results accurately is just as important as conducting the study carefully. In the Power Boost example, the formula was tested in experienced weight-lifters. The results may not have been the same if a group of nonathletes used this product, so the study cannot conclude that it will increase muscle size in everyone. Likewise, if the study measured only muscle size, the ad can't claim that strength is also increased. One way to ensure that experiments are correctly interpreted is to have the results reviewed by experts in the field who did not take part in the research that is being evaluated. This **peer-review** process is used in determining whether or not experimental results can be published in scientific journals. The reviewing scientists must agree that the experiments were well conducted and that the results were interpreted fairly. Nutrition articles that have undergone peer review can be found in journals such as *The American Journal of Clinical Nutrition*, *The Journal of Nutrition*, *The Journal of the American Dietetic Association*, *The New England Journal of Medicine*, and *The International Journal of Sport Nutrition*.

Placebo A fake medicine or supplement that is indistinguishable in appearance from the real thing. It is used to disguise the control and experimental groups in an experiment.

Single-blind study An experiment in which either the study participants or the researchers are unaware of who is in a control group or an experimental group.

Double-blind study An experiment in which neither the study participants nor the researchers know who is in a control group or an experimental group.

On the Side

Much of what we know today about the effects of starvation in humans was determined during World War II by conducting studies with conscientious objectors. These subjects were monitored physically and psychologically while they were starved and then re-fed. Today ethical and safety guidelines would prohibit this type of experiment.

Peer review Review of the design and validity of a research experiment by experts in the field of study who did not participate in the research.

TABLE 1.3
How Do We Study Nutrition?

Type of Study	Who It Studies	What It Can Tell Us	What the Limitations Are	Example
Epidemiology	Population groups	Patterns in food intake and health	Can determine only patterns, not what causes these patterns	By comparing the intake of saturated fat with blood cholesterol levels and the incidence of heart disease, researchers can see if the saturated fat in the diet is related to heart disease risk
Human intervention study	Individuals from within the population	The effect of a specific treatment such as a drug or diet on health or nutrition	Can be difficult to know whether the subjects are actually following the treatment plan	By decreasing the amount amount of fat in the diets of a group of women, researchers can see if it affects their risk of breast cancer
Human laboratory study	Individuals under controlled conditions in research facilities such as hospitals and universities	The effect of a specific treatment such as a drug or diet on health or nutrition	Expensive; hard to find subjects; can't keep subjects in the hospital for a long time, so can continue for only short periods of time	By feeding a high-protein diet, researchers can measure the effect of a high-protein diet on kidney function
Depletion-repletion study (a type of laboratory study)	Subjects in a controlled environment	Information about the functions and requirements of nutrients	Diet may be difficult to follow, and subjects may experience uncomfortable deficiency symptoms	By restricting vitamin C intake, researchers can study the symptoms of scurvy; by adding vitamin C back to the diet, they can determine how much is needed to eliminate symptoms
Balance study (a type of laboratory study)	Subjects in a controlled environment	Information about how much of a nutrient is needed in the diet to balance body losses	Diet may be difficult to follow, and collection of excretion products may be incomplete	By looking at the amount of protein needed to balance losses under different conditions, researchers can determine protein requirements
Animal study	Animals such as rats, mice, or pigs	Effect of diet on animal biology	Does not harm humans but may harm animals, and the results are not always directly applicable to humans	By feeding a vitamin A-deficient diet to pregnant animals, researchers can evaluate the effect of vitamin A deficiency during pregnancy
Cell study	Cells from humans or animals	The effect of nutrients on the biochemistry or molecular biology of individual cells	Results may not apply to the entire organism	By studying cells from genetically obese mice, researchers can identify obesity genes

Common sense can help you identify nutrition misinformation

Nutrition, like all science, continues to evolve. As new discoveries provide clues to the right combination of nutrients needed for optimal health, new nutrition principles are developed. Sometimes, established beliefs and concepts must give way to new discoveries. As knowledge increases, recommendations change. Consumers may find this frustrating because the experts seem to change their minds so often. One day you are told margarine is better for you than butter; the next day a report says that it is just as bad. Which should you believe? Who are the experts? How can you tell accurate from misleading nutrition information (Table 1.4)?

Just as scientists use the scientific method to expand their understanding of the world around us, each of us can use an understanding of how science is done to evaluate nutrition claims. Many of the nutrition claims we hear are very appealing, but they must be critically examined before they can be accepted. Some things that may tip you off to misinformation are if the claim sounds too good to be true, if it comes from an unreliable source, if it is selling a product, or if it is new or untested information.

Does the information make sense? The first question to ask yourself when evaluating a nutrition claim is, Does the information make sense? Some claims are too outrageous to be true. For example, if a product claims to increase your muscles without any exercise, common sense should tell you it is too good to be true. On the other hand, an article that tells you that adding exercise to your daily routine will with help you lose weight and increase your stamina is not so outrageous.

Where did the information come from? If the claim seems reasonable, look to see where it came from. Was it a personal testimony, a government recommendation, or advice from a health professional? Was it the result of a research study? Is it in a news story or an advertising promotion? Is it on television, in a magazine, or on a Web page? Generally stories that contain reliable information will tell you the government agency, university, or other source of the information.

On the Side

Fifteen years ago the supermarket was full of low-fat foods. We couldn't get enough of them. Today these have been replaced by low-carb foods. This demonstrates how susceptible consumers and manufacturers are to nutrition fads.

TABLE 1.4
Tips for Evaluating Nutritional Claims

- Think about it. Does the information presented make sense? If not, disregard it.

- Seek out the source. Where did the information come from? If it is based on personal opinions, be aware that one person's perception does not make something true.

- Consider credentials. What is the background of the researchers or authors? Are they at a university or government agency? If no credentials are listed, there is no way to determine if they are qualified to give this information.

- Assess the intent. Is the information helping to sell a product? Is it making a magazine cover or newspaper headline more appealing? If so, the claims may be exaggerated to help the sale.

- Be skeptical. If a statement claims to be based on a scientific study, think about who did the study, whether the study is one of a kind, and whether other studies show similar results. If it is one of a kind, it may be because no one else was able to duplicate the findings.

- Weigh the risks. Be sure the expected benefit of the product is worth the risk associated with using it.

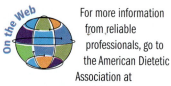

On the Side

Web sites sponsored by the government can be identified because they end in .gov. University-sponsored Web sites can be identified by addresses ending with .edu. Web sites sponsored by nonprofit organizations can be identified by addresses ending in .org. Internet addresses ending with .com are either privately sponsored or sponsored by a commercial for-profit organization.

On the Web

For more information from reliable professionals, go to the American Dietetic Association at **www.eatright.org**.

Individual testimonies are not proof. Just because someone says a product worked for him or her doesn't mean it will work for you. Claims that come from individual testimonies have not been tested by experimentation. So although the product worked for that one individual, there is no way to know if the product will work for others. For example, weight-loss products commonly show before and after photos of people who have successfully lost weight using the products. Their success is not a guarantee that the product will produce the same results for you or anyone else. These testimonials are not compared to a control group or subjected to scientific evaluation. Therefore, it cannot be assumed that similar results will occur in other people.

Information from government, nonprofit, and educational institutions is generally reliable. Government recommendations regarding healthy dietary practices are a reliable source of information. They are developed by committees of scientists who interpret the latest well-conducted research studies and use their conclusions to develop recommendations for the population as a whole. The information is designed to improve the health of the population. For example, these recommendations are used to develop food-labeling guidelines and are the basis of public health policies and programs. They are published in pamphlets and are available at government Web sites.

Information that comes from universities is supported by research and is also a reliable place to look for information. University research studies are usually published in peer-reviewed journals and are well scrutinized. Many universities also provide information that targets the general public. Nonprofit organizations such as the American Dietetic Association and the American Medical Association are also good source of nutrition information.

The author's credentials can help you tell if the information is valid. Knowing who is providing the information can help you decide whether or not to believe it. What are the credentials of the individuals providing the information? Where do they work? Do they have a degree in nutrition or medicine? If you are looking at an article or a Web site, check the credentials of the author. Care must be taken even when obtaining information from nutritionists. Although "nutritionists" and "nutrition counselors" may provide accurate information, the term nutritionist is not legally defined and is used by a wide range of people, from college professors with doctoral degrees from reputable universities to health food store clerks with no formal training. One reliable source of nutrition information is registered dietitians (RDs). Registered dietitians are nutrition professionals who have earned a 4-year college degree in a nutrition-related field and who have met established criteria to certify them in providing nutrition education and counseling.

Information that is selling a product may be less reliable

If a person or company will profit from the information presented, you should be wary. Claims that are part of an advertisement should be viewed skeptically, because advertisements are designed to increase sales and the company stands to profit from your believing the claim. Even information presented in newspapers and magazines and on television may be biased or exaggerated because it must help sell magazines or boost ratings (Figure 1.16). A well-designed, carefully executed, peer-reviewed experiment can be a source of misinformation if its results are interpreted incorrectly or exaggerated. For example, a study that shows that rats fed a diet high in vitamin E live longer than those consuming less vitamin E could be the basis of the headline "Vitamin E Supplements Increase Longevity." The fact that a diet high in vitamin E increased longevity does not mean that supplements will have the same effect. In addition, this study was done in rats. Can the result be extrapolated to human health? Just because rats consuming diets high in vitamin E live longer does not mean that the

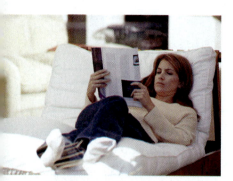

FIGURE 1.16

Headlines may exaggerate the facts to attract attention and sell magazines. (Javier Pierini/Getty/Brand X Pictures)

same is true for humans. This is also true of information on the Internet. If it comes from a site where you can buy something, the information is more likely to be biased toward the product or service.

Reliable information stands the test of time Often the results of a new scientific study are on the morning news the same day they are published in a peer-reviewed journal. Sometimes this information is accurate, but a single study is never enough to develop a reliable theory. Results need to be reproducible before they can be used as the basis for nutrition decisions. Headlines based on a single study should therefore be viewed skeptically. The information may be accurate, but there is no way to know because there has not been time to repeat the work and reaffirm the conclusions. If, for example, someone has found the secret to easy weight loss, you will undoubtedly see this information again if the finding is valid. If it is not, it will fade away with all the other weight-loss cures that have come and gone.

THINKING FOR YOURSELF

1. How healthy is your diet?
   a. How many different vegetables and fruits did you eat today? How about this week? If you average fewer than 5 a day, make some suggestions that would increase the fruit and vegetable variety in your diet.
   b. If you had a treat such as a doughnut or an extravagant dessert, did you balance it with some healthier choices at other times during the day or the next day? Suggest a healthy choice you could have to balance two of your favorite treats.
   c. Do you order supersize portions? If you do, try medium-size portions the next time you have fast food and see if you are full at the end of your meal.
   d. Do you ever eat foods right out of the package? If you do, it is hard to tell how much you really ate. Next time you grab the whole bag, pour it into a bowl before you put it in your mouth so you know just how much you are eating.

2. What determines your food choices?
   a. List four food items you ate today or yesterday. For each, indicate the factor or factors that influenced your selection of that particular food. For example, if you ate a candy bar before your noon class, did you choose it because the machine was available outside the lecture hall, because you didn't have enough money for anything else, because you just like candy bars, because you were depressed, because all of your friends were eating them, because they are good for you, or for some other reason?
   b. For each food, indicate what information you used in making the selection. For example, did you read the label on the product or consider something you read

or heard recently in the news media, or did you choose it simply because you like the taste?
   c. What three factors most often influence your food choices?
   d. What three types of information do you most often use to make your food choices?

3. Can you tell if this information is reliable?
   a. Examine a nutritional supplement ad provided by your instructor or select one from a health- or fitness-related magazine.
   b. Are the claims made about this product believable?
   c. Where did the information come from? Are the claims based on anecdotal reports of individual users? Is the information based on a government recommendation? Does it cite a university research study? If so, does the study seem well controlled? Are the results based on quantifiable measurements? Are the conclusions consistent with the results obtained? Are they published in a peer-reviewed journal?
   d. How might the fact that this is an ad affect the presentation of the information?
   e. On the basis of this ad, would you choose to take this supplement?

4. What type of information is on the Internet?
   a. Use an Internet search program to explore the types of nutrition information available on the Web. Search for the word nutrition.
   b. Make a list of four nonprofit organizations that you find. Why do these organizations have Web sites?
   c. Look at four Web sites that end in .com. Why do these companies have Web sites?

SUMMARY

1. Your diet affects your health. The foods you choose contain nutrients needed to keep you alive and healthy. The foods you choose determine which nutrients you consume. Poor choices can cause nutrient deficiencies and can contribute to chronic diseases as you age.

2. The typical diet in North America does not meet the recommendations for a healthy diet and contributes to the high incidence of chronic diseases such as diabetes, obesity, and heart disease.

3. Nutrients are grouped into six classes: carbohydrates, lipids, proteins, water, vitamins, and minerals. The right amounts of each of these is needed by the body for growth, maintenance and repair, and reproduction. Food also contains nonnutritive substances such as phytochemicals that may provide additional health benefits.

4. Nutrients provide energy, which is measured in calories. They provide structure to the body and regulate biochemical reactions and physiological processes to maintain homeostasis.

5. No food is good or bad, and no one food choice can make a diet healthy or unhealthy; each choice contributes to the diet as a whole.

6. A healthy diet includes a variety of nutrient-dense foods from each of the food groups as well as a variety of foods from within each group. It balances calorie and nutrient intake with needs and moderates choices to keep intakes of energy, fat, sugar, salt, and alcohol within reason. This diet will be rich in whole grains, fruits, and vegetables; high in fiber; moderate in fat, sugar, and sodium; and low in saturated fat, cholesterol, and *trans* fat.

7. The food choices we make are affected by many factors other than nutrition. They are affected by food availability; what we have learned to eat from our family, culture, and traditions; personal tastes; and what we think we should eat.

8. Nutrition uses the scientific method to determine the relationships between food and the nutrient needs of the body. The scientific method involves making observations of natural events, formulating hypotheses to explain these events, designing and performing experiments to test the hypotheses, and developing theories that explain the observed phenomenon based on the experimental results.

9. To be valid, a nutrition experiment must provide quantifiable measurements, use appropriate controls, choose the right type and number of experimental subjects, and interpret the results carefully.

10. Not all the nutrition information that comes to us is accurate. When judging nutrition claims, you need to consider whether the information makes sense, whether it came from a reliable source, whether the information is trying to sell a product, and whether it has been confirmed by multiple studies.

REVIEW QUESTIONS

1. What determines your nutrient intake?
2. What is malnutrition?
3. Give an example of overnutrition.
4. What are the six classes of nutrients?
5. To what class of nutrients do fiber, starch, cholesterol, and fatty acids belong?
6. List the energy-yielding nutrients.
7. What classes of nutrients are considered macronutrients?
8. What classes of nutrients are considered micronutrients?
9. List three functions provided by nutrients.
10. What is a phytochemical?
11. List three factors other than nutrient needs that influence what we eat.
12. Why is it important to choose a variety of foods?
13. How does moderation help maintain a healthy weight?
14. List the steps of the scientific method.
15. What is a control group?
16. What is a placebo?
17. What factors should be considered when judging nutrition claims?

REFERENCES

1. American Dietetic Association. Nutrition and you: trends 2002. Available online at www.eatright.org/Public/Media/PublicMedia_10240.cfm accessed April 28, 2004.

2. Institute of Medicine, Food and Nutrition Board. *Dietary Reference Intakes for Calcium, Phosphorus, Magnesium, Vitamin D, and Flouride.* Washington, D.C.: National Academy Press, 1997.

3. US Centers for Disease Control and Prevention. Physical Activity and Good Nutrition: Essential elements to prevent chronic diseases and obesity, 2004. Available online at www.cdc.gov/nccdphp/aag/pdf/aag_dnpa2004.pdf accessed July 31, 2004.

4. Weight-control information network Statistics related to obesity. Available online at www.niddk.nih.gov/health/nutrit/pubs/statobes.htm accessed July 31, 2004.

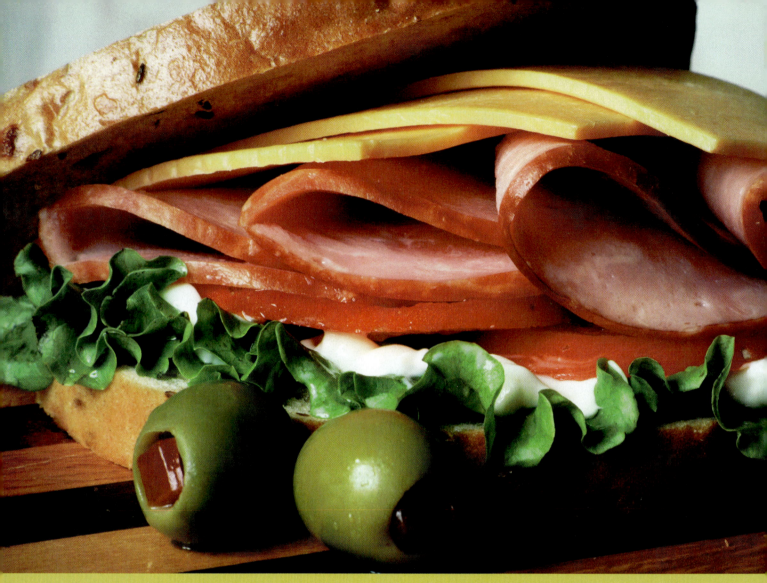

(Fotokat/Age Fotostock America, Inc.)

- There are many types of nutrition recommendations designed to promote health by guiding nutrient intake and food choices.
- The Dietary Reference Intakes are a set of reference values for the amounts of calories, nutrients, and food components needed in the diets of healthy people.
- The Food Guide Pyramid is a tool to plan diets that meet nutrition recommendations.
- Food labels provide information about the nutrient content of individual foods and how they fit into a healthy overall diet.
- The Dietary Guidelines for Americans are a set of nutrition and lifestyle recommendations that help consumers reduce the risks of chronic disease.
- The Exchange Lists are a food group system for planning and evaluating diets.
- Nutritional status can be assessed by evaluating your food intake, body size, and medical history.

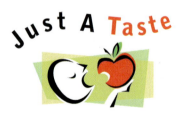

Just A Taste

Will you develop a deficiency disease if your diet does not meet the RDA?

Isn't all that bread at the bottom of the Food Guide Pyramid bad for you?

How do you know if your hot dog is high in fat?

How can you tell if you are meeting your nutrient needs?

Guidelines for a Healthy Diet

INTRODUCTION

The New York Times

U.S. Considers Food Labels with Whole-Package Data

By *Sherri Day*

Nov. 21, 2003—The Food and Drug Administration said yesterday that it was considering whether to require food companies to list nutrition information in its entirety, rather than by serving size, on packaged-food labels.

Currently, if a package contains more than one serving, consumers must multiply nutrition data by the number of servings to determine total calories, fat and carbohydrates. Some consumer groups and nutritionists have argued that such food labels are misleading and could cause consumers to take in more calories, sodium and fat than they realize. Now, it seems, the F.D.A. may agree.

To read the entire article, go to www.nytimes.com/pages/health/index.html.

Does the serving size listed on a package of food influence how much you eat? The answer is yes and no: sometimes we check the label to see what the recommended serving is, but more often than not, we eat until we are full or until the package is empty. Serving size is one of the many types of information the government supplies regarding what we are eating or what we should be eating. If the information provided is misleading, it could contribute to our less than healthy diet and the increasing incidence of diseases like obesity, diabetes, and heart disease in our population. What is the ideal way to provide consumers with information about their food? What types of information would help you choose a more healthful diet?

Nutrition Recommendations Promote a Healthy Population

For most of human history there were no guidelines about what to eat. People ate what was available, whether it was what was put in front of them or what was available in the local fields and forests. Today, there are many different guidelines regarding what we should eat. Some describe the amounts of individual nutrients we need and some recommend patterns of food intake that promote health and prevent disease. Many are made by government agencies responsible for promoting the well-being of the majority of healthy people in the population. Others come from special interest groups targeting specific segments of the population.

Governments have been making nutrition recommendations for 150 years

The U.S. government is not the first to provide nutrition recommendations. Some of the earliest nutrition recommendations were made in England in the 1860s, when the Industrial Revolution caused a rise in urban populations with large numbers of homeless and hungry people. The government developed a dietary standard based on the least expensive foods needed to keep people alive and maintain the work force. It wasn't until World War I that the British Royal Society decided that dietary standards should not only keep people alive but also keep them healthy. They therefore recommended that fruits and green vegetables be included in a healthy diet and that milk be included in the diets of all children.

Since these early recommendations, the governments of many countries have established their own sets of dietary standards based on the interpretations of their scientists and the nutritional problems and dietary patterns specific to their populations. The World Health Organization and the Food and Agriculture Organization of the United Nations have published dietary standards to promote health worldwide (see Appendix F).[1]

There are many types of nutrition recommendations in the United States

The original dietary standard in the United States was the Recommended Dietary Allowances (RDAs). First published in 1943, they were developed in response to the widespread food limitations created by World War II (Figure 2.1). Recommendations

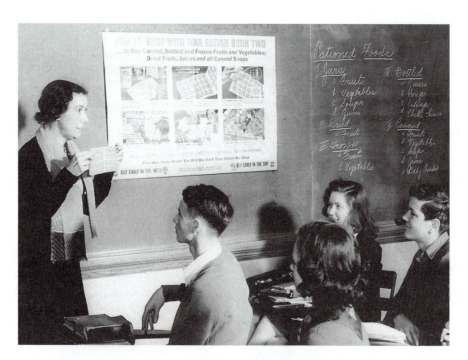

FIGURE 2.1

Food shortages during World War II prompted the U.S. government to establish dietary standards. (Office of War Information)

were made for the intake of energy and nutrients at risk for deficiency—protein, vitamins, and minerals. Levels of intake were recommended based on amounts that would prevent nutrient deficiencies.[2] Over the years since these first standards were developed, our knowledge of nutrient needs has increased and patterns of dietary intake and disease have changed. Overt nutrient deficiencies are now rare in the United States, while the incidence of diet-related chronic diseases such as heart disease, cancer, and obesity has increased. In response to these changes in our diet and health, the original RDAs have been replaced by a set of nutrient intake recommendations called the **Dietary Reference Intakes**, or **DRIs** for short.

In addition to the DRIs, there are a number of other types of recommendations that help Americans choose the foods that are needed to provide a healthy diet. The Food Guide Pyramid translates recommendations for nutrient intakes into food choices. A set of standards called the **Daily Values** has been established for use on food labels. These help Americans see how the nutrients provided by individual foods fit into an overall healthy diet. The Dietary Guidelines for Americans is a set of general recommendations about diet and lifestyle that show us how to combine other tools to choose a healthy diet and lifestyle.

Dietary Reference Intakes (DRIs) A set of reference values for the intake of nutrients and food components that can be used for planning and assessing the diets of healthy people in the United States and Canada.

Daily Value A nutrient reference value used on food labels to help consumers see how foods fit into their overall diets.

Dietary Reference Intakes Are Nutrient Intake Standards

The current standard for nutrient intake in the United States and Canada is the Dietary Reference Intakes (DRIs).[3] The DRIs provide recommendations for the amounts of energy, nutrients, and other food components that should be consumed by healthy people on an average daily basis. The amounts recommended by the DRIs are designed to promote health and reduce the incidence of chronic disease as well as prevent deficiencies.

DRI recommendations have been established for energy, vitamins, minerals, protein and amino acids, carbohydrates, fats, water, and electrolytes, and are planned for other food components that affect health, such as phytochemicals. The DRIs include several types of recommendations designed for different purposes. Values have been set for each gender and for various **life-stage groups**. These take into account the physiological differences that alter nutrient needs among men and women, infants, children, adolescents, adults, older adults, and pregnant and lactating women. The pregnancy and lactation life stages also include age categories to distinguish the unique nutritional needs of pregnancy and lactation in teenagers and older mothers (see Inside Cover).

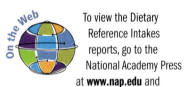 To view the Dietary Reference Intakes reports, go to the National Academy Press at **www.nap.edu** and search for Dietary Reference Intakes.

Life-stage groups Groupings of individuals based on stages of growth and development, pregnancy, and lactation that have similar nutrient needs.

The DRIs tell us how much is enough and not too much

DRI values that recommend specific amounts of nutrients for individuals include the **Recommended Dietary Allowances (RDAs)** and **Adequate Intakes (AIs)**. RDAs are based on experimental data and are set high enough to meet the needs of most people in the population. When there is not sufficient data to establish an RDA, an AI is set based on what healthy people typically eat. Either an RDA or an AI is established for each of the nutrients. These values are designed to be goals for individual intake, so you can use them to plan or evaluate your diet. For example, if you are concerned about your intake of iron, you can compare your intake with the RDA for iron for someone of your age and gender. If your intake meets the RDA, your risk of deficiency is very low. If your intake is below the RDA, you are at risk for a deficiency. The farther below the RDA your intake is, the greater the risk of a deficiency. The **Estimated Average Requirements (EARs)** are another set of DRI values that provide average recommendations for the population. EAR values are used in evaluating the adequacy of a population's food supply or typical intake, but they are not appropriate for evaluating an individual's intake.

Recommended Dietary Allowances (RDAs) Intakes that are sufficient to meet the nutrient needs of almost all healthy people in a specific life-stage and gender group.

Adequate Intakes (AIs) Intakes that should be used as a goal when no RDA exists. These values are an approximation of the average nutrient intake that appears to sustain a desired indicator of health.

Estimated Average Requirements (EARs) Intakes that meet the estimated nutrient needs of 50% of individuals in a gender and life-stage group.

⚠ **Tolerable Upper Intake Levels (ULs)**
Maximum daily intakes that are unlikely to pose risks of adverse health effects to almost all individuals in the specified life-stage and gender group.

Tolerable Upper Intake Levels (ULs) are the recommended limits for the maximum daily intake; the UL for a specific nutrient is the upper limit of what most people can consume without some adverse effect. For some nutrients the UL is set for total intake from all sources, including food, fortified foods, and supplements. For other nutrients, the UL refers to intake from supplements alone or from supplements and fortified foods. For many nutrients, there is no UL because there is not enough information available to determine the toxic level.

The DRIs recommend proportions of carbohydrate, fat, and protein

⚠ **Acceptable Macronutrient Distribution Range (AMDR)** A range of intake for carbohydrate, fat, or protein, expressed as a percentage of total energy intake, that is associated with reduced risk of chronic disease while providing adequate intakes of essential nutrients.

The DRIs also make recommendations for the proportions of carbohydrate, fat, and protein that make up a healthy diet. These are called the **Acceptable Macronutrient Distribution Ranges (AMDRs)**. The AMDRs are expressed as ranges because healthy diets can contain many different combinations of carbohydrate, protein, and fat.[4] According to the AMDRs a healthy diet for an adult can contain from 45 to 65% of calories from carbohydrate, 20 to 35% from fat, and 10 to 35% from protein. When calorie intake stays the same, changing the proportion of one of these will change the proportion of the others as well. So for example, in a diet that provides 2000 Calories with 50% of calories from carbohydrate, the other 50% will come from protein and fat. If the calories are kept the same but carbohydrate intake is decreased, the percentage of fat and/or protein will increase (Figure 2.2). The AMDRs allow flexibility in food choices to satisfy individual preferences while still providing a diet that minimizes disease risk. AMDR values have also been set for specific amino acids and fatty acids (see Inside Cover).

The DRIs estimate energy requirements for weight maintenance

⚠ **Estimated Energy Requirements (EERs)** The average energy intake predicted to maintain body weight in healthy individuals.

The recommendations for energy intake established by the DRIs are called **Estimated Energy Requirements (EERs)**. They provide equations that can be used to calculate the number of calories needed to keep weight stable in a healthy person. Variables in the calculations include the individual's age, gender, weight, height, and level of physical activity (see Inside Cover). Changing any of these variables changes the EER. For example, a 19-year-old girl who is 5'4" tall and weighs 127 pounds and gets no exercise needs to eat only 1950 Calories a day to maintain her weight. If she adds an hour of moderate activity to her daily routine, her EER will increase to 2410 Calories, and she will need to increase her food intake by about 460 Calories per day to maintain her weight. If she grows taller or gains weight, her calorie needs will also increase.

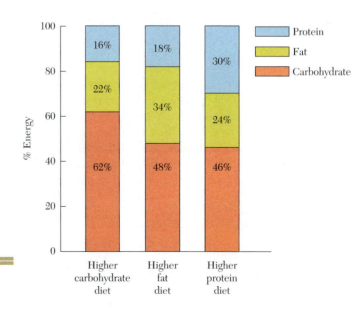

FIGURE 2.2

Changing the proportion of one of the energy-yielding nutrients in the diet changes the proportions of the others.

You can use the DRIs to make sure your diet is healthy

The different DRI values can be helpful in keeping your diet healthy. If you are concerned about your weight, you can use the EERs to calculate how many calories you should consume to keep your weight stable. If you are worried about getting enough calcium, you can check to see if your typical calcium intake meets the AI. If you are taking a supplement, you can use the RDA and UL values to be sure you are getting enough but not too much of the nutrients it contains. When using the DRIs, don't be concerned if your diet is below the recommended intake on any one particular day; the DRI values are meant to represent the average amount that most healthy people should eat over several days or even weeks, not each and every day.

You can also use the DRIs to plan your intake. For instance, if you know you need 1200 mg of calcium and that an 8-ounce glass of milk contains 300, you can calculate that you need to drink 4 glasses to meet the AI. However, using the DRIs to make all your food choices would be cumbersome and time consuming. Other types of recommendations are more useful for diet planning.

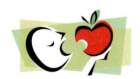

Eating less than the RDA does not mean you will develop a deficiency disease. But eating less than the recommended amount does mean that your risk of deficiency is greater.

The Food Guide Pyramid Is a Tool for Diet Planning

The Food Guide Pyramid is a guide for planning diets that meet nutrient requirements and recommendations for health promotion and disease prevention (Figure 2.3).[5,6] It was designed to help consumers make food choices that together add up to a healthy overall diet. The Pyramid is built around five food groups: Bread, Cereal, Rice, & Pasta; Vegetable; Fruit; Milk, Yogurt, & Cheese; and Meat, Poultry, Fish, Dry Beans, Eggs, & Nuts. Foods within each of these food groups supply similar nutrients. For example, foods in the Bread, Cereal, Rice, & Pasta Group provide carbohydrates and B vitamins; those in the Milk, Yogurt, & Cheese Group provide protein, calcium, riboflavin, and vitamin D. By choosing a variety of foods from each group according to the serving sizes and selection tips provided with the Pyramid, you

To learn more about the Food Guide Pyramid, go to the Food and Nutrition Information Center at **www.nal.usda.gov/fnic/** and click on Food Guide Pyramid.

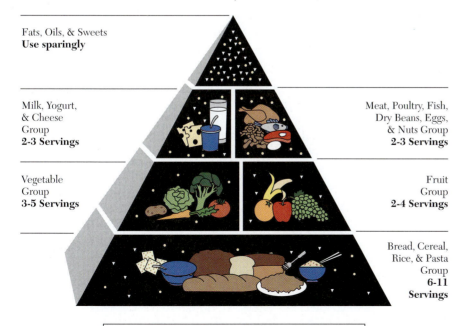

Food Guide Pyramid
A Guide to Daily Food Choices

Fats, Oils, & Sweets
Use sparingly

Milk, Yogurt, & Cheese Group
2-3 Servings

Meat, Poultry, Fish, Dry Beans, Eggs, & Nuts Group
2-3 Servings

Vegetable Group
3-5 Servings

Fruit Group
2-4 Servings

Bread, Cereal, Rice, & Pasta Group
6-11 Servings

Key
• Fat (naturally occurring and added)   ▼ Sugars (added)
These symbols show fats, oils, and added sugars in foods.

FIGURE 2.3

The Food Guide Pyramid. (USDA, 1992)

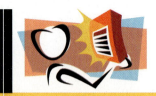

Off the Label: Watch Your Serving Size

How much cereal did you have for breakfast? Was it a cup, or was it more like 2 1/2 cups? The label on the box tells you that one cup has 200 Calories, but if you had two and a half times this amount, your breakfast had 500 Calories, not 200. Labels use standard serving sizes, but this doesn't mean it is the serving size you typically eat. For example, the label on the large bag of chips you buy to snack on during the Monday night football game says that a serving is one ounce or about 15 chips, but do you count the chips you eat while sitting in front of the TV? Fifteen chips is only a handful and will likely be gone before the first quarter ends. It may be helpful to occasionally weigh or measure out a serving to see how much it looks like on your plate or in your bowl or glass.

Another thing to watch is the number of servings in the container. Food manufacturers are required to follow standard serving size guidelines on the label, but they are not required to package products according to these standards. For example, the sports drink you guzzle after working out says a serving has only 100 Calories—certainly not enough to replace all the calories you just burned off at the gym. Look again. The serving size is 8 ounces, but the bottle contains 20 ounces. If you drink the whole bottle, you will be adding 250 Calories to your diet, mostly as added sugars. This is enough to replace the calories you would burn by jogging for about half an hour. People tend to eat in units; one doughnut, one packet, one bottle. You are unlikely to drink 8 ounces from the 20-ounce bottle and save the other 12 ounces for later.

Other serving sizes may be confusing because they tell you the serving that comes out of the box, not the serving that goes on your plate. For example, the serving size on a box of pasta is 2 ounces of dry pasta. What does 2 ounces of dry pasta look like once it is cooked? It turns out it is about a cup, but you can't tell this from reading the label. Some labels, such as the one shown here from falafel, do provide information on both the food as it comes out of

Falafel

Nutrition Facts		
Serving Size ¹/₄ cup (34g) dry mix		
(About 2¹/₂ Patties)		
Servings Per Container about 5 (dry)		

Amount Per Serving	As Packaged	As Prepared
Calories	100	230
Calories from Fat	10	140
		% Daily Value**
Total Fat 1g*	1%	24%
Saturated Fat 0g	0%	11%
Trans Fat 0g		
Cholesterol 0mg	0%	0%
Sodium 560mg	23%	23%
Total Carbohydrate 18g	6%	6%
Dietary Fiber 5g	21%	21%
Sugars 3g		
Protein 10g		
Vitamin A	0%	0%
Vitamin C	0%	0%
Calcium	4%	4%
Iron	10%	15%

the box and after it is prepared. This information can be helpful if you prepare the food according to package directions.

Food labels are a helpful tool in choosing foods to build a healthy diet if you use the information they provide.

can get adequate amounts of all the nutrients you need in the proportions recommended for a healthy diet.

The Pyramid's shape indicates the relative contributions of each food group

The large base of the Pyramid is made up of foods that come from grains: bread, cereal, rice, and pasta. Between 6 and 11 servings per day are recommended, depending on how many calories you need to maintain a healthy weight. In the next level of the Pyramid are two groups of foods that also come from plant sources: the Vegetable Group, of which three to five servings per day are recommended, and the Fruit Group, of which two to four servings per day are recommended. The next level, where the decreasing size of the Pyramid boxes reflects the smaller number of recommended servings, comprises two groups of foods that come primarily from animals: the Milk, Yogurt, & Cheese Group, of which two to three servings are recommended, and the Meat, Poultry, Fish, Dry Beans, Eggs, & Nuts Group, of which two to three servings a day are recommended. In the narrow tip of the Pyramid are Fats, Oils, & Sweets. These foods should be consumed sparingly because they are low in nutrient density.

Serving size recommendations ensure enough and not too much

The Food Guide Pyramid recommends a range of servings for each food group. The serving sizes within each group of the Pyramid are standardized. For instance, 1 serving from the Bread, Cereal, Rice, & Pasta Group is 1 slice of bread, 1 ounce of dry cereal, or 1/2 cup of cooked cereal, rice, or pasta (Table 2.1). To follow these recommendations, it is important to recognize that the Pyramid serving sizes may not be the same as what you consider a serving when you eat. So, if your dinner includes 2 cups of spaghetti (less than is often served in restaurants) and three slices of garlic bread, you have eaten at least 7 servings from the base of the Pyramid. If you need 1600 Calories to maintain your weight (Table 2.2), this one meal would exceed the recommended number of grain servings for the entire day. The large serving sizes that Americans have become accustomed to are thought to be one of the reasons for the growing rate of obesity in the United States.[7]

Following the Pyramid selection tips helps you choose a varied, nutrient-dense diet

Just choosing the specified number of servings from each group of the Food Guide Pyramid will not ensure an optimal diet if wise choices are not made. For example, if all your choices from the grain group at the base are from cookies, cakes, and white bread and the only vegetable you choose is french fries, it is unlikely that you will meet your nutrient needs or the recommendations for a healthy diet. However, if you pay attention to the selection tips provided along with the Pyramid, you will be choosing a varied, nutrient-dense diet (see Table 2.1). For example, the selection tip for the grain group suggests choosing whole grain breads, cereals, and grain products and limiting high-fat, high-sugar baked goods. The tip for the milk group endorses the use of low-fat dairy products and suggests limiting high-fat choices such as ice cream. These tips promote nutrient-dense choices. Others promote variety. For example, the selection tip for the vegetable group suggests including dark-green and deep-yellow vegetables in your choices. These all provide a vegetable source of vitamin A, but leafy green vegetables are higher in folate and iron. The tips for fruits recommend that some of your fruit choices be citrus or berries because they provide vitamin C. Choosing a varied diet is also important because there are interactions between different foods and nutrients. These interactions may be positive, enhancing nutrient utilization, or negative, inhibiting nutrient use. For example, having iron-fortified oatmeal along with a glass of orange juice can enhance the absorption of the iron, whereas having the same oatmeal with a glass of milk may reduce iron absorption. In a varied diet these interactions balance out. In addition, some foods may contain toxic substances such as pesticides, fertilizers, and natural toxins. If you always eat the same food, you will always be exposed to the same toxin. Choosing a variety of foods avoids an excess of any one of these substances.

The Pyramid meets individual needs and preferences

The Food Guide Pyramid is designed to be flexible enough to meet the needs and preferences of almost everyone (Figure 2.4). By varying the number of servings from each group, it can be used to plan diets for a wide range of calorie needs. For example, those who need 1600 Calories per day could meet their needs by using the low end of the range of daily servings: 6 bread servings, 3 vegetables, 2 fruits, etc. Someone who

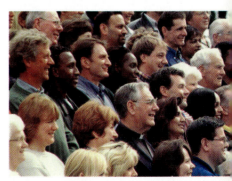

FIGURE 2.4

The Food Guide Pyramid is flexible enough to meet the needs and preferences of our diverse population. (Bob Thomas/Stone/Getty Images)

TABLE 2.1
Follow the Pyramid Selection Tips to Plan a Healthy Diet

Food Group/Serving Size	What Nutrients It Provides	Selection Tips
Bread, Cereal, Rice, & Pasta (6 to 11 servings) 1/2 cup cooked cereal, rice, or pasta 1 ounce dry cereal 1 slice bread, 1 tortilla 2 cookies 1/2 medium doughnut	B vitamins, fiber, iron, magnesium, zinc, complex carbohydrates	Choose whole-grain breads, cereals, and grains such as whole wheat or rye, oatmeal, and brown rice. Limit high-fat, high-sugar baked goods such as cakes, cookies, and pastries. Limit fats and sugars added as spreads, sauces, or toppings.
Vegetable (3 to 5 servings) 1/2 cup cooked or raw chopped vegetables 1 cup raw leafy vegetables 3/4 cup vegetable juice 10 french fries	Vitamin A, vitamin C, folate, magnesium, iron, fiber	Eat a variety of vegetables, including dark-green leafy vegetables like spinach and broccoli, deep-yellow vegetables like carrots and sweet potatoes, starchy vegetables such as potatoes and corn, and other vegetables such as green beans and tomatoes. Limit the fat you add to vegetables during cooking and at the table such as spreads and dressings.

Fruit
(2 to 4 servings)
1 medium apple, banana,
  or orange
1/2 cup chopped, cooked,
  or canned fruit
3/4 cup fruit juice
1/4 cup dried fruit
	Vitamin A, vitamin C, potassium, fiber	Choose fresh fruit, frozen without sugar, dried, or fruit canned in water or juice. If canned in heavy syrup, rinse with water before eating. Eat whole fruits more often than juices; they are higher in fiber. Regularly eat citrus fruits, melons, or berries rich in vitamin C. Only 100% fruit juice should be counted as fruit.

Milk, Yogurt, & Cheese (2 to 3 servings) 1 cup milk or yogurt 1 1/2 ounces natural cheese 2 ounces process cheese 2 cups cottage cheese 1 1/2 cups ice cream 1 cup frozen yogurt	Protein, calcium, riboflavin, vitamin D	Use low-fat or nonfat milk for healthy people over 2 years of age. Choose low-fat and nonfat yogurt, "part skim" and low-fat cheeses, and lower-fat frozen desserts like ice milk and frozen yogurt. Limit high-fat cheeses and ice cream.
Meat, Poultry, Fish, **Dry Beans, Eggs, & Nuts** (2 to 3 servings) 2–3 ounces cooked lean meat, fish, or poultry 2–3 eggs 4–6 tablespoons peanut butter 1 to 1 1/2 cups cooked dry beans 2/3 to 1 cup nuts	Protein, niacin, vitamin B_6, vitamin B_{12}, iron, zinc	Select lean meat, poultry without skin, and dry beans often. Trim fat, and cook by broiling, roasting, grilling, or boiling rather than frying. Limit egg yolks, which are high in cholesterol, and nuts and seeds, which are high in calories. Watch serving sizes; 3 ounces of meat is the size of an average hamburger.

Fats, Oils, & Sweets
(use sparingly)
Butter, mayonnaise, salad
  dressing, cream cheese,
  sour cream, jam, jelly
	Fat-soluble vitamins	Use unsaturated vegetable oils and margarines that list a liquid vegetable oil as first ingredient on the label. Substitute low-fat dressings and spreads.

Human Nutrition Information Service. *The Food Guide Pyramid.* Home and Garden Bulletin No. 252. Hyattsville, Md.: U.S. Department of Agriculture, 1992, 1996, revised.

TABLE 2.2
Choose the Right Number of Servings to Meet Your Calorie Needs*

	1600 Calories (sedentary women and some older adults)	2200 Calories (children, teenage girls, active women, and many sedentary men)	2800 Calories (teenage boys, many active men, and some very active women)
Bread, Cereal, Rice, & Pasta group	6	9	11
Vegetable group	3	4	5
Fruit group	2	3	4
Milk, Yogurt, & Cheese group	2–3†	2–3†	2–3†
Meat, Poultry, Fish, Dry Beans, Eggs, & Nuts group	(5 oz total)	(6 oz total)	(7 oz total)

*Assumes that food choices are mostly low fat and low calorie.
†Women who are pregnant or breastfeeding, teenagers, and young adults to age 24 need three servings.
Source: U.S. Department of Agriculture. *The Food Guide Pyramid.* Home and Garden Bulletin 252, 1992, revised 1996. The Food Guide Pyramid: A Tool for Diet Planning.

needs 2800 Calories per day should choose from the high end of the range for each food group: for instance, 11 breads, 5 vegetables, 4 fruits, and so on (see Table 2.2).

Because each food group contains a huge variety of food choices, a diet planned using the Pyramid can suit the preferences of people from diverse cultures and lifestyles. For example, a meal of tortillas, beans, and rice can provide the same number of servings from the same food groups as a meal of spaghetti, meatballs, and garlic bread (Figure 2.5). Special Pyramids designed around various ethnic diets have been

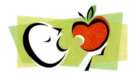

Bread is not an unhealthy choice, especially if it is a whole grain bread. And it turns out, bread and the other choices in the base of the Pyramid don't supply as much carbohydrate as you might think. Eating the recommended servings from the bottom group of the Food Guide Pyramid will provide between about 90 and 165 grams of carbohydrate, equivalent to about 20% of your calories for the day.

Food Guide Pyramid Servings

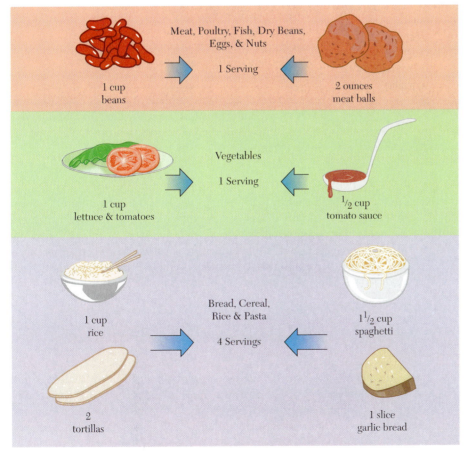

FIGURE 2.5

As shown by these two meals, many different choices can provide the same number of servings from the food groups of the Food Guide Pyramid.

PIECE IT TOGETHER

Using the Food Guide Pyramid To Choose a Healthy Diet

For the first time in his life, Jarad is living on his own. His diet is beginning to seem monotonous and he realizes that it is time to pay more attention to the kinds of foods he eats. To evaluate his food choices, he records everything he consumes for 1 day and compares it with the number of servings recommended by the Food Guide Pyramid.

Food	Serving Size	No. of Servings	Food Group
Breakfast			
Cornflakes	3/4 cup	1	Grain
Whole milk	3/4 cup	3/4	Milk
Orange juice	3/4 cup	1	Fruit
Coffee	1 cup		
with cream	1 Tbsp		Fats and sweets
and sugar	1 tsp		Fats and sweets
Snack			
Doughnut	1	2	Grain
Lunch			
Hamburger			
Bun	1 whole	2	Grain
Beef patty	2 oz	1	Meat
Onions	1 Tbsp	1/8	Vegetable
Mayonnaise	1 Tbsp		Fats and sweets
French fries	25 pieces	2 1/2	Vegetable
Milk shake	12 fluid oz	1 1/2	Milk
Snack			
Soda	1 can		Fats and sweets

Food	Serving Size	No. of Servings	Food Group
Dinner			
Lasagna			
Noodles	1 cup	2	Grain
Tomato sauce	1/2 cup	1	Vegetable
Ground beef	4 oz	2	Meat
Cheese	1 oz	2/3	Milk
Soda	1 can		Fats and sweets
Ice cream	1 cup	2/3	Milk
Snack			
Apple	1 medium	1	Fruit

DOES JARAD'S DIET MEET THE MINIMUM NUMBER OF SERVINGS RECOMMENDED BY THE FOOD GUIDE PYRAMID?

▼

Recommended Servings	Servings in Jarad's Diet
Bread, Cereal, Rice, & Pasta (6–11 servings)	7
Vegetable (3–5 servings)	~3 1/2
Fruit (2–4 servings)	2
Milk, Yogurt, & Cheese (2–3 servings)	~3
Meat, Poultry, Fish, Dry Beans, Eggs, & Nuts (2–3 servings)	3

Jarad consumes adequate numbers of servings from all the food groups, but is he eating a healthy diet? To find out, you need to compare his diet to the selection tips of the Food Guide Pyramid.

developed to focus on food choices that meet the needs of different cultures (Appendix H). By modifying the number of servings, the Pyramid can also be used for groups with special needs. For example, it is recommended that pregnant and lactating women, children, adolescents, and adults under 25 years of age consume three servings from the milk group. Modifications of the Food Guide Pyramid have been developed for vegetarians (Chapter 6), pregnant women (Chapter 12), young children, and older adults (Chapter 13).

The Pyramid is being revised to promote better choices

The Food Guide Pyramid is not the first food guide to be used in the United States. The first one was published in 1917 and called "How to Select Foods."[8] It consisted of five food groups: milk and meat, cereals, vegetables and fruits, fats and fat foods, and sugars and sugary foods. Since then, many different food guides have been developed

HOW MANY OF HIS CHOICES FROM THE BASE OF THE PYRAMID ARE FROM WHOLE GRAINS?

None of his grain choices are from whole grains. Having a whole wheat bagel instead of a doughnut or having a whole grain cereal like shredded wheat for breakfast will add a whole grain to his day.

HOW MANY OF HIS CHOICES ARE HIGH IN ADDED SUGARS?

He adds sugar to his coffee and drinks 2 cans of soda, which is mostly sugar. Other foods that are high in added sugar include the doughnut and milkshake. Foods high in added sugar are typically low in nutrient density.

DOES HIS DIET PROVIDE A VARIETY OF VEGETABLES AND INCLUDE DARK GREEN LEAFY AND DEEP YELLOW VEGETABLES?

No. The only vegetables he eats are french fries, a few onions on his burger, and the tomato sauce in the lasagna at dinner. It is hard to judge variety on the basis of a single day, but he eats no dark green, leafy vegetables such as kale or spinach and no deep yellow vegetables such as carrots or squash. An occasional serving of french fries is fine, but it is important to also include green and yellow-orange vegetables in the diet because they contain nutrients that are missing from potatoes.

DOES HE CHOOSE FRESH FRUIT AND INCLUDE A CITRUS FRUIT IN HIS DIET?

He has a fresh apple and the orange juice he drinks for breakfast is a citrus fruit.

DOES HE CHOOSE LOW-FAT DAIRY PRODUCTS AND LEAN MEATS?

He drinks whole milk, adds cream to his coffee, and has cheese, a milkshake, and ice cream—all full-fat dairy products. His meat choices, beef in the fast food burger and in the lasagna, are unlikely to be lean.

HOW WOULD MORE NUTRIENT-DENSE CHOICES AFFECT THE ENERGY CONTENT OF HIS DIET?

Your answer:

To increase the variety and nutrient density of his diet, Jarad decides to try having lunch at a local sandwich shop that assembles sandwiches to order.

SUGGEST A SANDWICH ORDER THAT INCLUDES SELECTIONS FROM AT LEAST THREE FOOD GUIDE PYRAMID FOOD GROUPS AND FOLLOWS THE SELECTION TIPS FOR THESE GROUPS.

Your answer:

and each has focused on the important nutrition issues of the time. Today, with the incidence of nutrition-related diseases on the rise and nutrition surveys showing us that Americans are not following the recommendations of the Pyramid, its structure is being reconsidered. A revised Pyramid is expected to be released in 2005 (see www.wiley.com/college/grosvenor).

This doesn't mean that the original Food Guide Pyramid gives poor nutrition advice. The Pyramid graphic shows us what foods fit into each group and how many servings of each we should have. The selection tips provide important information on making healthy choices from each food group. The problem is, many of us do not follow these recommendations. Even though the selection tips tell us to choose whole rather than refined grains, the average American consumes only one serving of whole grains per day. The Pyramid recommends 2–4 servings of fruit, but the average person eats less than 2 each day, and almost half of us don't even consume one piece of fruit daily. We also fall short of the 2 to 3 servings of dairy products recommended. The average American eats only 1 1/2 dairy servings daily; only 12% of teenage girls and 14% of women consume

On the Side

During the depression of the 1930's a food guide was released that consisted of 12 food groups and focused on responding to food scarcities. In 1943, influenced by World War II, a food guide called the "Basic Seven" was released. In 1956, the seven food groups were condensed to the "Basic Four" and presented in the USDA publication *Essentials of an Adequate Diet.*

the recommended amounts.[9] We eat too many foods that are high in added sugar and we consume servings that are way out of proportion with recommendations. To better address these issues, the reconstructed Pyramid will address how much to eat to avoid weight gain, provide better information on choosing healthy types of fats and carbohydrates, and offer more direction on choices from within the food groups.

Food Labels Can Help You Make Wise Food Choices

How do you know if a food you choose is a good source of vitamin C or how much fiber it contains? You can find this information, and more, on the food label. Standardized food labels provide information about the nutrient composition of foods and about how a food fits into the overall diet.[10] These labels must appear on almost all packaged foods. Raw fruits, vegetables, fish, meat, and poultry are not required to carry individual labels. However, grocery stores are asked to voluntarily provide nutrition information for the raw foods most frequently eaten in the United States. The information can appear on large placards or in consumer pamphlets or brochures.

All labels contain basic product information such as the name of the product, the contents, and the name and place of business of the manufacturer, packager, or distributor. In addition, most food labels contain a "Nutrition Facts" panel and a list of the food's ingredients. Some products may also include claims about their health or nutritional benefits; these claims are also regulated.

Foods in packages too small to fit the labeling information and those produced by small businesses are exempt from labeling regulations. The foods you choose in a restaurant also come without a label, but if a claim is made about a food's nutritional content or health benefits such as "low fat" or "heart healthy," the eating establishment must provide nutritional information about this food when requested.[11]

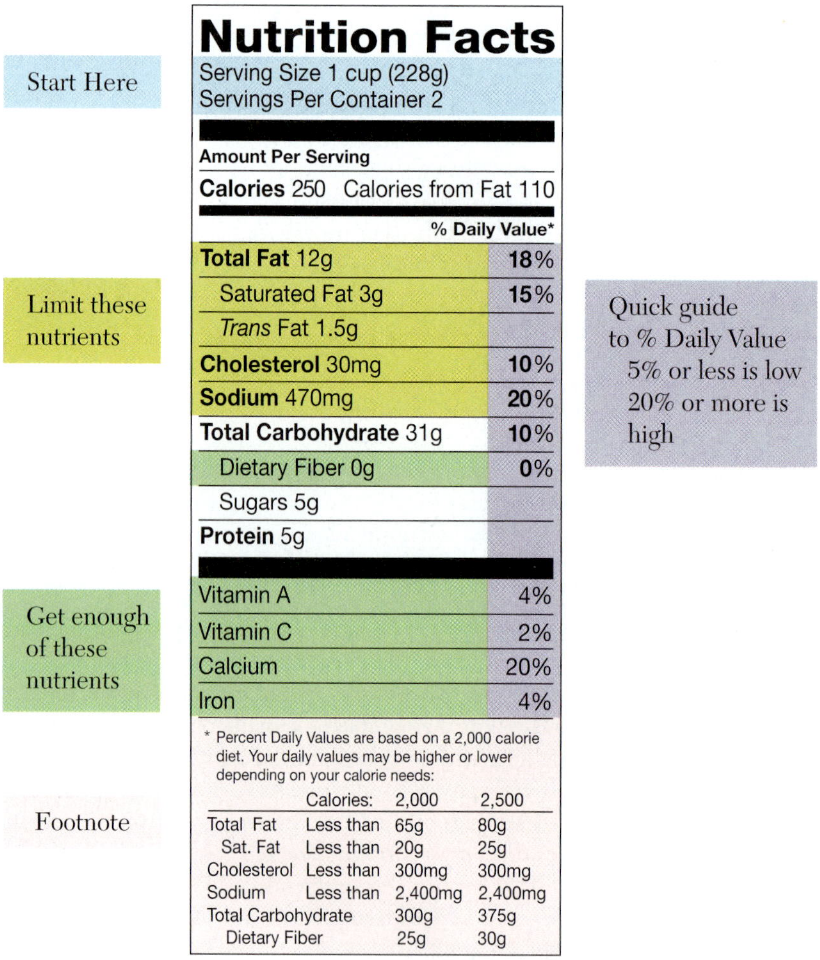

FIGURE 2.6

The Nutrition Labeling and Education Act of 1990 required standardization of the information on food labels. This label from macaroni and cheese illustrates how the information on the label can be used to make wise food choices.

Start Here

Limit these nutrients

Get enough of these nutrients

Footnote

Quick guide to % Daily Value 5% or less is low 20% or more is high

Nutrition Facts	
Serving Size 1 cup (228g)	
Servings Per Container 2	
Amount Per Serving	
Calories 250 Calories from Fat 110	
	% Daily Value*
Total Fat 12g	**18%**
Saturated Fat 3g	**15%**
Trans Fat 1.5g	
Cholesterol 30mg	**10%**
Sodium 470mg	**20%**
Total Carbohydrate 31g	**10%**
Dietary Fiber 0g	**0%**
Sugars 5g	
Protein 5g	
Vitamin A	4%
Vitamin C	2%
Calcium	20%
Iron	4%

* Percent Daily Values are based on a 2,000 calorie diet. Your daily values may be higher or lower depending on your calorie needs:

		Calories:	2,000	2,500
Total Fat	Less than		65g	80g
Sat. Fat	Less than		20g	25g
Cholesterol	Less than		300mg	300mg
Sodium	Less than		2,400mg	2,400mg
Total Carbohydrate			300g	375g
Dietary Fiber			25g	30g

The "Nutrition Facts" list the amounts of calories and nutrients per serving

The nutrition information section of the food label is entitled "Nutrition Facts" (Figure 2.6). In this section, the serving size is given based on a standard list of serving sizes. The serving size on the label is followed by the number of servings per container, the total Calories, and the Calories from fat in each serving.

Using standard serving sizes allows consumers to compare products. For example, comparing the calories in different types of crackers is easy because all packages must list information for a serving size of about 30 grams and tell you the number of crackers per serving. The next section of the nutrition facts panel lists the amounts of nutrients contained in a serving and, for most, the percent of the Daily Value they provide.

Daily Values tell you how one food fits into your total diet

Ice cream is high in fat, but is it so high that having a bowl as an afternoon snack will tip your daily fat intake into the overload zone? Checking out the percent Daily Value for fat listed on the label can give you an idea of what portion of the recommended maximum it provides.

The Daily Values are a set of standards developed for food labels to compare the amount of a nutrient in a food to recommendations for the amount of that nutrient in a healthy diet (Table 2.3). The Daily Values are used to calculate the percent Daily

On the Side

Having a lunch that includes a cup of pasta? According to the Food Guide Pyramid you are having 2 servings of pasta, but based on the Nutrition Facts label you are eating only 1 serving.

TABLE 2.3
The Daily Values Put Amounts in Perspective

Nutrient	Daily Value	Amount in 2000 Calorie Diet	Amount in 2500 Calorie Diet
Total fat	< 30% of calories	65 g	80 g
Saturated fat	< 10% of calories	20 g	25 g
Total carbohydrate	60% of calories	300 g	375 g
Dietary fiber	11.5 g/1000 Cal	25 g	30 g
Protein	10% of calories	50 g	63 g
Cholesterol	< 300 mg	< 300 mg	< 300 mg
Sodium	< 2400 mg	< 2400 mg	< 2400 mg
Potassium	3500 mg	3500 mg	3500 mg

Nutrient	Daily Value*	Nutrient	Daily Value*
Vitamin A	5000 IU[†]	Vitamin E	30 IU[†]
Biotin	300 μg	Riboflavin	1.7 mg
Vitamin C	60 mg	Niacin	20 mg
Vitamin B$_6$	2.0 mg	Vitamin B$_{12}$	6 μg
Thiamin	1.5 mg	Chromium	120 μg
Folic acid	400 μg	Phosphorus	1000 mg
Pantothenic acid	10 mg	Selenium	70 μg
Vitamin K	80 μg	Calcium	1000 mg
Iodine	150 μg	Magnesium	400 mg
Molybdenum	75 μg	Manganese	2 mg
Iron	18 mg	Zinc	15 mg
Vitamin D	400 IU[†]	Chloride	3400 mg
Copper	2 mg		

*Based on National Academy of Sciences' 1968 Recommended Dietary Allowances.
[†]The Daily Values for some fat-soluble vitamins are expressed in International Units (IU). The DRIs use a newer system of measurement (see Appendix D).

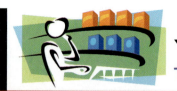

Your Choice: Choosing Off the Menu

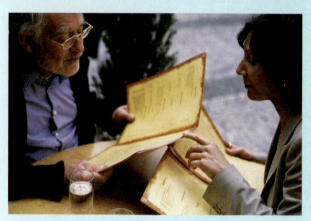

(Corbis Images)

Treating yourself to an occasional dinner out doesn't have much of an effect on your total diet, no matter what you order for your meal. But for many Americans, eating out is more than an occasional treat. Today, more than ever we are eating away from home. This is a problem because restaurant meals are usually higher in calories, fat, and cholesterol than meals we eat at home.[1] Our eat-on-the-run lifestyle has made choosing healthy foods from restaurant menus an important skill—but it can be a challenge.

Some healthy choices are easy, even at restaurants. If you are looking for a low-fat meal, skip the fried fish and have it broiled instead. Minimize sauces and spreads (like the honey butter on your corn bread) that add fat, sugar, and calories. Use less salad dressing by asking that it be served on the side. Be conscious of portion sizes. Those served in restaurants are often much larger than what we prepare at home. You don't have to finish everything—take it home for tomorrow's lunch.

Other restaurant choices are more difficult to make. Choices that sound like part of a healthy diet are not always what they seem. What's in that house special turkey tetrazzini, beef lo mein, or fajita wrap? Without the chef's recipe, it is impossible to know. The amounts of specific nutrients are usually not given on menus, and the ingredients can be a mystery. Even when you know what ingredients are usually in a dish like eggplant parmesan, you can never be sure how much oil or salt was used. Even an order of plain old green beans might come floating in butter.

Many restaurants and fast-food establishments have responded to consumer concern about healthy diets with healthier choices. Menus often highlight healthy items by making claims about nutrient content, such as low-fat tostados, low-salt lo mein, or reduced-calorie lasagna. The food labeling laws that regulate packaged foods also apply to menus, so the definition of these terms must match those used on food labels. For example, if you order low-fat tostados, the term "low fat" should mean the same as it does on labeled packaged foods—that it contains 3 grams or less of fat per serving.

Menus may also include statements that give general dietary guidance or make specific claims about the relationship between a nutrient and a disease or health condition. For example, the salad section may start with the general statement that "eating five fruits and vegetables a day is an important part of a healthy diet."[2] The description of a dish that is low in fat, saturated fat, and cholesterol might carry a claim that diets low in saturated fat and cholesterol may reduce the risk of heart disease. To carry a health claim, menu items must contain a significant amount of at least one of six key nutrients (vitamin A, vitamin C, iron, calcium, protein, or fiber) and cannot contain a food substance at a level that increases the risk of a disease or health condition.

Claims about the nutrient content and healthfulness of food items on the menu must be backed up with appropriate material when requested. This information can be on the menu or in accompanying nutrition information available upon request. It can be presented in any format, such as printed in a notebook or recited by the staff, and needs to provide information about only the nutrient or nutrients to which the claim is referring. Restaurants do not have to provide nutrition information about items that do not carry nutrient content or health claims or that are referred to in general dietary messages.

When choosing from a menu, look for items that fit into an overall healthy diet—and are also things you enjoy. Remember that a high-fat or high-calorie meal now and then doesn't make your overall diet unhealthy. But, if you eat out frequently, these meals make up a greater part of your overall diet and should be chosen carefully. Use nutrient content claims and health claims to choose items that meet your dietary and health needs.

References
1. USDA, Agricultural Service, 1997. Results from USDA's 1994–1996 Continuing Survey of Food Intakes by Individuals and 1994–1996 Health Knowledge Survey. ARS Food Surveys Research Group. Available online at www.barc.usda.gov/bhnrc/foodsurvey/home/htm/Accessed February 28, 2004.
2. Kurtzweil, P. Today's special nutrition information. *FDA Consumer* 31(May–June): 21–25, 1997.

Value listed in the Nutrition Facts panel. The percent Daily Value is the amount of the nutrient in the food as a percentage of the recommendation for a 2000-Calorie diet. For example, if a food provides 10% of the Daily Value for vitamin C, then the food provides 10% of the recommended daily intake for vitamin C in a 2000-Calorie diet. For some nutrients, such as total fat and saturated fat, the Daily Value is a maximum recommended amount. So, for example, if a food contains 15% of the Daily Value for saturated fat, then it contains 15% of the maximum amount recommended for a 2000-Calorie diet. Food labels must list the percent Daily Value for total fat, saturated fat, cholesterol, sodium, total carbohydrate, and dietary fiber as well as for vitamin A, calcium, vitamin C, and iron.

Because the Daily Values are a single standard for almost everyone, they may overestimate the amount of a nutrient needed for some groups, but they do not underestimate the requirement for any group, except pregnant and lactating women. Products intended for use by infants and children under the age of 4 years have a different set of labeling regulations (see Chapter 13).

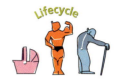

The ingredient list tells you what's in your food

The ingredients section of the label lists the contents of the product in order of their prominence by weight. For example, many juice drinks are mostly water and sugar. The label in Figure 2.7 shows that water and a sweetener are the first two ingredients. An ingredient list is required on all products containing more than one ingredient. Food additives, including food colors and flavorings, must be listed among the ingredients.

Food labels may include claims about nutrient content

Looking for low-cholesterol foods? You may not even need to look at the Nutrition Facts. In addition to the required nutrition information, food labels often highlight specific characteristics of a product that might be of interest to the consumer, such as "low in cholesterol" or "high in fiber." Standard definitions for these descriptors have been established by the Food and Drug Administration (FDA). For example, any product labeled "fat free" contains less than 0.5 gram of fat per serving. The specific definition of each of these descriptors is given in Table 2.4.

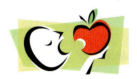

The Nutrition Facts on packaged foods lists the grams of fat per serving as well as the proportion of the recommended fat intake provided by a serving of the food. You can use this information to see if your hot dog is high in fat. Low-fat hot dogs have less than 3 grams of fat per serving, but a regular hot dog may have 12 to 15 grams of fat. This is about a quarter of the total amount of fat you should have for the entire day.

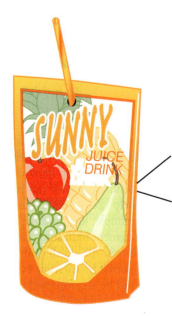

INGREDIENTS: Water, high fructose corn syrup, pear and grape juice concentrates, citric acid, water extracted orange and pineapple juice concentrates, natural flavor

FIGURE 2.7

The first ingredient listed for this juice drink is water, meaning the greatest proportion of the weight of the product is water. The second ingredient is high fructose corn syrup, which is used as a sweetener.

The exchanges are designed so that each serving within a list contains approximately the same number of calories and grams of carbohydrate, protein, and fat. For instance, a serving from the fruit list, whether it is a serving of grapes or a pear, provides about 60 Calories, 15 grams of carbohydrate, no protein, and no fat. A serving from the starch list, whether it is bread, potatoes, or pasta, will provide about 80 Calories, 15 grams of carbohydrate, 3 grams of protein, and 0 to 1 gram of fat. The food groupings of the Exchange Lists differ from the Food Guide Pyramid groups because the lists are designed to meet specific carbohydrate, protein, fat, and energy criteria, whereas the Pyramid groups are based on sources of specific nutrients without attention to their calorie content. For example, a potato is included in the starch exchange list because its carbohydrate, protein, and fat content are comparable to those in bread, but in the Food Guide Pyramid a potato is in the Vegetable Group because it is a good source of vitamins, minerals, and fiber. Also, the serving sizes may differ from those in the Food Guide Pyramid or used on food labels.

There Are Many Other Guidelines for Health Promotion

In addition to the recommendations and guidelines discussed in the previous sections, there are a number of other types of recommendations made to promote a healthy diet and lifestyle. One of these is the Healthy People Initiative, which is a health promotion program that includes nutrition in its recommendations. Other nutrition recommendations are made by special interest groups, which make recommendations for reducing the risks of specific diseases such as heart disease and cancer.

The Healthy People Initiative is a set of public health objectives

The U.S. Public Health Service, along with hundreds of private and public organizations, has developed a set of public health objectives called Healthy People. The first set, Healthy People 2000, developed in 1990, was directed toward the year 2000. The most recent objectives, Healthy People 2010, target the current decade. The purpose of Healthy People 2010 is to promote health and prevent illness, disability, and premature death. To achieve this it defines two overarching goals: increase quality and years of healthy life and eliminate health disparities. These goals served as a guide for developing objectives that can be used to measure progress. Healthy People 2010 contains 467 objectives designed to improve the health of all people in the United States by promoting healthy behaviors, protecting health, assuring access to quality health care, and strengthening community prevention.[14] Many of the objectives of Healthy People 2010 address improving the nutritional status of the population (see Appendix G). For instance, Healthy People is working toward reducing the number of cancer and heart disease deaths and the prevalence of obesity in adults by promoting active lifestyles and diets low in fat and sodium and high in fiber. It promotes a reduction in growth retardation in children by encouraging healthy feeding practices, including breast feeding for infants. Other nutrition-related objectives are designed to improve the delivery of nutrition information and services.

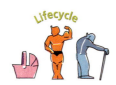

Lifecycle

Other recommendations are designed to reduce risks for particular diseases

In addition to guidelines for a healthy diet for the general population, recommendations are also made specifically for people who have or are at risk for particular diseases. For instance, the American Heart Association and the American Institute for Cancer Research have published guidelines for groups at risk for heart disease and cancer, respectively (see Appendix G). These groups base their recommendations on sound scientific literature, but because of their special interest in preventing a specific disease, their recommendations may differ slightly from one another in emphasis and focus. For example, to reduce the risk of heart disease, the guidelines developed by the American Heart Association include a recommendation to restrict dietary cholesterol to less than 300 mg per day, whereas the recommendations of the American Institute for Cancer Research, which are designed to reduce the incidence of cancer, do not comment on cholesterol intake but recommend a reduction in the consumption of cured and smoked meats because of a correlation with cancer.

Are You Meeting Your Nutritional Needs?

All of the guidelines for a healthy diet tell us how much of each nutrient the average person needs to stay healthy, and how to plan a diet to meet these needs. But how can you tell if you are meeting your needs? To evaluate your nutritional health, you can compare your intake to the recommendations for a healthy diet. In addition, you need to take into account your health history and genetic background.

Nutritional assessment can evaluate an individual's nutritional health

Are you losing weight? Gaining weight? Do you have a history of heart disease in your family? Are you at risk for a nutrient deficiency because you can't get to the store, can't afford to buy healthy foods, or don't know what to eat or how to cook? All of this information and more is needed to assess your **nutritional status**. Nutritional status refers to your state of health as it is affected by your intake and utilization of nutrients. Assessing nutritional status can help determine whether the dietary choices you are making are meeting your nutrient needs and minimizing your risks of chronic disease.

Nutritional status is determined by doing an individual nutritional assessment. This requires a review of past and present dietary intake, an assessment of body size, an evaluation of genetic risk factors, and a physical examination, including a review of your medical history and laboratory test results. Even with all these tools, diagnosing a nutritional deficiency or excess is not always clear cut. Estimates of dietary intake are not always accurate, and symptoms may be indistinguishable from other medical conditions.

Nutritional status State of health as it is influenced by the intake and utilization of nutrients.

Compare your intake to recommendations to see if your diet is adequate A good place to start when evaluating your nutritional status is to determine what you typically eat. This can be done by recording your food as you consume it or by recalling what you ate in the past. An accurate food record includes everything you eat and drink, along with descriptions of cooking methods and brand names of products. Since food intake varies from day to day, to reflect your typical intake it is beneficial to keep track of it for more than 1 day. Most food records are kept for 2 to 7 days, including at least 1 weekend day, because we tend to eat differently on weekends.

Once you have a record of what you ate, you can compare your intake to recommendations. To get a general picture of dietary intake, you could compare your food choices with a guide for diet planning such as the Food Guide Pyramid. For example, did you consume the recommended number of servings of milk each day? For a more complete assessment of overall diet quality you could calculate your Healthy Eating Index, which compares your food choices to the recommendations of the Dietary Guidelines and Food Guide Pyramid. It scores 10 components of the diet; 5 measure how well your diet complies with the serving recommendation of the Food Guide Pyramid and the other 5 score the diet based on how well it complies with the recommendations of the Dietary Guidelines regarding total fat, saturated fat, cholesterol, sodium, and variety. Each component has a maximum score of 10, so an individual who follows all of the guidelines would have a Healthy Eating Index score of 100.

For a more complete analysis of your diet, you can use food composition tables or a computer database to calculate your intake of energy and nutrients (see The Nutrient Composition of Foods supplement for an abbreviated list). These values can then be

On the Side

It's not easy to accurately figure out what people eat. When asked to write down everything they eat, people often change their food choices to conform to what they think is a "good diet" or even skip certain foods to avoid the inconvenience of writing them down. Asking people to recall what they ate also has problems. Can you remember what you had for breakfast, lunch, and dinner yesterday?

On the Web

To calculate your Healthy Eating Index, go to the Center for Nutrition Policy and Promotion at **www.usda.gov/cnpp** and click on Healthy Eating Index.

PIECE IT TOGETHER

Is Diet the Problem?

Alison is 20 years old and has just started college. Recently she has been feeling tired and has had difficulty concentrating in class. She goes to the health clinic, where she is weighed and measured. A physician does a physical examination and asks about her medical history. Blood and urine samples are collected for laboratory analysis, and she is referred to a dietitian to assess her dietary intake.

ASSESSING BODY SIZE, APPEARANCE, AND MEDICAL HISTORY

The physician notes that she appears thin and pale. She is 5 feet 4 inches tall and weighs 114 pounds. She recalls that a year ago she weighed 120 pounds and hasn't been trying to lose weight. Although her body weight is in the normal range, her unintentional weight loss is a concern.

COMPARING INTAKE TO RECOMMENDATIONS

Alison tells the dietitian that she stopped eating red meat last year. Using information from a diet record, the dietitian enters her diet into a computer program. A portion of the analysis is shown below.

Nutrient	Value	Goal %
Calories	1500	68%
Protein	46 g	100%
Vitamin C	110 mg	146%
Vitamin A	1028 µg	147%
Iron	6 mg	33%
Calcium	1300 mg	130%

BASED ON THIS COMPUTER PRINTOUT, WHAT NUTRIENTS DO NOT MEET RECOMMENDATIONS?

Alison consumes more than the recommended amounts of vitamin A, vitamin C, and calcium. Her calorie intake is less than the recommended amount and, since she is losing weight, is not enough to maintain her body weight. Her iron intake is well below the recommendation for young women.

LABORATORY TESTS

The results of her blood test indicate that blood hemoglobin level is 11.2 g per 100 ml of blood and that her hematocrit, which measures the total volume of blood cells, is 35 ml per 100 ml of blood.

LOOK UP THE NORMAL VALUES FOR HEMOGLOBIN AND HEMATOCRIT IN APPENDIX C. ARE HER VALUES IN THE NORMAL RANGE?

Her values for both hemoglobin and hematocrit are below normal.

ARE HER SYMPTOMS DUE TO LOW IRON INTAKE?

Hemoglobin is the oxygen-carrying protein in red blood cells, and hematocrit is an index of how many red blood cells she has. Low hemoglobin and hematocrit indicate that her ability to deliver oxygen to cells is reduced, which could be the cause of her tiredness and difficulty concentrating. Iron is needed to make hemoglobin. The low hemoglobin may be due to low iron intake, high iron needs, or an increase in iron losses. Since her diet history indicates that her iron intake is low, this is very likely to be the cause of her symptoms.

SHOULD SHE BE CONCERNED ABOUT THE NUTRIENTS SHE IS CONSUMING IN EXCESS OF HER GOAL? USE THE DRI TABLES TO DETERMINE IF THEY ARE LIKELY TO POSE A RISK.

Your answer:

To assess the nutrient content of foods in your diet, go to the USDA's Nutrient Data Laboratory at
www.nal.usda.gov/fnic/foodcomp/search/

compared to the recommended amounts for someone of your age, gender, and life-stage. Performing this analysis with a computer is fast and accurate. A program can calculate the nutrients for each day or average them over several days. It can also compare nutrient intake to recommended amounts (Figure 2.11). However, the information generated by computer diet analysis is useful only if the foods are entered correctly and the results are interpreted within the context of other parameters of nutritional assessment.

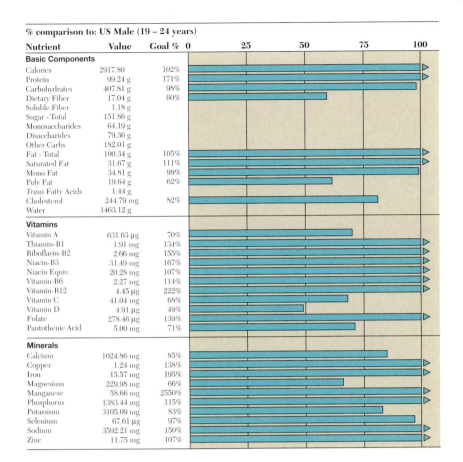

% comparison to: US Male (19 – 24 years)							
Nutrient	**Value**	**Goal %**	**0**	**25**	**50**	**75**	**100**
Basic Components							
Calories	2917.80	102%					
Protein	99.24 g	171%					
Carbohydrates	407.81 g	98%					
Dietary Fiber	17.04 g	60%					
Soluble Fiber	1.18 g						
Sugar - Total	151.86 g						
Monosaccharides	64.19 g						
Disaccharides	79.36 g						
Other Carbs	182.01 g						
Fat - Total	100.34 g	105%					
Saturated Fat	31.67 g	111%					
Mono Fat	34.81 g	99%					
Poly Fat	19.64 g	62%					
Trans Fatty Acids	1.44 g						
Cholesterol	244.79 mg	82%					
Water	1463.12 g						
Vitamins							
Vitamin A	631.63 μg	70%					
Thiamin-B1	1.91 mg	134%					
Riboflavin-B2	2.66 mg	155%					
Niacin-B3	31.49 mg	167%					
Niacin Equiv.	20.28 mg	107%					
Vitamin-B6	2.27 mg	114%					
Vitamin-B12	4.45 μg	222%					
Vitamin C	41.04 mg	68%					
Vitamin D	4.91 μg	49%					
Folate	278.46 μg	139%					
Pantothenic Acid	5.00 mg	71%					
Minerals							
Calcium	1024.86 mg	85%					
Copper	1.24 mg	138%					
Iron	15.57 mg	195%					
Magnesium	229.98 mg	66%					
Manganese	58.66 mg	2550%					
Phosphorus	1383.44 mg	115%					
Potassium	3105.09 mg	83%					
Selenium	67.61 μg	97%					
Sodium	3592.21 mg	150%					
Zinc	11.75 mg	107%					

FIGURE 2.11

To be meaningful, the information from a computer diet analysis must be accurately interpreted. This printout shows 1 day's intake for a 19- to 24-year-old male. The "Value" column gives the total amount of each nutrient consumed that day, and the "Goal %" column compares this amount to dietary standards. For example, this individual's vitamin C intake for the day is only 68% of the recommended goal. For some nutrients, such as vitamin C, the goal is a target for average daily intake. For these nutrients a goal % that is consistently below 100% indicates an increased risk of inadequate intake.

Compare your body size to standards to see where you fit Evaluating nutritional health also involves assessing your height and weight. These measurements can be compared with population standards (see Appendix B) or used to monitor changes in your size over time (Figure 2.12). Measurements significantly above or below the standard could indicate a nutritional deficiency or excess. However, this information should be evaluated only within the context of your personal and family history. For example, children who are small for their age may have a nutritional deficiency or may simply have inherited their small body size. Individuals who weigh less than the standard may be adequately nourished if they have never weighed more than their current weight and are otherwise healthy.

Your nutrient needs are affected by your current health and medical history The optimal diet for you depends on who you are, what your genetic background is, and how healthy you are. Nutrient needs change through your life cycle as you grow and mature. Pregnant women have increased needs to support the development of a healthy child. Young infants have higher calorie and protein needs per unit body weight than at any other time of life. The needs of older adults change as their body composition changes and as the ability to digest and absorb certain nutrients declines. Your health also affects your nutrient needs. For example, someone who has kidney disease should consume a different amount of protein than someone who has healthy kidneys. A careful physical examination with a review of your personal and family medical history can detect the symptoms of and risk factors for nutrition-related diseases.

Your genetic background affects your risk for nutrition-related diseases Just as your potential to be 6 feet tall is affected by how tall your parents are, your risk of developing some nutrition-related diseases is affected by the genes you inherit. If your mother died of a heart attack at age 50 years, you have a

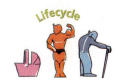

FIGURE 2.12

Measures of height, weight, and body circumference are important in assessing an individual's nutritional health. (Andy Levin/ Photo Researchers)

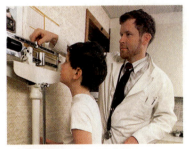

Lifecycle

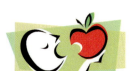

If your intake comes close to the RDA or AI for each nutrient, you are not losing or gaining excessive amounts of weight, and you have no symptoms of a nutrient deficiency, then you are most likely meeting all your nutrient needs.

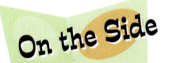

Does your hair reflect your diet? Hair analysis has been suggested as a means of assessing body mineral levels. However, because many factors, including exposure to environmental contaminants, shampoos, and hair treatments, affect the mineral content of hair, this analysis may not provide much useful information about mineral status in the body.

higher-than-average risk of developing heart disease (see Chapter 5). If you have a family history of diabetes, you have an increased risk of developing this disease. If both of your parents are overweight, it increases the chances that you too will have a weight problem. Therefore, genetic background is an important consideration when assessing your nutritional status and the diet that is best for you.

Laboratory tests can measure nutrient levels and assess the risk of chronic disease Measures of nutrients, their by-products, or their functions in your blood, urine, and body cells can help detect nutrient deficiencies and excesses (see Appendix C). For instance, levels of iron and iron-carrying proteins in the blood can be used to determine if you have iron deficiency anemia. The rate of certain biochemical reactions in your blood or cells can be used to assess the adequacy of certain vitamins. Only measures that reflect body status are useful in nutritional assessment.

Some laboratory tests can help evaluate your risk for nutrition-related chronic diseases (see Appendix C). For instance, heart disease risk can be assessed by measuring levels of cholesterol in the blood. Measuring the amount of glucose in the blood can be used to diagnose diabetes. More sophisticated medical tests can be used to obtain additional information about the risk and progression of nutrition-related diseases. For example, procedures are available to determine the extent of coronary artery blockage in an individual with heart disease or to assess bone density in someone at risk for osteoporosis.

Assessment can also evaluate the nutritional health of the population

Assessing the nutritional health of the population is important for establishing public health policy. By surveying the food supply and the population, we can find out what foods are available to the population (the supply) and what foods are purchased (food disappearance). By knowing which foods disappear from the food supply we can get a rough idea of what people are eating (Figure 2.13). This information can be used to identify possible nutrient deficiencies and excesses in the population. Nutritional problems can then be prevented or eliminated by public health measures such as nutrition education, food assistance programs, or the addition of a specific nutrient to the food supply.

Other types of surveys collect more specific information on individual food intake and health. These are helpful in identifying relationships between dietary intake and health and disease. For example, these surveys have helped us recognize that Ameri-

FIGURE 2.13

Food disappearance data can identify population trends in food intake such as the increase in the consumption of lower-fat milks and the decrease in whole milk consumption that has occurred over the last 50 years. (USDA Economic Research Service. Major trends in the U.S. food supply, 1909–1999, *Food Review* 23:12, 2000. Available online at www.ers.usda.gov/epubs/pdf/foodrevw/jan2000/.)

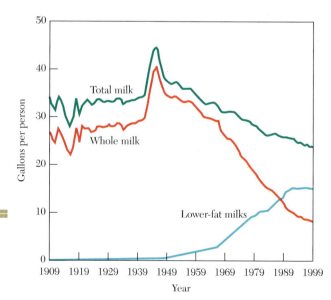

cans do not consume enough fruits and vegetables, that our intake of added sugars has increased, and that the incidence of obesity has been on the rise in all age groups. In the United States, these types of surveys are conducted periodically and are used to monitor the nutritional health of the population and identify ways that the diet can be improved.

THINKING FOR YOURSELF

1. What do you eat? To find out, make a form similar to the sample shown here or use one provided by your instructor to keep a food diary of everything you eat for 3 days. Since you may eat differently on weekends, record for 2 weekdays and 1 weekend day. To make sure you don't forget anything, carry your record with you and record food as it is consumed. This record will be used in Thinking for Yourself exercises throughout this book to focus on particular nutrients. Make the record as complete as possible by using the following tips:
   a. Include all food and drink, and be as specific as possible. For example, did you eat a chicken breast or thigh?
   b. Estimate as carefully as possible the portion size that you ate: for example, 1/2 cup of rice, 10 potato chips, 2 ounces of tofu, and 6 ounces of milk.
   c. Record the preparation or cooking method. For example, was your potato peeled? Was your chicken skinless? Was it baked or fried?
   d. Include anything added to your food, such as butter, ketchup, or salad dressing.
   e. Don't forget snacks, beverages, and desserts.
   f. If the food is from a fast-food chain, list the name.
   g. You may have to break down mixed dishes into their ingredients. For example, a tuna sandwich can be listed as 2 slices of whole wheat bread, 1 tablespoon of mayonnaise, and 3 ounces of tuna packed in water.

Sample Food Record

Food or Beverage	Kind/ How Prepared	Amount
Chicken salad sandwich		
Wheat bread		2 slices
Chicken	Skinless breast	1/2 cup
Mayonnaise	Low-fat	1 Tbsp
Diet cola		1 can

2. How does your diet stack up against the Food Guide Pyramid?
   a. Make a form similar to the sample shown here or use one provided by your instructor to list the foods and amounts from one day of your food record.
   b. Next to each food, list the Food Guide Pyramid food group to which it belongs.

   c. In the next column list the number of Food Guide Pyramid servings or fractions of servings it provides. For mixed foods, list all ingredients separately and identify the food groups and serving sizes that apply.

Sample Food Guide Pyramid Serving Record

Food	Amount	Pyramid Group	No. of Servings
2 Egg rolls			
Wrappers	2	Grain	1
Carrots	1/2 cup	Vegetable	1
Pork	1 oz	Meat	1/2
Peanut oil	1 Tbsp	Fats and sweets	
Rice	1/2 cup	Grain	1

   d. How many servings from each food group did you consume?
   e. Does your diet meet the guidelines for number of servings from each group of the Food Guide Pyramid? If not, what types of food(s) do you need to add to or eliminate from your diet?
   f. Are your food choices consistent with the selection tips described in Table 2.1? How might you modify your food choices to more closely follow these suggestions?

3. Do you understand food labels?
   a. From your kitchen cupboard or the grocery store, select three packaged foods with food labels.
   b. What is the percent of calories from fat in each of these foods?
   c. How many grams of carbohydrate, fat, and fiber are in a serving of each?
   d. How does each of these foods fit into your overall daily diet with regard to total carbohydrate? total fat? dietary fiber?
   e. If you consumed a serving of each of these three foods, how much more fat could you consume during the day without exceeding the recommendations? How much more total carbohydrate and fiber should you consume that day to meet recommendations for a 2000-Calorie diet?

4. What is your Healthy Eating Index? Calculate your Healthy Eating Index by going to the interactive Healthy Eating Index at www.usda.gov/cnpp/.

SUMMARY

1. Nutrition recommendations made to the public for health promotion and disease prevention are based on available scientific knowledge. The current nutrient intake standards in the United States are the Dietary Reference Intakes (DRIs). They provide recommendations for intakes of nutrients and other food components that will avoid deficiencies and excesses and prevent chronic diseases in the majority of healthy persons.

2. The Recommended Dietary Allowances (RDAs) and Adequate Intakes (AIs) are DRI recommendations for amounts of nutrients that will meet the needs of most healthy individuals in the population. The Estimated Average Requirements (EARs) are the average requirements of the population; these are used to evaluate and plan nutrient intakes for population groups. The Tolerable Upper Intake Levels (ULs) provide a guide for a safe upper limit of intake. Recommendations for healthy proportions of carbohydrate, protein, and fat in the diet are given as Acceptable Macronutrient Distribution Ranges (AMDRs). Estimated Energy Requirements (EERs) provide a recommendation for energy intakes that will maintain body weight.

3. The Food Guide Pyramid is a tool for planning diets that meet recommendations. It recommends servings from each of five major food groups. The pyramid shape reflects the relative proportions of each food group that should be included in the diet. The number of servings is given as a range so it can be used by individuals with different energy needs. Following the selection tips for each group will help you make varied nutrient-dense choices and ensure a healthy diet. A new Pyramid is under construction.

4. Food labels follow a standard format and are designed to provide consumers with the information they need to make wise food choices. They use a standard called the Daily Value. Nutrient amounts expressed as a percent of the Daily Values show how a food fits into the recommendations for a healthy diet.

5. The Dietary Guidelines for Americans, 2000, makes dietary and lifestyle recommendations that help Americans "Aim for Fitness" by targeting body weight and physical activity, "Build a Healthy Base" by encouraging healthy food choices and food safety, and "Choose Sensibly" by limiting certain dietary components. These recommendations promote good health and help reduce the risk of chronic diseases that are common in developed countries today. It instructs consumers on how to use the Food Guide Pyramid and food labels as tools to meet these guidelines.

6. The Exchange Lists are used to plan individual diets that provide specific amounts of energy, carbohydrate, protein, and fat.

7. An individual's nutritional status is assessed by evaluating dietary intake, examining clinical parameters such as body size, and interpreting laboratory values within the context of a medical history. The population's nutritional health is monitored by measuring what foods are available, what foods are consumed, and how nutrient intake is related to overall health.

REVIEW QUESTIONS

1. Explain the following DRI standards: RDA, AI, EAR, UL, AMDR, EER.
2. What is the reason for using a food guide shaped like a pyramid?
3. List the food groups of the Food Guide Pyramid.
4. What is meant by nutrient density? Give an example.
5. Why are standard serving sizes used on food labels?
6. How do the Daily Values help consumers determine how foods fit into their overall diets?
7. What determines the order in which food ingredients are listed on a label?
8. What are the three tiers of the Dietary Guidelines?
9. How are the Exchange Lists used in planning diets?
10. What is nutritional status?
11. List the components of individual nutritional assessment.

REFERENCES

1. FAO/WHO/UNU. *Energy and Protein Requirements.* WHO Technical Report Series, no. 724. Geneva: World Health Organization, 1985.
2. National Research Council, Food and Nutrition Board. *Recommended Dietary Allowances,* 10th ed. Washington, DC: National Academy Press, 1989.
3. Institute of Medicine, Food and Nutrition Board. *Dietary Reference Intakes for Thiamin, Riboflavin, Niacin, Vitamin B-6, Folate, Vitamin B-12, Pantothenic Acid, Biotin, and Choline.* Washington, DC: National Academy Press, 1998.
4. Institute of Medicine, Food and Nutrition Board. *Dietary Reference Intakes for Energy, Carbohydrates, Fiber, Fat, Protein, and Amino Acids.* Washington, DC: National Academy Press, 2002.
5. U.S. Department of Agriculture. *The Food Guide Pyramid, Revised 2000.* Available online at www.nal.usda.gov/fnic/Fpyr/pyramid.html.
6. Goldberg, J. P., Belury, M. A., Elam, P., et al. The obesity crisis: don't blame it on the Pyramid. *J. Am. Diet. Assoc.* 104:1141–1147, 2004.

7. Young, L. R., and Nestle, M. The contribution of expanding portion size to the obesity epidemic. *Am. J. Public Health* 92:246–249, 2002.

8. International Food Information Council. Food insight. We've come a long way: looking back at food guides and recommendations. Available online at www.ific.org/foodinsight/1999/nd/foodguidefi699.cfm/Accessed July 6, 2004.

9. Cleveland, E., Cook, J. E., Wilson, J. W., et al. Pyramid servings data from the 1994 CSFII data ARS Food Survey research. Available online at www.barc.usda.gov/bhnrc/foodsurveys/home.html/Accessed May 30, 2004.

10. Food and Drug Administration, Center for Food Safety and Applied Nutrition. Labeling claims. Available online at www.cfsan.fda.gov/~dms/lab-ind.html/Accessed February 2, 2004.

11. U.S. Food and Drug Administration, Center for Food Safety and Applied Nutrition. Food labeling: a guide for restaurants and other retail establishments. Questions, August, 1995; revised February 1996. Available online at www.cfsan.fda.gov/~frf/qaintro.html/Accessed March 13, 2004.

12. U.S. Department of Agriculture, U.S. Department of Health and Human Services. *Nutrition and Your Health: Dietary Guidelines for Americans*, 5th ed. Item number 147-G. Hyattsville, MD: U.S. Government Printing Office, 2000.

13. *Exchange Lists for Meal Planning*, Alexandria, VA: The American Diabetes Association, Inc., and the American Dietetic Association, 2003.

14. National Center for Health Statistics. About healthy people 2010. Available online at www.cdc.gov/nchs/about/otheract/hpdata2010/abouthp.htm/Accessed December 10, 2003.

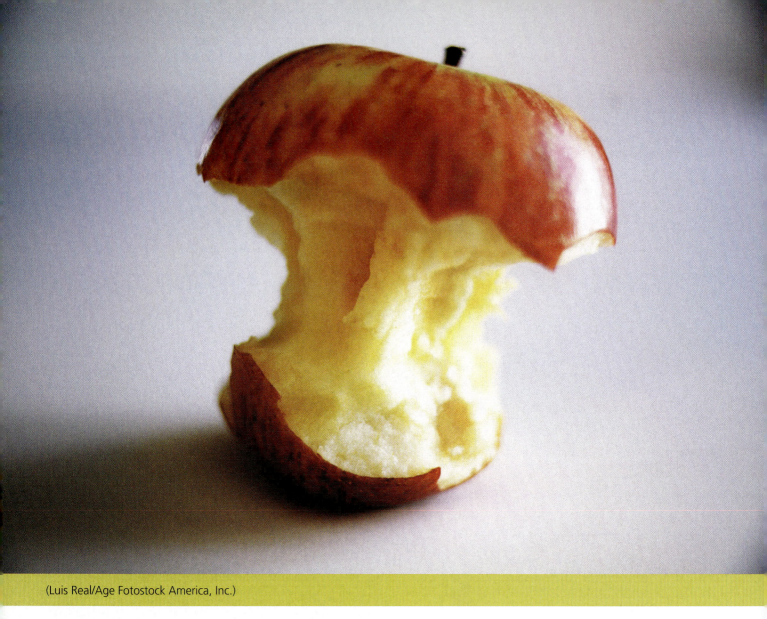

CHAPTER 3 CONCEPTS

- All plant and animal life is made up of cells, which form tissues that compose the organs and organ systems of a living organism.
- The food we eat is digested in the gastrointestinal tract and its nutrients are absorbed into the body.
- Hormones released into the blood and enzymes released into the gastrointestinal tract facilitate the digestion of food and the absorption of nutrients.
- Digestion begins in the mouth. Food is then swallowed and moves down the esophagus to the stomach for storage and further digestion.
- The small intestine is the primary site of digestion and absorption.
- Water-soluble materials are absorbed into the blood. Most fat-soluble materials are absorbed into the lymph.
- Changes in the gastrointestinal tract can alter digestion and absorption and affect nutritional status.
- Nutrients delivered to the cells can be used to produce energy in the form of ATP and to synthesize molecules for immediate use or for storage.
- Materials that are not absorbed pass into the large intestine and are excreted in feces. The waste products generated inside the body by metabolism are eliminated via the lungs, skin, and kidneys.

Just A Taste

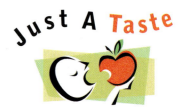

Why does your mouth water at the sight or smell of food?

Why are you hungry very soon after eating some meals while others stick with you longer?

Is it healthy to have bacteria living in your gastrointestinal tract?

The Digestive System: ③
From Meals to Molecules

INTRODUCTION

WebMD Feature Archive

Bariatric Surgery: A Radical Obesity Fix

By *Catherine Guthrie*

Dec. 18, 2000—Two years ago, Rhonda Bailey was fat and miserable. The 38-year-old bore 245 pounds on her 5-foot-1 frame. Squeezing into a restaurant booth, airplane seat, or amusement park ride was unimaginable. Walking made her joints stiff and sore. She leaned heavily on a cane to get from the handicapped parking space to her desk at work.

Today, Bailey is literally half the woman she used to be. Over the past 18 months, she has shed 50% of her body weight. Her waist shrunk from a size 26 to a size six. Now, at 125 pounds, the Southern California resident jogs daily, bicycles with her stepdaughter, and rejoices in her ability to do life's little things—like tying her shoes—without asking her husband for help. Bailey's secret isn't the latest fad diet or radical weight loss drug. She owes her slimmed-down body to gastric-bypass surgery. The procedure is just one of several weight loss operations that fall under the heading of bariatric surgery.

As obesity rates creep skyward, so do the number of Americans turning to surgery as a weight loss tool.

To read the rest of this article, go to www.my.webmd.com/content/article/14/1689_51239.htm.

Bariatric surgery is used to treat obesity. It reduces the size of the stomach to the size of your thumb so it can't hold as much. It also reroutes the intestines so less of what is eaten can be absorbed. After this surgery, people can't eat as much and can't absorb as much, so they lose weight.

Was this surgery a cure for Rhonda's obesity? She has lost weight, but not without consequences. Her digestive tract has been permanently altered and so has her ability to get the nutrients she needs. She can no longer eat a large meal or absorb all the nutrients from that meal. If she does overeat she may experience pain, sweats, chills, and nausea.

Even when she is careful to eat small meals, diarrhea can be a problem. Bypassing part of her intestines also put her at risk for a number of vitamin deficiencies. Understanding how the gastrointestinal tract functions will help you grasp the consequences of this type of surgery as well as appreciate how important this organ system is for obtaining nutrients.

Our Complex Bodies Are Built from Simpler Units

⚠️ **Atoms** The smallest units of an element that still retain the properties of that element.

⚠️ **Chemical bonds** Forces that hold atoms together.

⚠️ **Molecules** Units of two or more atoms of the same or different elements bonded together.

⚠️ **Organic molecules** Molecules that contain two or more carbon atoms.

⚠️ **Inorganic molecules** Substances that do not contain carbon-to-hydrogen bonds.

⚠️ **Cells** The basic structural and functional units of plant and animal life.

⚠️ **Organ** A discrete structure composed of more than one tissue that performs a specialized function.

When it comes down to it, we are all made of **atoms**. Atoms can be linked by **chemical bonds** to form **molecules**. The carbohydrates, lipids, proteins, and vitamins in our diet and in our bodies are **organic molecules**. Water and minerals are **inorganic molecules**. These molecules are organized to form **cells**, the smallest unit of plant and animal life (Figure 3.1). These cells are then grouped to provide different structures and functions in the body.

Cells form tissues, tissues form organs, organs form organ systems

In any living system, whether a sunflower, a cow, or a human being, molecules are organized into cells. Cells that are similar in structure and function form tissues. The human body contains four types of tissue: muscle, nerve, epithelial, and connective. These tissues are organized in varying combinations into **organs**. Organs such as the heart, the stomach, and the kidneys are discrete structures that perform specialized functions in the body (Figure 3.2).

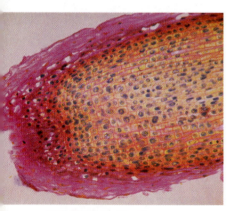

FIGURE 3.1

All living things are made up of cells. This photo shows the cells that make up the root tip of an onion plant. Various types of cells make up all the tissues of the human body. (© Lester V. Bergman/Corbis Images)

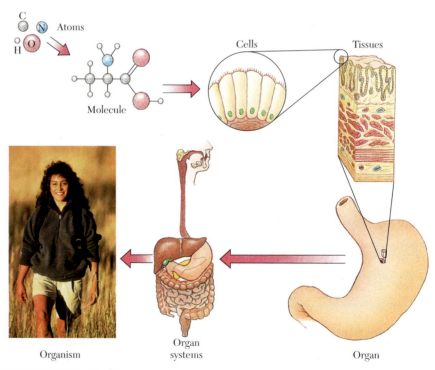

FIGURE 3.2

The organization of life begins with atoms that form molecules, which are then organized into cells to form tissues, organs, organ systems, and organisms. (Brian Bailey/Stone/Getty Images)

TABLE 3.1
What Do Organ Systems Do?

Organ System	What It Includes	What It Does
Nervous	Brain, spinal cord, and associated nerves	Responds to stimuli from the external and internal environments; conducts impulses to activate muscles and glands; integrates activities of other systems
Respiratory	Lungs, trachea, and air passageways	Supplies the blood with oxygen and removes carbon dioxide
Urinary	Kidneys and their associated structures	Eliminates wastes and regulates the balance of water, electrolytes, and acid in the blood
Reproductive	Testes, ovaries, and their associated structures	Produces offspring
Cardiovascular	Heart and blood vessels	Transports blood, which carries oxygen, nutrients, and wastes
Lymphatic/Immune	Lymph and lymph structures, white blood cells	Defends against foreign invaders, picks up fluid leaked from blood vessels, transports fat-soluble nutrients
Muscular	Skeletal muscles	Provides movement and structure
Skeletal	Bones and joints	Protects and supports the body, provides a framework for the muscles to use for movement
Endocrine	Pituitary, adrenal, thyroid, pancreas, and other ductless glands	Secretes hormones that regulate processes such as growth, reproduction, and nutrient use
Integumentary	Skin, hair, nails, and sweat glands	Covers and protects the body; helps control body temperature
Digestive	Mouth, esophagus, stomach, intestines, pancreas, liver, and gallbladder	Ingests and digests food, absorbs nutrients into the blood, eliminates unabsorbed food residue and other waste products

Adapted from E. N. Marieb. *Human Anatomy and Physiology*, 5th ed. Redwood City, California: Benjamin/Cummings Publishing Co., 2000.

Most organs do not function alone but are part of organ systems. The organ systems in humans include the nervous system, respiratory system (lungs), urinary system (kidneys and bladder), reproductive system, cardiovascular system (heart and blood vessels), lymphatic/immune system, muscular system, skeletal system, endocrine system (hormones), integumentary system (skin and body linings), and digestive system (Table 3.1). An organ may be part of more than one organ system. For example, the pancreas is part of the endocrine system as well as the digestive system.

Organ systems work together to digest, absorb, and utilize nutrients

The digestive system is the organ system primarily responsible for the movement of nutrients into the body; however, several other organ systems are also needed to regulate these processes and use the nutrients. The endocrine system secretes **hormones** that help regulate how much we eat and how quickly food and nutrients travel through the digestive system. The nervous system sends nerve signals that help control the passage of food through the digestive tract. The cardiovascular system transports nutrients to individual cells in the body. The urinary, respiratory, and integumentary systems eliminate wastes generated within the body.

Hormones Chemical messengers that are produced in one location, released into the blood, and elicit responses at other locations in the body.

The Digestive System Digests Food and Absorbs Nutrients

⚠ Digestion The process of breaking food into components small enough to be absorbed into the body.

⚠ Absorption The process of taking substances into the interior of the body.

⚠ Fatty acids Chains of carbon atoms that are often present as components of larger molecules known as triglycerides, which we commonly call fats.

⚠ Feces Body waste, including unabsorbed food residue, bacteria, mucus, and dead cells, which is excreted from the gastrointestinal tract by passing through the anus.

⚠ Gastrointestinal tract A hollow tube consisting of the mouth, pharynx, esophagus, stomach, small intestine, large intestine, and anus, in which digestion and absorption of nutrients occur.

⚠ Lumen The inside cavity of a tube, such as the gastrointestinal tract.

The digestive system provides two major functions: **digestion** and **absorption**. Most food must be digested in order for the nutrients it contains to be absorbed into the body. For example, a slice of bread does not travel through the digestive system intact. First it is broken apart, releasing its carbohydrate, protein, and fat. Most of the carbohydrate is digested to sugars, the protein to amino acids, and the fat to **fatty acids**. Sugars, amino acids, and fatty acids can be absorbed. The fiber from the bread cannot be digested and therefore is not absorbed into the body. Fiber and other unabsorbed substances pass through the digestive tract and are excreted in the **feces**.

The gastrointestinal tract is a long, hollow tube

The main part of the digestive system is the **gastrointestinal tract**. It is also referred to as the GI tract, gut, digestive tract, intestinal tract, or alimentary canal. It can be thought of as a hollow tube, about 30 feet in length, that runs from the mouth to the anus. The organs of the gastrointestinal tract include the mouth, pharynx, esophagus, stomach, small intestine, large intestine, and anus (Figure 3.3). The inside of the tube that these organs form is called the **lumen**. Food within the lumen of the gastrointestinal tract is not technically inside the body because it has not been absorbed. Therefore, if you swallow something that cannot be digested, such as an unchewed raisin or corn kernel, it will pass through your digestive tract and exit in the feces without ever being broken down or entering your blood or cells. Only after substances are transferred into the cells that line the intestine by the process of absorption are they actually "inside" the body. The amount of time it takes for food to pass through the length

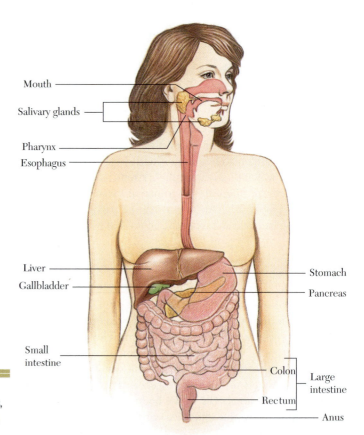

FIGURE 3.3

The digestive system consists of the organs of the gastrointestinal tract: the mouth, pharynx, esophagus, stomach, small intestine, large intestine, and anus, as well as a number of accessory organs: the salivary glands, liver, gallbladder, and pancreas.

Mouth
Salivary glands
Pharynx
Esophagus
Liver
Gallbladder
Small intestine
Stomach
Pancreas
Colon
Large intestine
Rectum
Anus

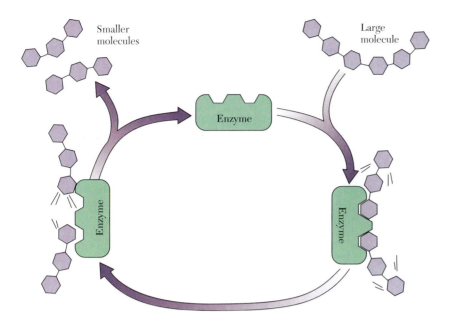

Smaller molecules

Large molecule

Enzyme

Enzyme

Enzyme

FIGURE 3.4

Enzymes speed up chemical reactions without themselves being altered by the reaction. In this example, an enzyme breaks a large molecule into two smaller ones.

of the GI tract from mouth to anus is referred to as **transit time**. The shorter the transit time, the more rapid the passage through the digestive tract. In a healthy adult, transit time is about 24 to 72 hours. It is affected by the composition of the diet, physical activity, emotions, medications, and illnesses.

Digestive tract secretions aid digestion

The digestive process is aided by substances that are secreted into the digestive tract from cells lining the digestive tract and from a number of accessory organs. One of these substances is **mucus**. It moistens, lubricates, and protects the digestive tract. **Enzymes** are another component of digestive system secretions. Enzymes are protein molecules that speed up chemical reactions without themselves being consumed or changed by the reactions (Figure 3.4). In the digestive tract, enzymes break down food into absorbable units. Different enzymes are needed for the breakdown of different food components. For example, enzymes called amylases digest carbohydrate but have no effect on fat, and enzymes called lipases digest fat but have no effect on carbohydrate.

The digestive system also releases hormones. Hormones are chemical messengers that are secreted into the blood by one organ to regulate body functions elsewhere. In the gastrointestinal tract, hormones regulate the rate at which food moves through the system by sending signals that help prepare different parts of the GI tract for the arrival of food. For example, a hormone called cholecystokinin signals the pancreas and gallbladder to secrete digestive substances into the GI tract.

The wall of the gastrointestinal tract has four layers

The wall of the gastrointestinal tract contains four layers (Figure 3.5). The layer lining the lumen, which is in contact with the gut contents, is the **mucosa**. Because mucosal cells are in direct contact with churning food and harsh digestive secretions, they live only about 2 to 5 days. The dead cells are sloughed off into the lumen, where some components are digested and absorbed and the rest are excreted in the feces. Mucosal cells reproduce rapidly to replace those that die. To allow for this rapid replacement, the mucosa has high nutrient requirements and is one of the first parts of the body to be affected by nutrient deficiencies. Surrounding the mucosa is a layer of connective tissue containing nerves and blood vessels. This layer provides support, delivers nutrients to the mucosa, and provides the nerve signals that control secretions and muscle contractions. Layers of smooth muscle—the type over which we do not have voluntary

Transit time The time between the ingestion of food and the elimination of the solid waste from that food.

Mucus A viscous fluid secreted by glands in the gastrointestinal tract and other parts of the body. It acts to lubricate, moisten, and protect cells from harsh environments.

Enzymes Protein molecules that accelerate the rate of specific chemical reactions without being changed themselves.

Mucosa The layer of tissue lining the gastrointestinal tract and other body cavities.

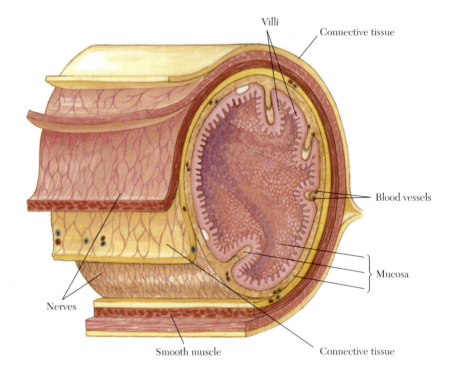

Villi

Connective tissue

Blood vessels

Mucosa

Connective tissue

Smooth muscle

Nerves

FIGURE 3.5

This cross-section through the wall of the small intestine shows the four tissue layers: mucosa, connective tissue, smooth muscle layers, and outer connective tissue layer.

⭐ **Antigen** A foreign substance (almost always a protein) that, when introduced into the body, stimulates an immune response.

⭐ **Antibodies** Proteins produced by cells of the immune system that destroy or inactivate foreign substances in the body.

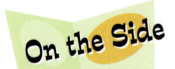

When you receive a vaccination or immunization you are receiving a small dose of harmless antigen, such as an inactivated or killed virus. It does not make you sick but is seen as foreign, and your body produces antibodies to that antigen. Then, if you are exposed to the same antigen again, your immune system remembers how to make the specific antibody, and you are able to quickly fight off the infection. Antibodies are discussed more in Chapter 6.

control—surround the connective tissue. The contraction of smooth muscles in the GI tract mixes food, breaks it into smaller particles, and propels it through the digestive tract. The final, external layer is also made up of connective tissue and provides support and protection.

The gastrointestinal tract protects us from infection

The gastrointestinal tract is an important part of the immune system, which protects the body from foreign invaders. It limits the absorption of toxins and disease-causing organisms. If an invading substance, or **antigen**, does get past the intestinal cells, the immune system has a number of weapons that can destroy it. Some of these are cells and some are chemicals released into the blood. The different types of white blood cells make up the cells of the immune system. Many of these reside in the gastrointestinal tract, so a foreign substance or harmful organism that enters the body through the mucosa can be destroyed quickly. The first types of cells to come to the body's defense are called phagocytes. They will target any invader and act by engulfing and destroying foreign substances. These cells also release chemicals that signal other immune system cells called lymphocytes to come join the fight. Lymphocytes are very specific about what they will attack. Some lymphocytes bind directly to a specific invader or antigen and destroy it. This type of lymphocyte helps eliminate cancer cells, foreign tissue, and cells that have been infected by viruses and bacteria. Other lymphocytes produce and secrete protein molecules called **antibodies**. Antibodies bind to invading antigen and help to destroy it. Each antibody is designed to fight off only one specific type of antigen. Once the body has made antibodies to a specific antigen, it remembers and is ready to fight that antigen any time it enters the body.

Our immune system protects us from many invaders without our even being aware of it. Unfortunately, the response of the immune system to a foreign substance is also responsible for allergic reactions. An allergic reaction occurs when the immune system produces antibodies to a substance that is present in our diet or environment. For example, a food allergy occurs when proteins present in food are seen as foreign and trigger an immune response. The immune response causes symptoms that range from hives to life-threatening breathing difficulties.

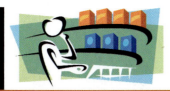

Your Choice: When Food Is the Foe

Food provides nourishment along with interesting tastes and smells that stir our senses. However, for someone with a food allergy, unfamiliar foods and flavors must be considered with caution. Food allergies occur when the immunological components of the digestive tract become confused and see a particular food as an invader rather than a source of nutrition. Once you have developed a food allergy, exposure to the offending food can cause uncomfortable and even deadly reactions. How does food become the foe?

The first time a food is consumed, it does not trigger an allergic reaction, but in a susceptible person, this begins the process. As the food travels down the digestive tract it is mechanically broken apart, exposed to acid, and chemically digested, but tiny fragments of undigested protein remain. These fragments are absorbed into the body. In susceptible individuals this triggers the production of a particular type of antibody. This antibody binds to cells called mast cells. When the offending food is eaten again, the food proteins bind to the antibody and trigger the mast cells to release chemicals, such as histamine, that cause redness and swelling and other symptoms of an allergic reaction. The tiny protein fragments that cause allergies are not destroyed by cooking, broken down by stomach acid, or digested by enzymes. They are able to cross the gastrointestinal lining and travel through the bloodstream.[1]

The symptoms of a food allergy change depending on where in the digestive tract and the body these protein fragments trigger the release of histamine. For example, when the food enters the mouth the allergic person may experience an itching or tingling sensation on the tongue or lips. As it travels down to the stomach and intestines the food may cause vomiting and cramps. After it is absorbed and travels through the bloodstream, these protein fragments may cause a drop in blood pressure, hives, and when it reaches the lungs, asthma.

Food allergies affect about 1.5% of adults and up to 6% of children under 3 years of age. They are responsible for 150 deaths each year.[1] Foods that most commonly cause allergies in adults include seafood, peanuts, tree nuts, fish, and eggs. In children allergies to eggs, milk, peanuts, soy, and wheat are most common. The best way to avoid allergic symptoms is to choose foods that are free of ingredients that trigger an immune response. This sounds easy, but it can be difficult to identify all the ingredients in foods. Reading food labels is essential, but many of the foods we eat don't come out of a package. For most of us, trying a new entrée at a restaurant or going to a potluck dinner is an adventure in eating, but for those with food allergies, it is a potential danger. Careful reconnaissance is required before a new food can be considered safe.

Reference
1. Formanek, R. Food allergies: when food becomes the enemy. *FDA Consumer*, July/Aug, 2001. Available online at www.fda.gov/fdac/features/2001/401 food.html/Accessed Nov. 17, 2003.

Food Must Be Digested for Nutrients to Be Absorbed

To be used by the body, food must be consumed and digested, and the nutrients must be absorbed and transported to the cells of the body. Because most foods are mixtures of carbohydrate, fat, and protein, the digestive tract is designed to allow the digestion of all of these components without competition among them. The following sections of this chapter will trace a meal through all these processes, from the body's anticipation of food to the elimination of waste products.

Digestive activity begins with the sights, sounds, and smells of food

Imagine slices of oven-roasted turkey served on fresh baked whole grain bread accompanied by a crisp apple and a tall glass of cold milk. Is your mouth watering? You don't even need to put something in your mouth for activity in the digestive tract to begin. As the meal is being prepared, sensory input such as the sight of a turkey being lifted out of the oven, the clatter of the table being set, and the smell of freshly baked bread may make your mouth water and your stomach begin to secrete digestive substances.

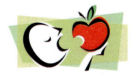

You can't digest food without putting it in your mouth, but you can get the juices flowing. Just looking at or smelling appetizing food can send signals to your salivary glands to make your mouth water and to your stomach to secrete gastric juice.

This response occurs when the nervous system signals the digestive system to ready itself for a meal.

Digestion begins in the mouth

Take a bite (Figure 3.6). The mouth is the point at which food enters the digestive tract. The presence of food in the mouth stimulates the flow of **saliva** from the salivary glands (see Figure 3.3). Saliva moistens food and carries dissolved food molecules to the taste buds. Signals from the taste buds along with the smell of food allow us to experience the full flavor of food. Saliva helps digest food because it contains the enzyme salivary amylase, which begins breaking starches into sugars. Saliva also helps protect against tooth decay because it washes away food particles and contains substances that inhibit the growth of bacteria that may cause tooth decay.

Chewing food is important for digestion. Chewing breaks food into small pieces and thereby increases the surface area that is in contact with digestive juices. Adult humans have 32 teeth, specialized for biting, tearing, grinding, and crushing foods. The tongue helps mix food with saliva and aids chewing by constantly repositioning food between the teeth. Chewing also breaks apart fiber that traps nutrients. If the fiber is not broken, some nutrients cannot be absorbed. For example, the peel of an apple is a source of vitamins and minerals; these nutrients cannot be absorbed without first being released from the fiber in the peel.

Swallowing occurs in the pharynx

The meal that entered the mouth as a turkey sandwich, apple, and milk has now been formed into a bolus, a ball of chewed food mixed with saliva. From the mouth, the bolus moves into the **pharynx**, the part of the gastrointestinal tract responsible for swallowing. The pharynx is shared by the digestive tract and the respiratory tract: food passes through the pharynx on its way to the stomach, and air passes on its way to and from the lungs. During swallowing, the air passages are blocked by a valve-like flap of tissue called the epiglottis, so food goes to the stomach, not the lungs. Sometimes eating too quickly or talking while eating can interfere with the closing of the epiglottis and food can pass into an upper air passageway. It is usually dislodged with a cough, but if it becomes stuck it can block the flow of air and cause choking. A quick response is required to save the life of a person whose airway is completely blocked. The Heimlich maneuver, which forces air out of the lungs with a sudden application of pressure to the upper abdomen, can blow an object out of the blocked air passage (Figure 3.7).

Swallowed food travels down the esophagus to the stomach

The **esophagus** passes through the diaphragm, a muscular wall separating the abdomen from the chest cavity where the lungs are located, to connect the pharynx and stomach. In the esophagus the bolus of food is moved along by rhythmic contractions of the smooth muscles, a process called **peristalsis**. The contractions of peristalsis are strong enough that even food swallowed while you are standing on your head will reach your stomach. This contractile movement, which is controlled automatically by the nervous system, occurs throughout the gastrointestinal tract, pushing the food bolus along from the pharynx through the large intestine.

To move from the esophagus into the stomach, food must pass through a **sphincter**, a muscle that encircles the tube of the digestive tract and acts as a valve. When the sphincter muscle contracts, the valve is closed (Figure 3.8). The gastroesophageal sphincter, located between the esophagus and the stomach, prevents foods from moving back out of the stomach. Occasionally, materials do pass out of the stomach through this valve. The pain of heartburn is caused when some of the acidic stomach contents leak up and out of the stomach into the esophagus, causing a burning sensation. Vomiting is the result of reverse peristalsis that causes the sphincter to relax and allow the food to pass upward out of the stomach toward the mouth.

Saliva A watery fluid produced and secreted into the mouth by the salivary glands. It contains lubricants, enzymes, and other substances.

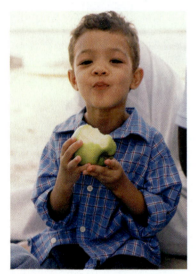

FIGURE 3.6

By the time you take a bite, the sights, smells, sounds, or thoughts of food have already triggered activity in your digestive tract. (Ann Ackerman/Taxi/Getty Images)

Pharynx A funnel-shaped opening that connects the nasal passages and mouth to the respiratory passages and esophagus. It is a common passageway for food and air and is responsible for swallowing.

Esophagus A portion of the gastrointestinal tract that extends from the pharynx to the stomach.

Peristalsis Coordinated muscular contractions that move food through the gastrointestinal tract.

Sphincter A muscular valve that helps control the flow of materials in the gastrointestinal tract.

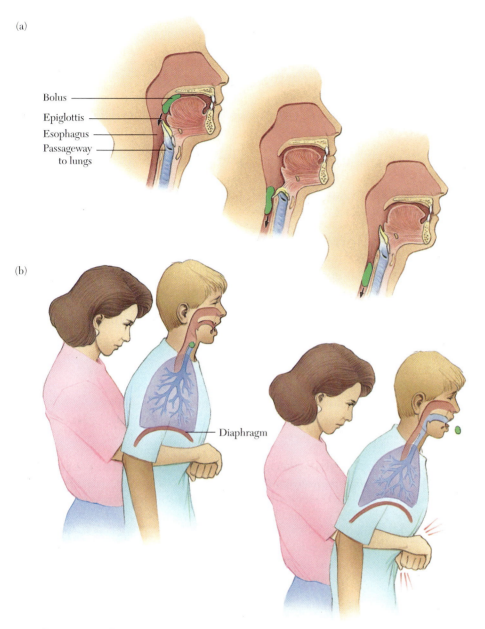

(a)

Bolus
Epiglottis
Esophagus
Passageway to lungs

(b)

Diaphragm

FIGURE 3.7

(a) When a bolus of food is swallowed, it pushes the epiglottis down over the opening to the air passageways. (b) If food does become lodged in the air passageways, it can be dislodged by the Heimlich maneuver, illustrated here.

The stomach mixes and stores food and begins protein digestion

The stomach is an expanded portion of the gastrointestinal tract that serves as a temporary storage place for food. While held in the stomach, the bolus is mixed with highly acidic stomach secretions to form a semiliquid food mass called chyme. The mixing of food in the stomach is aided by an extra layer of smooth muscle in the stomach wall. While most of the gastrointestinal tract is surrounded by two layers of muscle, the stomach contains a third layer, allowing for powerful contractions that thoroughly churn and mix the stomach contents. Some digestion takes place in the stomach, but, with the exception of some water, alcohol, and a few drugs such as aspirin and acetaminophen (Tylenol), very little absorption occurs here.

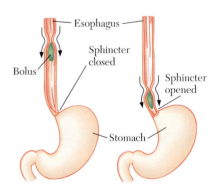

Esophagus
Sphincter closed
Bolus
Sphincter opened
Stomach

FIGURE 3.8

The rhythmic contractions of peristalsis propel food down the esophagus, through the open sphincter, and into the stomach.

Gastric juice contains acid and enzymes Stomach secretions called gastric juice are produced by gastric glands in the lining of the stomach. One of the components of gastric juice is hydrochloric acid. This acid kills most of the bacteria present in food. It also stops the activity of the carbohydrate-digesting enzyme salivary amylase and helps begin the digestion of protein by unfolding proteins and activating the enzyme **pepsin**. The digestion of the starch from the bread stops in your stomach, and digestion of the protein from the turkey, milk, and bread begins. The protein of the stomach wall is protected from the acid and pepsin by a thick layer of mucus. If the mucus layer is penetrated, pepsin and acid can damage the underlying tissues and cause **peptic ulcers**, erosions of the stomach wall or some other region of the gastrointestinal tract. One of the leading causes of ulcers is infection of the stomach lining by acid-resistant bacteria called *Helicobacter pylori*. These bacteria damage the gastrointestinal tract wall and destroy the protective mucosal layer.[1]

Nerves and hormones regulate stomach motility and secretions How much your stomach churns and how much gastric juice is released is regulated by signals from both nerves and hormones. These signals originate from three different sites—the brain, stomach, and small intestine. The thought, smell, sight, or taste of food causes the brain to send nerve signals that stimulate gastric secretion, preparing the stomach to receive food (Figure 3.9). Food entering the stomach then also stimulates secretions and motility by stimulating local nerve signals, sending signals to the brain, and by stimulating **gastrin** secretion. Gastrin is a hormone that triggers the release of gastric juice and increases stomach motility.

Food entering the small intestine triggers hormonal and nervous signals that can decrease stomach motility and secretions. This slows the release of food into the intestine, ensuring that the amount of chyme entering the small intestine does not exceed the ability of the intestine to process it.

The size and composition of the meal affect stomach emptying Chyme normally empties from the stomach in 2 to 6 hours. The rate of stomach emptying is determined by the size and composition of the meal and is controlled by signals from the small intestine. To move from the stomach to the small intestine, chyme must pass through the pyloric sphincter. This sphincter helps regulate the rate at which food enters the intestine. The small intestine stretches as it fills

⚠ **Pepsin** A protein-digesting enzyme produced by the stomach. It is secreted in the gastric juice in an inactive form and activated by acid in the stomach.

⚠ **Peptic ulcer** An open sore in the lining of the stomach, esophagus, or small intestine.

⚠ **Gastrin** A hormone secreted by the stomach mucosa that stimulates the secretion of gastric juices.

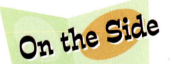

On the Side

Over half of the world's population is infected with the bacterium *Helicobacter pylori*. It causes ulcers in the stomach and esophagus, and long-term infection is associated with the development of gastric cancer. But not everyone who is infected will develop any symptoms. The good news for those who do is that 2 weeks of antibiotic therapy can kill the bacteria, allowing the ulcer to heal.

FIGURE 3.9

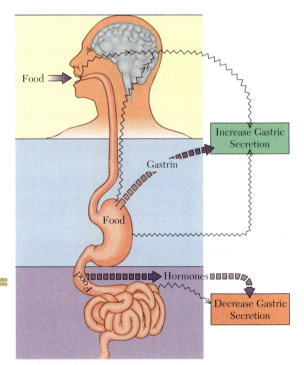

The sight, smell, and taste of food cause the brain to signal an increase in gastric secretions. When food enters the stomach, gastric secretions are stimulated by the stretching of local nerves, signals sent to the brain, and the release of gastrin. As food enters the small intestine, gastric secretions are inhibited by nervous and hormonal signals. In this diagram the zigzag arrows represent nerve signals, and the dashed arrows represent hormonal signals.

with food; this distension inhibits stomach emptying. A large meal takes longer to completely leave the stomach than a small meal, and a solid meal leaves the stomach more slowly than a liquid meal. The nutritional composition of a meal also affects how long it stays in the stomach. The meal of a sandwich, apple, and milk that we have been following through the GI tract contains protein, carbohydrate, and fat and is partly solid and partly liquid. It will leave the stomach in an average amount of time, about 4 hours. A higher-fat meal would stay in the stomach the longest because fat slows stomach emptying. A meal that is primarily protein will leave more quickly than a high-fat meal, and a meal of mostly carbohydrate will leave the fastest. Because the nutrient composition of a meal affects how quickly it leaves your stomach, it affects how soon after eating you feel hungry again. Thus, what you choose for breakfast can affect when you become hungry for lunch. Toast and coffee will leave your stomach far more quickly than a larger meal with more protein and some fat, such as a bowl of cereal with low-fat milk and toast with peanut butter. Factors besides food composition also can affect gastric emptying. For example, sadness and fear tend to slow emptying, while aggression tends to increase gastric motility and speed emptying.

The reason some meals stick with you longer relates to the amount of carbohydrate, fat, and protein they contain. A high-fat, high-protein meal such as fried chicken with buttered corn bread will empty from your stomach slowly and keep you full longer than a high carbohydrate meal of rice and steamed vegetables.

The small intestine is the site of most digestion and absorption

The small intestine is a narrow tube about 20 feet in length. It is divided into three segments. The first 12 inches are the duodenum, the next 8 feet are the jejunum, and the last 11 feet are the ileum. The small intestine is the main site of digestion of food and absorption of nutrients.

Digestive secretions from accessory organs aid digestion

In the small intestine, secretions from the **pancreas** and **gallbladder** as well as from the intestine itself aid digestion. The pancreas secretes pancreatic juice, which contains bicarbonate and digestive enzymes. The bicarbonate neutralizes the acid in the chyme, making the environment in the small intestine neutral or slightly basic rather than acidic as it is in the stomach. This neutrality allows enzymes from the pancreas and small intestine to function. Pancreatic amylase continues the job of breaking starches into sugars that was started in the mouth by salivary amylase. Pancreatic protein-digesting enzymes, including trypsin and chymotrypsin, continue to break protein into shorter and shorter chains of amino acids. Intestinal digestive enzymes, found attached to or inside the cells lining the small intestine, aid the digestion of sugars into single sugar units and the digestion of short amino acid chains into single amino acids.

The gallbladder stores and secretes **bile**, a substance produced in the liver that is necessary for fat digestion and absorption. Bile secreted into the small intestine mixes with fat and breaks it into smaller globules, allowing pancreatic enzymes, called **lipases**, to more efficiently access the fat and digest it. The bile and digested fats then form small droplets that facilitate the absorption of fat into the mucosal cells.

Absorption occurs by passive and active mechanisms

The small intestine is the primary site of absorption for water, vitamins, minerals, and the products of carbohydrate, fat, and protein digestion. To be absorbed, these nutrients must pass from the lumen of the GI tract into the mucosal cells lining the tract and then into the blood or lymph. Several different mechanisms are involved (Figure 3.10). Many nutrients can cross into the mucosa by diffusion, which is the movement of substances from an area of higher concentration to an area of lower concentration. In this case nutrients move from the lumen, where their concentration is high, into the cells of the intestine, where their concentration is lower. In **simple diffusion**, substances pass freely across cell membranes and no energy is required. Vitamin E and fatty acids are absorbed by simple diffusion. Water is also absorbed by diffusion. The diffusion of water is called **osmosis**. In osmosis there is a net movement of water in a direction that will balance the concentration of dissolved substances on either side of a membrane. For example, if there is a high concentration of sugar in the lumen of the

Pancreas An organ that secretes digestive enzymes and bicarbonate into the small intestine during digestion.

Gallbladder An organ of the digestive system that stores bile, which is produced by the liver.

Bile A substance made in the liver and stored in the gallbladder. It is released into the small intestine to aid in fat digestion and absorption.

Lipases Fat-digesting enzymes.

Simple diffusion The movement of substances from an area of higher concentration to an area of lower concentration. No energy is required.

Osmosis The diffusion of water across a membrane to equalize the concentration of dissolved substances on both sides.

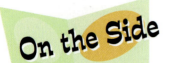

The protein in our cells could be digested by the same enzymes that digest the protein in our food, but they aren't. One reason is that digestive enzymes like pepsin and trypsin are produced in inactive forms so they can't harm the glands that produce them. They are activated only after they are in the lumen of the GI tract, which is protected by a layer of mucus.

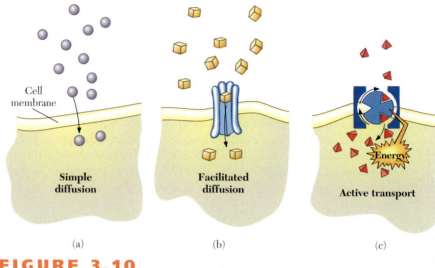

(a) (b) (c)

FIGURE 3.10

Nutrients are absorbed from the lumen across the cell membrane into the cell by several mechanisms. (a) Simple diffusion, which requires no energy, is shown here by the purple balls that move across the membrane from an area of higher concentration to an area of lower concentration. (b) Facilitated diffusion, which requires no energy, is shown here by the yellow cubes that move across the membrane from an area of higher concentration to an area of lower concentration with the help of a carrier. (c) Active transport, which requires energy and a carrier, is shown here by the red pyramids that move across the membrane from an area of lower concentration to an area of higher concentration.

Facilitated diffusion The movement of substances across a cell membrane from an area of higher concentration to an area of lower concentration with the aid of a carrier molecule. No energy is required.

Active transport The transport of substances across a cell membrane with the aid of a carrier molecule and the expenditure of energy.

Villi (villus) Fingerlike protrusions of the lining of the small intestine that increase the absorptive surface area.

Microvilli Minute brushlike projections on the mucosal cell membrane that participate in the digestion and absorption of foodstuffs.

Lymph vessel or **lacteal** A tubular component of the lymphatic system that carries fluid away from body tissues. Lymph vessels in the intestine are known as lacteals and can transport large particles such as the products of fat digestion.

intestine, water will actually move from the mucosal cells into the lumen. As the sugar is absorbed, and the concentration in the lumen decreases, water will move back into the mucosal cells by osmosis.

Some nutrients cannot pass freely across cell membranes; they must be helped across by carrier molecules in a process called **facilitated diffusion**. They still move from an area of higher concentration to one of lower concentration, and no energy is needed for their transport. The sugar fructose found in the apple is absorbed by facilitated diffusion.

Substances unable to be absorbed by simple or facilitated diffusion must enter the body by **active transport**, a process that requires both a carrier molecule and energy. This use of energy allows substances to be transported from an area of lower concentration to an area of higher concentration. The sugar glucose from the breakdown of starch in the bread and amino acids from the protein in the milk, turkey, and bread are absorbed by active transport. Active transport allows these nutrients to be absorbed even when they are present in higher concentrations inside the mucosal cells than in the lumen. More specific information about the absorption of the products of carbohydrate, fat, and protein digestion will be discussed in Chapters 4, 5, and 6, respectively.

The small intestine has a huge surface area for absorbing nutrients

The structure of the small intestine is specialized to allow maximal absorption of the nutrients. In addition to its length, the small intestine has three other features that increase the area of its absorptive surface (Figure 3.11). First, the intestinal walls are arranged in circular or spiral folds, which increase the surface area in contact with nutrients. Second, its entire inner surface is covered with fingerlike projections called **villi** (singular, villus). And finally, each of these villi is covered with tiny **microvilli**, often referred to as the brush border. Together these features provide a surface area that is about the size of a tennis court (300 m^2 or 3229 ft^2). Each villus contains a blood vessel and a **lymph vessel** or **lacteal**, which are located only one cell layer away from the nutrients in the intestinal lumen. Nutrients must cross the mucosal cell layer to reach the bloodstream or lymphatic system for delivery to the tissues of the body.

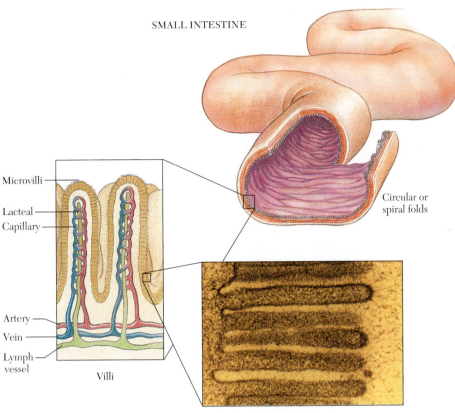

SMALL INTESTINE

Circular or spiral folds

Microvilli

Lacteal
Capillary

Artery

Vein

Lymph vessel

Villi

Microvilli

FIGURE 3.11

The small intestine contains folds, villi, and microvilli, which increase the absorptive surface area. (S. Ito and D. W. Fawcett/Visuals Unlimited)

The large intestine is the last chance for absorption

Materials that have not been absorbed in the small intestine enter the large intestine through a sphincter. This sphincter prevents material from the large intestine from reentering the small intestine. The large intestine is about 5 feet long and includes the **colon** and **rectum**. Although most absorption occurs in the small intestine, water and some vitamins and minerals are also absorbed in the colon. Peristalsis here is slower than in the small intestine. Water, nutrients, and fecal matter may spend 24 hours in the large intestine, in contrast to the 3 to 5 hours it takes material to move through the small intestine. This slow movement favors the growth of bacteria. These bacteria, called the **intestinal microflora**, are permanent beneficial residents of this part of the gastrointestinal tract. They break down unabsorbed portions of food, such as the fiber, producing nutrients that the bacteria themselves can use or, in some cases, that can be absorbed into the body. For example, the microflora synthesize small amounts of some B vitamins and vitamin K, some of which can be absorbed. As the microflora break down food, they produce gas, which causes flatulence. In normal adult humans, between 200 and 2000 ml of gas is produced per day.

Materials not absorbed in the colon are excreted as waste products in the feces. The feces are a mixture of undigested unabsorbed matter, dead cells, secretions from the GI tract, water, and bacteria. The amount of bacteria varies but can make up more than half the weight of the feces. The amount of water in the feces is affected by fiber and fluid intake. Fiber retains water, so when adequate fiber and fluid are consumed, feces have a high water content and are easily passed. When inadequate fiber or fluid is consumed, feces are hard and dry, and constipation can result.

The end of the colon is connected to the rectum, where feces are stored prior to defecation. The rectum is connected to the **anus**, the external opening of the digestive tract. The rectum and anus work with the colon to prepare the feces for elimination. Defecation is regulated by a sphincter that is under voluntary control. It allows the

Colon The largest portion of the large intestine.

Rectum The portion of the large intestine that connects the colon and anus.

Intestinal microflora Microorganisms that inhabit the large intestine.

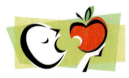

It is normal and healthy to have bacteria living in your colon. Although you're not aware of their presence, you miss them when they are gone. For example, taking antibiotics to kill harmful bacteria often also kills the beneficial bacteria in our gut, causing diarrhea.

Anus The outlet of the rectum through which feces are expelled.

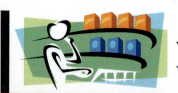

Your Choice: Should You Feed Your Flora?

Bacteria growing in your gut? Sounds bad, but the large intestine of a healthy adult is home to 300 to 500 different species of bacteria. In fact, the number of bacterial cells living in your gut is about 10 times greater than the total number of cells in your entire body.[1] The type and number of bacteria in your gastrointestinal tract are affected by both your diet and your health. In turn, the type and amount of bacteria in your GI tract can affect your health.

Most of the time these microflora provide beneficial effects. They break down non-digestible dietary substances; improve the digestion and absorption of essential nutrients; synthesize vitamins, some of which can be absorbed; and metabolize harmful substances, such as ammonia, thus reducing their concentration in the blood. They are important for intestinal immune function, proper growth and development of cells in the colon, and optimal intestinal motility and transit time.[2] A strong population of healthful bacteria can also inhibit the growth of harmful bacteria. If the wrong bacteria take over, they can cause diarrhea, infections, and perhaps an increased risk of cancer. Should we be supplementing our diet with beneficial bacteria or eating certain foods to promote the growth of these good bugs?

The recognition that intestinal bacteria are important to human health is not new. In the early 1900s, Nobel Prize–winning Russian scientist Eli Metchnikoff observed that Bulgarian peasants who consumed large quantities of yogurt and other fermented milk products lived long healthy lives. He proposed that the bacteria in these foods positively affected the microflora in the colon and "prevented intestinal putrification" and helped "maintain the forces of the body."[3] Modern research continues to support Metchnikoff's hypothesis that the bacteria in fermented dairy products, which include *Bifidobacterium* and *Lactobacillus*, provide health benefits.

Today, the consumption of products, such as yogurt, that naturally contain these bacteria and supplements containing live bacteria are referred to as probiotic therapy. Probiotics are living organisms which when consumed in adequate amounts confer a health benefit on the host. When consumed, some of these organisms survive passage through the upper GI tract and live temporarily in the colon before they are excreted in the feces. Some of the health benefits of probiotics are well documented. For example, they improve the digestion of the sugar lactose in lactose-intolerant people (see Chapter 4). They have been shown to prevent diarrhea associated with antibiotic use and to reduce the duration of diarrhea due to intestinal infections and other causes.[4,5] Probiotic bacteria have also been found to have beneficial effects on immune function in the intestine.[6] They have been shown to reduce the production of toxic substances in the colon and inhibit the activity of enzymes that produce carcinogens.[1] Although probiotics have not been clearly demonstrated to reduce the risk of colon cancer in humans, studies in animals have shown that they can prevent the formation and growth of cancerous cells in the colon.[7] There is also some evidence that probiotics may have other beneficial effects, including relief from constipation, reduction of allergic symptoms, and reduction of blood cholesterol levels.

One problem with probiotics is that when they are no longer consumed, the added bacteria are rapidly washed out of the colon. However, a healthy population of bacteria can be promoted by consuming substances that encourage the growth of particular types of bacteria. These substances, called prebiotics, pass undigested into the colon and stimulate the growth and/or activity of certain types of bacteria. Prebiotics are currently sold as dietary supplements and are added to commercially prepared tube feeding formulas to promote gastrointestinal health.

Our understanding of probiotics and prebiotics is expanding. We know that the risks of using these products are negligible, but their specific health benefits are still being investigated. Soon we may be able to take probiotics, instead of antibiotics, to eliminate hazardous bacteria in our intestines. And we may be paying attention to what we are feeding our flora—as well as ourselves.

References
1. Bengmark, S. Ecological control of the gastrointestinal tract: the role of probiotic flora. *Gut* 42:2–7, 1998.
2. Guarner, F., and Malagelada, J.R. Gut flora in health and disease. *Lancet* 361:512–519, 2003.
3. Metchnikoff, E. *The Prolongation of Life.* New York: GP Putnam's Sons, 1908.
4. D'Souza, L., Rajkumar, C., Cooke, J., and Bulpitt, C.J. Probiotics in prevention of antibiotic associated diarrhea: meta–analysis. *BMJ* 324:1361–1366, 2002.
5. Martineau, P.R., de Vrese, M., Cellier, C.J., and Schrezenmeir, J. Protection from gastrointestinal diseases with the use of probiotics. *Am. J. Clin. Nutr.* 73(suppl):430S–436S, 2001.
6. Isolauri, E., Sütas, Y., Kankaanpää, P., et al. Probiotics: effects on immunity. *Am. J. Clin. Nutr.* 73(suppl):444S–450S, 2001.
7. Brady, L. J., Gallaher, D.D., and Busta, F.F. The role of probiotic cultures in the prevention of colon cancer. *J. Nutr.* 130:410S–414S, 2000.

In food prepara
dings, and gravie
When a starch-thi
ating a gel. Many
fied food starch, v
stable gel.

Fiber canno

digestible carbohyc
in the small intesti
consumed in the d
all health.[2] Some
sources, this is call
meal is classified as
other sources and
this is called functi
oat bran added du
tional fiber. Total f
dietary fiber and fu

Fibers are cl
tract Fiber inclu

physical and physi
solutions in the int
the gastrointestinal
gested by bacteria
fatty acids, small q
found around and
ples, beans, and sea
luloses. Pectin is fc
when making jams
and stabilizers in p
from separating. T
in food processing
arabic, gum karaya
Agar, carrageenan,
ers and stabilizers (
to mimic the textu

Fibers that can
fecal matter. These
These fibers pass
crease the amount
from the structural
bran, rye bran, an
cellulose, some her
are considered fibe

Some starch

fined as fiber, there
tract. This **resistan**
is not digested bec
cooking and proce
starch more digest
resistant starch rea
starch helps prever
feces. Foods high i
potatoes, rice, and

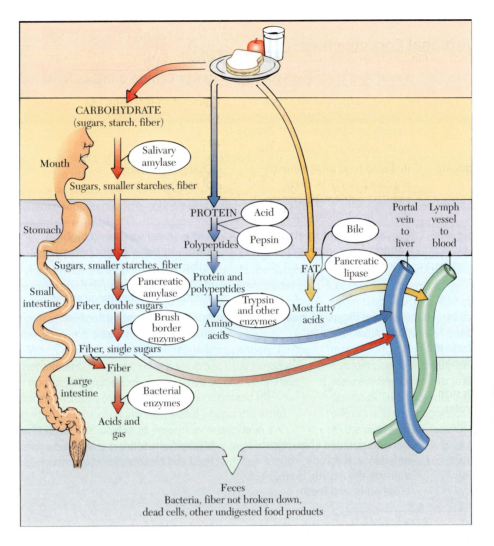

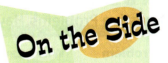

FIGURE 3.12

This overview of the digestion and absorption of a meal illustrates the digestion of carbohydrates into smaller starches and eventually single sugars, the breakdown of proteins into shorter amino acid chains called polypeptides and eventually into amino acids, and the digestion of fats into fatty acids, most of which must be absorbed into the lymph.

feces to be eliminated at convenient and appropriate times. The digestion and absorption of carbohydrate, fat, and protein are summarized in Figure 3.12.

Alterations in the GI Tract Can Affect Digestion and Absorption

Each of the organs and processes of the digestive system is necessary for the proper digestion of food and absorption of nutrients. Alterations in the GI tract due to illness or injury can affect your ability to obtain nutrients from food. Life stage, such as pregnancy, infancy, and old age, also affects the physiology of the digestive tract. Some digestive problems and their causes, consequences, and solutions are given in Table 3.2.

Digestive system problems and discomforts are common

Almost everyone experiences digestive discomforts from time to time, limiting the types of food that can be consumed. For example, dental problems can make it difficult to chew. When food is poorly chewed, contact between digestive enzymes and the nutrients in food is reduced, thereby limiting absorption.

FIGURE 4.7

Complex carbohydrates are made [...]
or branching chains of monosacch[...]

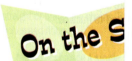

On the S[...]

Cassava, which is also calle[...]
manioc and yucca root, orig[...]
in South America. Today it is [...]
mostly in Africa, Indonesia, a[...]
Southeast Asia. You may thi[...]
have never had cassava, bu[...]
have ever had tapioca pud[c]
have. Tapioca is made from [...]
cassava root. Some varietie[s]
cassava contain high levels [...]
compound that can be conv[...]
into poisonous cyanide in th[...]
To prevent poisoning, the ca[...]
can be boiled or soaked be[...]
cooked or made into flour.

⚠ **Oligosaccharides** Short-ch[...]
carbohydrates containing 3 to 10[...]

⚠ **Polysaccharides** Carbohyc[...]
containing many sugar units link[...]

⚠ **Glycogen** A carbohydrate [...]
many glucose molecules linked [...]
highly branched structure. It is t[...]
form of carbohydrate in animals[...]

⚠ **Starch** A carbohydrate ma[...]
glucose molecules linked in stra[...]
branching chains. The bonds tha[...]
glucose molecules together can [...]
by human digestive enzymes.

PIECE IT TOGETHER

Losing Weight on a Low-Carbohydrate Diet

Josh is 5' 10" tall and weighs 200 pounds, about 25 pounds more than he would like to. At the recommendation of a friend he decides to try a low-carbohydrate weight-loss diet. The diet allows an unlimited amount of his favorite breakfast foods— bacon, eggs, and sausage. He can also have all the beef, chicken, fish, and cheese he wants but can't have fruit, bread, cereal, pasta, milk, and starchy vegetables. He can have limited amounts of low-carbohydrate vegetables such as lettuce, spinach, and tomatoes. The goal is to keep his intake of carbohydrates below 20 grams per day. Josh's typical day's intake while following the diet is given below.

> **Breakfast:** 3 scrambled eggs with 3 sausage links and coffee
>
> **Lunch:** 3 fried chicken thighs from KFC and water
>
> **Snack:** 2 hard boiled eggs
>
> **Dinner:** 8 ounces of barbecued steak, and a lettuce and tomato salad with oil and vinegar

Josh is overjoyed with his rapid weight loss. But after only a week he is feeling tired, has a headache, and is bored with his food choices. He misses having sandwiches for lunch and potatoes alongside his steak. He is tempted to have some toast with his breakfast.

WHAT WOULD JOSH NEED TO EAT TO EXCEED THE 20-GRAM CARBOHYDRATE LIMIT?

▼

To exceed the 20-gram carbohydrate limit, all Josh would need to eat is 2 slices of bread (30–40 grams), or a small potato (30 grams), 1/2 cup of spaghetti (20 grams), a banana (30 grams), 1/2 cup of baked beans (26 g), or 2 glasses of milk (24 grams).

HOW DOES THE AMOUNT OF CARBOHYDRATE IN THIS DIET COMPARE TO THE RDA?

▼

The RDA for carbohydrate is 130 grams per day. Consuming less than this may cause proteins to be used to synthesize glucose and will limit the amount of carbohydrate available to break down fat, leading to ketone formation. Although the ketones inhibit Josh's appetite, they may be the cause of his headaches.

HOW MANY CALORIES IS JOSH EATING WHILE FOLLOWING THIS DIET?

▼

Even though Josh can eat as much as he wants of allowed foods he is only consuming about 1700 Calories a day. Before starting the diet Josh was eating about 2800 Calories a day to maintain his weight.

JOSH HAS A FAMILY HISTORY OF HEART DISEASE. SHOULD HE BE CONCERNED ABOUT HIS FAT INTAKE?

▼

His diet now has about 114 grams of fat, which is 60% of his calories. This is well above the acceptable range for fat intake of 20 to 35%. He is also eating 33 grams of saturated fat, which is 17% of his calories. Diets high in saturated fat increase the risk of heart disease. The recommendation is 10% or less of calories from saturated fat. His diet includes over 1300 mg of cholesterol; the recommendation is 300 mg or less per day.

DO YOU THINK YOU JOSH SHOULD CONTINUE TO EAT THIS DIET AS A WAY TO MAINTAIN HIS WEIGHT LOSS?

▼

Your answer:

⚠ **Glucagon** A hormone made in the pancreas that stimulates the breakdown of liver glycogen and the synthesis of glucose to increase blood sugar.

Glucagon raises blood glucose

A few hours after eating, the glucose levels in the blood—and consequently glucose available to the cells—begins to decrease. This triggers the pancreas to secrete the hormone **glucagon** (see Figure 4.14). Glucagon signals liver cells to break down glycogen into glucose, which is released into the bloodstream bringing glucose levels back to normal. Glucagon also stimulates the synthesis of new glucose molecules from 3-carbon molecules, most of which come from the breakdown of amino acids from body proteins.

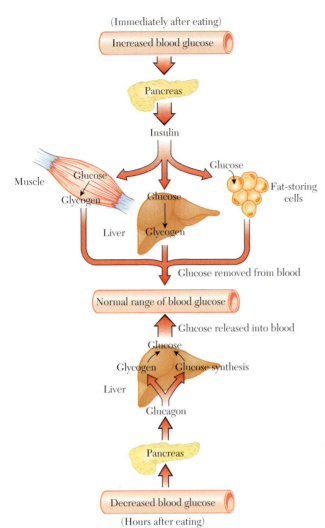

FIGURE 4.14

Blood glucose is regulated by hormones secreted by the pancreas. Immediately after a meal, when blood glucose increases, insulin is released and stimulates the uptake and storage of glucose. Several hours after a meal, when blood glucose levels begin to decrease, glucagon is released and stimulates the breakdown of glycogen into glucose and the synthesis of new glucose from 3-carbon molecules.

Diabetes Occurs When Glucose Levels Stay Too High

Diabetes mellitus is characterized by consistently high levels of blood glucose due to either a lack of insulin or an unresponsiveness of body cells to insulin (Figure 4.15). Over 18 million people in the United States have diabetes; more than 5 million of these do not know that they have the disease. The incidence is higher among minority groups, particularly African Americans, Hispanic Americans, and Native Americans.[7]

Diabetes is a serious disease. Uncontrolled diabetes damages the heart, blood vessels, kidneys, eyes, and nerves. It is the leading cause of blindness in adults and accounts for 40% of all new cases of kidney failure and over 60% of non-traumatic lower-limb amputations.[7] In the United States today diabetes is a major public health problem, accounting for about $132 billion in direct medical costs and indirect costs due to disability, lost work, and premature death. There are three types of diabetes: type 1, type 2, and gestational diabetes, which occurs during pregnancy.

For more information on diabetes go to the American Diabetes Association at **www.diabetes.org** and the National Diabetes Education Program at **www.ndep.nih.gov/**

Type 1 diabetes occurs when the body doesn't make insulin

Type 1 diabetes is an autoimmune disease in which the body's own immune system destroys the insulin-secreting cells of the pancreas. Therefore insulin is no longer made in the body. Type 1 diabetes is usually diagnosed before the age of 30. It accounts for only 5 to 10% of diagnosed cases of diabetes. It is not known what causes the immune

Type 1 diabetes A form of diabetes that is caused by the autoimmune destruction of insulin-producing cells in the pancreas, usually leading to absolute insulin deficiency; previously known as insulin-dependent diabetes mellitus or juvenile-onset diabetes.

FIGURE 4.15

Blood glucose levels are used to diagnose diabetes. After an 8-hour fast, normal blood glucose is less than 100 mg/100 ml. Prediabetes is defined as a fasting blood glucose between 100 and 125 mg/100 ml, and diabetes is defined as a fasting blood glucose of 126 mg/100 ml or above. Blood glucose measured 2 hours after consuming 75 g of glucose is normally less than 140 mg/100 ml. Prediabetes is defined as a blood glucose level between 140 and 199 mg/100 ml 2 hours after a glucose load and diabetes is defined as a blood glucose of 200 mg/100 ml or above 2 hours after a glucose load. (American Diabetes Association at www. diabetes.org/diabetescare/ supplement/98/s2.htm)

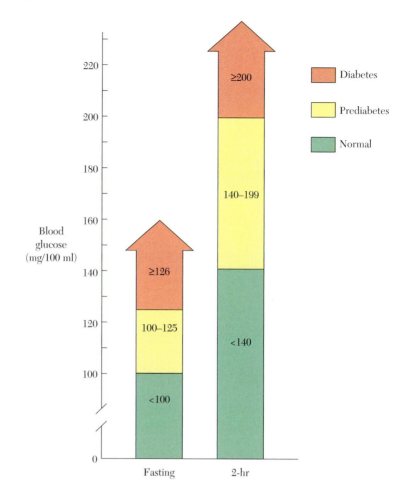

Type 2 diabetes A form of diabetes that is characterized by insulin resistance and relative (rather than absolute) insulin deficiency; previously known as noninsulin-dependent diabetes mellitus or adult-onset diabetes.

system to malfunction and attack its own cells but genetics, viral infections, exposure to toxins, and abnormalities in the immune system may play a role. In people with type 1 diabetes, levels of glucose in the blood remain high while many of the body's cells are starving for glucose because without insulin glucose cannot enter certain cells. Weight loss occurs with diabetes because glucose cannot enter cells so they are starved for energy. Fat is broken down for energy and ketones are produced. Some ketones are used as fuel, but when they are produced more rapidly than they can be used or excreted they cause a potentially fatal increase in the acidity of the blood called ketoacidosis.

Type 2 diabetes occurs when insulin doesn't function properly

Type 2 diabetes is the more common form of diabetes; it accounts for 90 to 95% of all cases. It is usually the result of a decrease in the sensitivity of cells to insulin; insulin is present, often in high levels, but the cells don't respond to it normally. As a result, only limited amounts of glucose can enter the cells and blood glucose levels rise. Type 2 diabetes is believed to be due to a combination of genetic and lifestyle factors. Risk is increased in individuals who are overweight, in those who have a body type with more fat in the abdominal region, and in those with a family history of diabetes. This form of diabetes usually appears in persons over the age of 40, but lifestyle and dietary factors in the United States such as inactivity and excess body weight have contributed to an increasing incidence among younger individuals. Type 2 diabetes often occurs as part of a combination of diseases called metabolic syndrome. This syndrome includes obesity, elevated blood pressure, high levels of blood lipids, and.insulin insensitivity; it is thought to be related to being overweight and physically inactive.

In addition, many people in the United States today have blood glucose levels that are higher than normal but not high enough for a diagnosis of diabetes. People with this condition, called pre-diabetes, have an increased risk of developing type 2 diabetes, as well as heart disease and stroke. Progression to diabetes among those with pre-diabetes is not inevitable. Studies suggest that weight loss and increased physical activity among people with pre-diabetes can prevent or delay diabetes and may return blood glucose levels to normal.

Gestational diabetes occurs during pregnancy

A third form of diabetes, called **gestational diabetes**, occurs in some women during pregnancy. The high levels of glucose in the mother's blood increase the risk of complications for the unborn child (see Chapter 12). Gestational diabetes is thought to be caused by the hormonal changes that occur during pregnancy. It usually disappears once the pregnancy is complete and hormones return to nonpregnant levels. However, individuals who have had gestational diabetes are at increased risk for developing type 2 diabetes later in life.[5]

Gestational diabetes A form of diabetes that occurs during pregnancy and resolves after the baby is born.

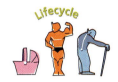

Diabetes has short-term symptoms and long-term complications

The symptoms of diabetes result from high glucose levels in the blood and the inability to use glucose normally. Cells that require insulin to take up glucose are starved for glucose, whereas cells that can use glucose without insulin are exposed to damaging high levels.

Early diabetes symptoms include thirst, frequent urination, and blurred vision
Many of the early symptoms of diabetes are a direct result of the effects of high blood glucose. Excessive thirst and frequent urination occur because as blood glucose levels rise the kidneys work to excrete the extra glucose and as a result also excrete extra fluid, increasing the volume of urine. Blurred vision occurs when excess glucose enters the lens of the eye, drawing in water and causing the lens to swell. Weight loss can also be an early symptom of diabetes as cells are unable to use glucose.

In the long term, diabetes damages organs and tissues throughout the body
Despite its few early symptoms, diabetes has serious long-term complications. These include damage to the heart, blood vessels, kidneys, eyes, and nerves. This damage is thought to be a result of prolonged exposure to high levels of blood glucose. When glucose is high it can bind to proteins and alter cell function, contributing to blood vessel damage and abnormalities in blood cell function. Damage to the large blood vessels leads to an increased risk of heart disease and stroke. Heart disease is a major complication and the leading cause of premature death among people with diabetes.[7] Changes in small blood vessels and nerves lead to kidney failure, blindness, and nerve dysfunction. For example, accumulation of glucose in the eye damages small vessels in the retina, leading to blindness (Figure 4.16). High

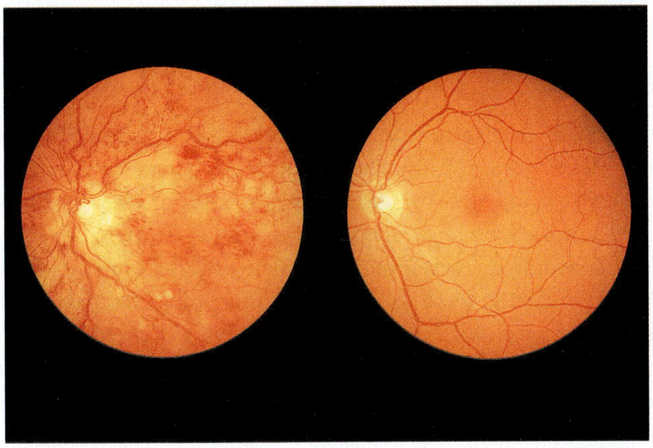

FIGURE 4.16

(left) Damaged blood vessels in the retina caused by diabetes. (right) Normal blood vessels in the retina of the eye. (© SBHA/Stone)

glucose levels cause kidney failure by damaging kidney cells and small blood vessels in the kidney. Exposure to high glucose also affects the function of peripheral nerves, often causing numbness and tingling in the feet. In addition to these problems, infections are more common in diabetes because high blood glucose levels favor microbial growth; these are usually the cause of amputations of the toes, feet, and legs.

Diabetes treatment involves diet, exercise, and medication

The goal in treating diabetes is to maintain blood glucose levels within the normal range so the damage caused by high levels is prevented. Pocket-size meters are available so that people with diabetes can easily measure their blood glucose levels to assure they are within the normal range. Maintaining blood glucose in the normal range requires a program of diet, exercise, and, in many cases, medication.

Dietary treatment involves modifying intake to control the amount of carbohydrate consumed at any given time to prevent large fluctuations in blood glucose levels.[8] Carbohydrate consumption must be coordinated with medication and exercise schedules so that glucose and insulin are available in the proper proportions at the same time to maintain normal blood glucose levels. The diet must be adequate in energy, protein, and micronutrients. To help delay the onset of heart disease, the diet should meet the recommendations of no more than 30% of energy from fat, with no more than 10% from saturated fat. Weight management is an important component of diabetes treatment because excess body fat increases the resistance of body cells to insulin. For overweight individuals, weight loss can help bring blood glucose levels into the normal range.[8]

Exercise is an important component of diabetes management because exercise increases the sensitivity of body cells to insulin. Because exercise can reduce blood glucose levels by making insulin more efficient, individuals with diabetes are encouraged to maintain regular exercise patterns. A change in the amount of exercise an individual participates in may change the amount of insulin required.

Drug treatments include insulin injections and oral medications to lower blood glucose (Figure 4.17). In type 1 diabetes, insulin is not made in the body so it must be provided. Insulin must be injected because it is a protein that would be broken down in the gastrointestinal tract if taken orally. In type 2 diabetes, if blood glucose cannot be normalized with diet and exercise, medications that increase insulin production, decrease glucose production by the liver, enhance insulin action, or slow carbohydrate digestion may be prescribed. In some cases of type 2 diabetes, injected insulin is needed to achieve normal blood glucose levels.

Adherence to this type of treatment regimen can keep blood glucose levels in the normal range and reduce the complications of diabetes. To promote diabetes education and reduce the disability and death associated with this disease, the National Institutes of Health and the Centers for Disease Control and Prevention have established the National Diabetes Education Program. This program is designed to increase public awareness of the seriousness of diabetes, promote better management among individuals with diabetes, and improve the quality of and access to health care.[9]

Hypoglycemia is low blood sugar

Hypoglycemia is low blood glucose that causes symptoms including irritability, nervousness, sweating, shakiness, anxiety, rapid heartbeat, headache, hunger, weakness, and sometimes seizures and coma. It can occur in diabetics as a result of over-medication or an imbalance between insulin level and carbohydrate intake. People with diabetes learn to recognize the symptoms of hypoglycemia and treat it by consuming a quickly absorbed source of carbohydrate, such as a glass of juice or a few pieces of hard candy. Following this with a meal within about 30 minutes will keep glucose from dropping again.

In individuals without diabetes, hypoglycemia can result from abnormalities in the production of or response to insulin or other hormones. There are two forms of hypo-

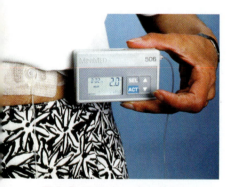

FIGURE 4.17

Insulin pumps, such as the one shown here, are no bigger than a deck of cards. They can be set to deliver the right amount of insulin to keep blood sugar normal. The insulin is pumped through a narrow, flexible plastic tube that ends with a needle inserted just under the skin. (© Russell D. Curtis/Photo Researchers)

⭐ **Hypoglycemia** A low blood glucose level, usually below 40 to 50 mg of glucose per 100 ml of blood.

glycemia. Reactive hypoglycemia occurs in response to the consumption of high-carbohydrate foods. The rise in blood glucose from the carbohydrate stimulates insulin release. However, too much insulin is secreted, resulting in a rapid fall in blood glucose to an abnormally low level. The treatment for reactive hypoglycemia is a diet that prevents rapid changes in blood glucose. Small, frequent meals low in simple carbohydrates and high in protein and fiber are recommended. A second form of hypoglycemia, fasting hypoglycemia, is not related to food intake. In this disorder, abnormal insulin secretion results in episodes of low blood glucose levels. This condition is often caused by pancreatic tumors.

The Type of Carbohydrate Determines its Health Effects

Are carbohydrates good for you or bad for you? The consumption of carbohydrates has been blamed for a host of chronic health problems, from obesity and diabetes to dental caries and hyperactivity. Meanwhile, guidelines for a healthy diet are recommending that Americans base their diet on carbohydrate-rich foods in order to reduce their disease risk. This incongruity relates to the health effects of different types of dietary carbohydrates: A dietary pattern that is high in whole sources of carbohydrates, such as whole grains, fruits, and vegetables, has been associated with a lower incidence of a variety of chronic diseases, whereas diets high in refined carbohydrates, such as added sugars and refined grains, may contribute to chronic disease risk.[10]

Carbohydrates increase the risk of dental caries

The most significant health problem associated with carbohydrate intake is **dental caries**, or tooth cavities. It is one of the most common childhood diseases in the United States: 85% of people 18 years of age and older have had caries.[11] Cavities are caused when bacteria that live in the mouth form colonies on the tooth surface known as plaque. If the plaque is not brushed, flossed, or scraped away the bacteria metabolize carbohydrate from the food we eat, producing acid. The acid can then dissolve the enamel and underlying structure of the teeth, forming cavities. Bacteria can metabolize both naturally occurring and added refined sugars and starches. Some types of food are more cavity causing than others. Simple carbohydrate, particularly sucrose, is the most rapidly used food source for bacteria and therefore easily produces tooth-damaging acids. But starchy foods that stick to the teeth can also promote tooth decay. Foods such as sticky candies, cereals, crackers, cookies, raisins, and other dried fruits tend to remain on the teeth longer, providing a continuous supply of nutrients to decay-causing bacteria. Other foods, such as chocolate, ice cream, and bananas, are rapidly washed away from the teeth and therefore are less likely to promote cavities. Limiting sugar intake can help prevent dental caries, but other dietary factors and proper dental hygiene are important even if the diet is low in sugar. Frequent snacking increases contact time by providing a continuous food supply for the bacteria. Sucking on hard candy or slowly sipping soda also increases exposure. Dairy products, sugarless gums (sweetened with sugar alcohols), and fluoride reduce caries formation. Brushing teeth after eating reduces cavity risk no matter what food was consumed (Figure 4.18).

Dental caries The decay and deterioration of teeth caused by acid produced when bacteria on the teeth metabolize carbohydrate.

Hyperactivity is due more to circumstances than to sugar intake

The consumption of sugary foods has been blamed for hyperactivity in children (see Chapter 13). The increase in blood glucose after a meal high in simple carbohydrates has been hypothesized to provide the energy for the excessive activity of a hyperactive child. However, research on sugar intake and behavior has failed to support this hypothesis.[12] Hyperactive behavior that is observed after sugar consumption is likely the

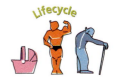
Lifecycle

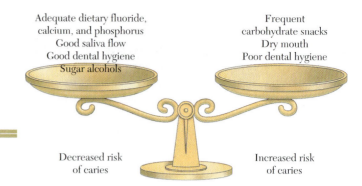

Adequate dietary fluoride,
calcium, and phosphorus
Good saliva flow
Good dental hygiene
Sugar alcohols

Frequent
carbohydrate snacks
Dry mouth
Poor dental hygiene

Decreased risk
of caries

Increased risk
of caries

FIGURE 4.18

Your risk of tooth decay is a balance between factors that protect your teeth from damage and reduce bacterial growth and those that promote bacterial acid production.

result of other circumstances. For example, the excitement of a birthday party rather than the sugar in the birthday cake is more likely the cause of hyperactive behavior. Hyperactivity might also be caused by lack of sleep, over-stimulation, caffeine consumption, the desire for more attention, or lack of physical activity.

Carbohydrate alone does not cause weight gain

For more information on low-carbohydrate diets go to the Weight control network at www.niddk.nih.gov/health/nutrit/win.htm

Cut carbs and lose weight, right? Low-carbohdrate diets are a current weight-loss craze. The rationale behind the use of a low-carbohydrate diet for weight loss is that foods high in carbohydrate stimulate the release of insulin, which is a hormone that promotes energy storage. It is suggested that the more insulin you make, the more fat you will store. High glycemic index foods, which increase blood sugar and then stimulate insulin release, are therefore hypothesized to shift metabolism toward fat storage. In contrast, a low-carbohydrate diet causes less of a rise in insulin and therefore is suggested to promote fat loss. Recent studies on the effectiveness of low-carbohydrate diets for weight loss show that these diets do promote weight loss.[13] Some of the reason for this is that when carbohydrate intake is low ketones are produced—these help suppress appetite, so the dieter eats less. In general people who are consuming low-carbohydrate diets are also consuming low-energy diets. The weight loss on these diets, as with other weight-loss diets, is caused by consuming less energy than the body expends, rather than the metabolic effects of insulin.

The popularity of low-carbohydrate diets makes people think that carbohydrates are fattening. In fact, carbohydrates provide 4 Calories per gram; less than half the 9 Calories per gram provided by fat. However, this is not to say that if carbohydrates are consumed in excess, they won't add pounds. Anytime energy is consumed in excess of requirements regardless of the source of the excess, weight will increase. But carbohydrate is no more fattening than fat or protein. In fact, excess carbohydrate in the diet is less efficient at producing body fat than excess fat in the diet (see Chapter 7). Unrefined carbohydrates might even help reduce energy intake because the fiber in these foods adds bulk to the gastrointestinal tract and is digested and absorbed more slowly causing you to feel full longer and after consuming less.

Carbohydrates are not fattening. They add fewer calories to the diet per gram than fat. A high-carbohydrate diet will cause weight gain if you are eating more calories than you are using, but so will a high-protein diet. So, when you reach for that low-carb bar, check out how many calories it is adding to your day.

There is evidence that in some people an abnormal craving for carbohydrate-rich foods contributes to their weight problems. Carbohydrate craving is a component of a variety of disorders including obesity, premenstrual syndrome, bulimia, depression, and seasonal affective disorder.[14,15] One theory proposed to explain carbohydrate craving is that these individuals have an abnormality in the regulation of brain levels of the neurotransmitter serotonin. This abnormality causes them to seek carbohydrate like a drug to increase serotonin levels, which improves their mood.

Fiber is good for your heart, but sugar is not

Some carbohydrates help protect you from heart disease, but others may increase your risk. There is evidence that a diet high in sugar can raise blood lipid levels and thereby increase the risk of heart disease.[1,16] On the other hand, diets high in whole grains and fiber have been found to reduce the risk of heart disease.[17,18] Fiber-rich foods provide

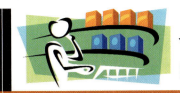

Your Choice: Low-Carbohydrate Bread?

Man cannot live by bread alone—especially if he is on a low-carb diet. But what about low-carbohydrate bread? The food industry has responded to the increasing popularity of low-carbohydrate diets by providing a host of low-carbohydrate products ranging from low-carbohydrate bread to low-carbohydrate beer and chips. Are these products really low in carbohydrate? Should you be eating them?

How much carbohydrate is in a slice of low-carb bread? The answer depends on who made the bread. The FDA has not defined the term "low carbohydrate," so at the moment the definition is up to the manufacturer. Some of these products are only slightly lower in carbohydrate than regular bread, whereas others have taken a significant bite out of the total carbohydrate. A small slice of regular bread has about 15 grams of carbohydrate; low-carb bread has anywhere from 3 to 10 grams per slice depending on how it is made and how it is sliced. Often, the low-carb bread is sliced very thinly.

To make a low-carb product, the carbohydrate in the original recipe has to be replaced with something. Low-carbohydrate bread is often prepared by replacing some of the wheat flour with soy protein. The resulting bread is lower in carbohydrate and higher in protein and has about 60 Calories a slice—the same amount as a regular slice of

bread. Low-carbohydrate chips also contain more protein and less carbohydrate than the traditional fare but again about the same number of calories. Low-carb beer is made by a process similar to that of light beer—the carbohydrates are broken down by enzymes in the brewing process; the resulting beer contains fewer calories, less carbohydrate, and more water than regular beer.

Should you be choosing low-carb products? Many people swear that a low-carbohydrate diet is the only way they can lose weight. For them, the craving for some starch may be satisfied by a low-carb slice. If having this option helps them achieve a healthy weight, it is a good thing. But, low carb does not mean low calorie. The plethora of low-carbohydrate products flooding the market is reminiscent of the low-fat products that dominated the shelves in the 1990s. Like the low-fat cookies and low-fat ice cream that we gobbled up a decade ago, low-carbohydrate products cannot be consumed in unlimited amounts without weight gain. The headlines affirm that the low-fat fad didn't trim the American waistline—we are fatter than ever. So, if you are going to choose low-carb products, do so as part of a healthy diet that meets your nutrient needs without exceeding your calorie needs.

---

micronutrients and phytochemicals—some of which may be protective against heart disease. A high-fiber diet may also reduce blood cholesterol levels. One of the reasons for this is that fiber binds cholesterol and **bile acids**, which are made from cholesterol, in the digestive tract. Normally, bile acids secreted into the GI tract are absorbed and reused. When bound to fiber, they are excreted in the feces rather than being absorbed. The liver must then use cholesterol from the blood to synthesize new bile acids. This provides a mechanism for eliminating cholesterol from the body and reducing blood cholesterol levels (Figure 4.19). Soluble fibers from legumes, oats, guar gum, pectin, flax seed, and psyllium (a grain used in bulk-forming laxatives such as Metamucil) are effective at reducing cholesterol, but insoluble fibers such as wheat bran and cellulose are not.[19] Soluble fiber may also reduce blood cholesterol by inhibiting cholesterol synthesis in the liver or by increasing the removal of cholesterol from the blood.[1,20]

A diet high in refined carbohydrates may increase diabetes risk

Bingeing on sugary snacks doesn't give you diabetes, but if you do it too often, it might increase your risk. There is some evidence that populations that eat a diet high in refined starches and added sugars may have an increased risk of developing type 2 diabetes.[21] These foods have a high glycemic index, meaning that blood sugar rises rapidly after eating them. In response to this rise in blood sugar, more insulin is produced. It is hypothesized that over the long term, the high demand for insulin eventually wears out the insulin-producing cells in the pancreas. Diets lower in simple carbohydrates and refined starches cause a more gradual rise in blood sugar and therefore a lower insulin demand.

⭐ **Bile acids** Emulsifiers present in bile that are synthesized by the liver from cholesterol.

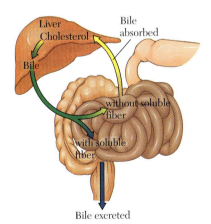

FIGURE 4.19

When the diet is low in soluble fiber, bile, which contains cholesterol and bile acids made from cholesterol, is absorbed and returned to the liver. When soluble fiber is present, it binds cholesterol and bile acids so they are excreted rather than absorbed.

TABLE 4.1
How Much Carbohydrate Do You Eat?

If you want to know the number of calories from carbohydrate in a food or a diet:
- Determine the number of grams of carbohydrate
- Multiply the grams of carbohydrate by 4 Calories per gram
  For example: A diet that contains 130 grams of carbohydrate

  130 grams $\times$ 4 Calories per gram = 520 Cal from carbohydrate

If you want to know the percent of calories from carbohydrate in this food or diet:
- Determine the total calories
- Divide calories from carbohydrate by total calories and multiply by 100 to express as a percent
  For example: A diet contains 2000 total Cal and 520 Cal of carbohydrate

  520 Cal $\div$ 2000 Cal = .26 $\times$ 100 = 26% carbohydrate

ketosis. This amount of carbohydrate provides only 520 Calories; that's 26% of the energy in a 2000-Calorie diet (Table 4.1). It is the equivalent of a breakfast of a cup of juice, two slices of toast with jelly, and a bowl of cereal with half a banana and milk; or a snack of a 20-ounce bottle of soda and a candy bar (Figure 4.21). Most people consume well in excess of this amount over the course of a day. In fact, a diet that includes only this much carbohydrate and meets calorie needs would be very high in protein and fat.

On the Side

What do advertising claims such as "only 5 grams net carbs" mean? What's a net carb? There is no official definition of net carbs but usually these are calculated by subtracting the grams of fiber and sometimes other carbohydrates from the grams of total carbohydrates in a food.

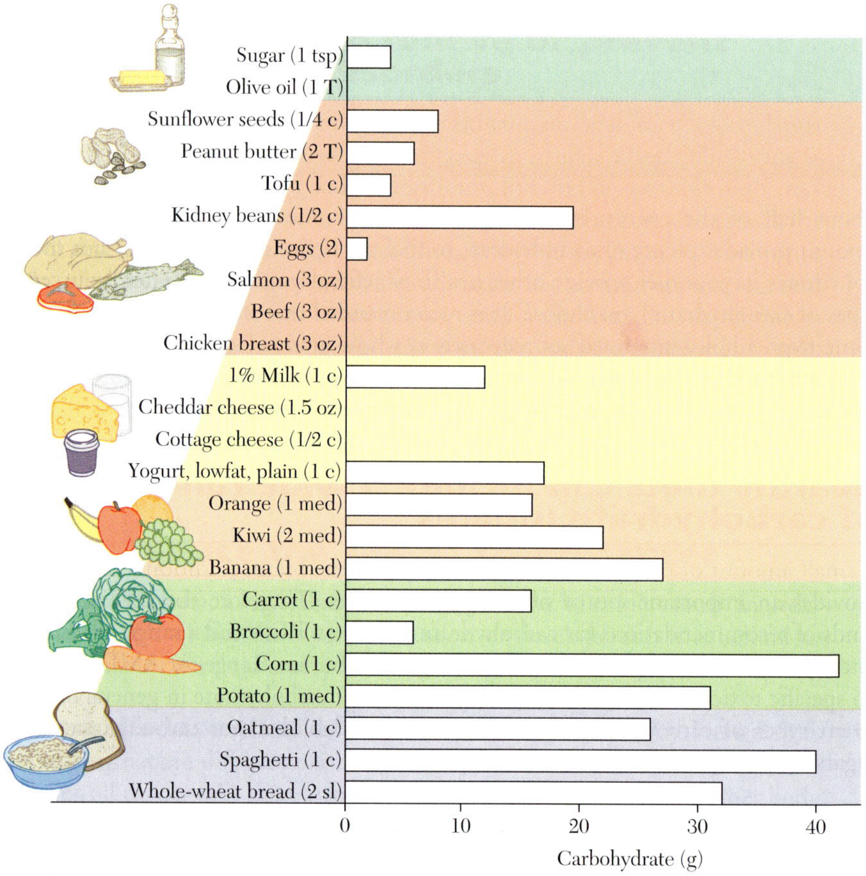

FIGURE 4.21

Carbohydrate content from selections from each group of the Food Guide Pyramid. The Bread, Cereal, Rice, & Pasta Group; the Vegetable Group; and legumes from the Meat, Poultry, Fish, Eggs, Dry Beans, & Nuts Group are the best sources of high-fiber, unrefined carbohydrates. The Fruit Group and the Milk, Yogurt, and Cheese Group contain good sources of unrefined sugars.

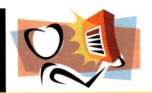

Off the Label: Finding Fiber

Consumers often choose brown breads and colored pasta in an effort to increase the fiber in their diet. The color of a product, however, often reveals little about the fiber content. Better places to look are the list of ingredients and the Nutrition Facts section of the food label.

On the ingredient list of breads, cereals, pastas, crackers, and other grain products, the term "whole" before the name of the grain indicates that the bran layer is still present in the food. Wheat flour, used to describe refined white flour made from wheat, is often confused with whole wheat flour. Only when whole wheat flour is the first ingredient, as it is in the label shown here from whole wheat bread, is the product made with mostly wheat flour containing the bran layer. The first ingredient on the "wheat bread" label shown in the figure is enriched wheat flour, rather than whole wheat flour. For products containing oats, the term "rolled" indicates that the whole oat grain has been used. Don't be fooled by the term "multigrain." It means the product contains more than one kind of grain, but the grains aren't necessarily whole grains, so check the ingredients. Fiber added to processed foods can also be identified from the list of ingredients. Insoluble fibers, such as the wheat bran added to the wheat bread shown here, are usually added to decrease the energy content of a product or to meet consumer demands for a high-fiber product. The soluble fiber oat bran is also added for these reasons, but most added soluble fibers, such as pectins and gums, are used to thicken and stabilize foods and rarely contribute a significant amount of fiber.

The Nutrition Facts section of a food label provides information about how much dietary fiber is in a product and how it fits into the recommendations for an overall diet. It lists the total amount of dietary fiber contained in a serving of the product; the amounts of soluble and insoluble fiber are not mandatory, but some manufacturers choose to include them. The percent Daily Value, based on the Daily Value for fiber of 25 grams for a 2000-Calorie diet, is also listed. For example, the whole wheat bread shown here contains 2 grams of fiber per slice, which is 8% of the Daily Value of 25 grams. Foods that contain 20% or more of the Daily Value for fiber per serving can state on the label that they are "high in dietary fiber." Products containing 10 to 19% of the Daily Value can state that they are "a good source of dietary fiber" (see Table 4.4).

Food labels may also carry health claims related to fiber and chronic disease risk. Grain products, fruits, and vegetables that contain at least 2.5 grams of fiber per serving and are low in fat may claim to reduce the risk of cancer. Fruits, vegetables, and grain products that are low in total fat, saturated fat, and cholesterol and that contain at least 0.6 gram of soluble fiber per serving, and foods that contain at least 0.75 gram of soluble fiber per serving from whole oats or psyllium husks, may claim to reduce the risk of heart disease.

Although whole grain breads are usually brown in color, the dark color may also be due to ingredients such as molasses that contribute no fiber. The green, orange, and red colors of some pasta products are due to the addition of such vegetable extracts as spinach, carrot, or tomato. These vegetables may add some nutrients but the amount of fiber they contribute is insignificant. So, when looking for fiber, look beyond the color of the products you choose, and read the label.

Whole Wheat Bread

Nutrition Facts
Serving Size 1 Slice (27g)
Servings Per Container 17
Calories 70
 Calories from Fat 10

Amount/Serving	%DV*	Amount/Serving	%DV*
Total Fat 1g	**2%**	**Total Carb.** 12g	**4%**
Sat. Fat 0g	**0%**	Dietary Fiber 2g	**8%**
Cholesterol 0mg	**0%**	Sugars 2g	
Sodium 10mg	**0%**	**Protein** 2g	

Vitamin A 0% • Vitamin C 0% • Calcium 4% • Iron 4%
Thiamin 4% • Riboflavin 2% • Niacin 4%

*Percent Daily Values (DV) are based on a 2,000 calorie diet. Your daily values may be higher or lower depending on your calorie needs:

	Calories:	2,000	2,500
Total Fat	Less than	65g	80g
Sat Fat	Less than	20g	25g
Cholesterol	Less than	300mg	300mg
Sodium	Less than	2,400mg	2,400mg
Total Carbohydrate		300g	375g
Dietary Fiber		25g	30g

NOT A SODIUM FREE FOOD

INGREDIENTS: WHOLE WHEAT FLOUR, WATER, SWEETENERS (HIGH FRUCTOSE CORN SYRUP, MOLASSES), WHEAT GLUTEN, SOYBEAN OIL, CONTAINS 2% OR LESS OF THE FOLLOWING: YEAST, DOUGH CONDITIONERS (MONO & DIGLYCERIDES, ETHOXYLATED MONO & DI-GLYCERIDES, CALCIUM STEAROYL-2-LACTYLATE), YEAST NUTRIENTS (CALCIUM SULFATE, MONO- CALCIUM PHOSPHATE), CALCIUM PROPIONATE (A PRESERVATIVE).

Wheat Bread

Nutrition Facts
Serving Size 1 Slice (28g)
Servings Per Container 20
Calories 80
 Calories from Fat 15

Amount/Serving	%DV*	Amount/Serving	%DV*
Total Fat 1g	**2%**	**Total Carb.** 13g	**4%**
Sat. Fat 0g	**0%**	Dietary Fiber 1g	**4%**
Cholesterol 0mg	**0%**	Sugars 2g	
Sodium 190mg	**8%**	**Protein** 2g	

Vitamin A 0% • Vitamin C 0% • Calcium 4% • Iron 4%
Thiamin 4% • Riboflavin 4% • Niacin 4%

*Percent Daily Values (DV) are based on a 2,000 calorie diet. Your daily values may be higher or lower depending on your calorie needs:

	Calories:	2,000	2,500
Total Fat	Less than	65g	80g
Sat Fat	Less than	20g	25g
Cholesterol	Less than	300mg	300mg
Sodium	Less than	2,400mg	2,400mg
Total Carbohydrate		300g	375g
Dietary Fiber		25g	30g

INGREDIENTS: ENRICHED WHEAT FLOUR, (WHEAT FLOUR, BARLEY MALT, NIACIN, IRON, THIAMIN MONONITRATE, RIBOFLAVIN), WATER, WHOLE WHEAT FLOUR, SWEETENERS, (HIGH FRUCTOSE CORN SYRUP, MOLASSES, HONEY), WHEAT BRAN, YEAST, SOYBEAN OIL, CONTAINS 2% OR LESS OF THE FOLLOWING: SALT, DOUGH CONDITIONERS (MONOGLYCERIDES, SODIUM STEAROYL LACTYLATE), YEAST NUTRIENTS (AMMONIUM SULFATE, CALCIUM SULFATE), CALCIUM PROPIONATE (A PRESERVATIVE).

carbohydrate is 60% of the energy. For a 2000-Calorie diet, this represents 300 grams of carbohydrate ([2000 Cal x 0.6] ÷ 4 Cal/g of carbohydrate = 300 g). The Daily Value for fiber is 25 grams in a 2000-Calorie diet. No Daily Value has been established for sugars, but labels can help identify products that are high in sugars. The number of grams of sugars is listed in the Nutrition Facts, but no distinction is made between added and naturally occurring sugars. For example, the fructose found naturally in unsweetened frozen strawberries, and that added as high-fructose corn syrup in soft drinks, are both listed as sugars. In a food such as canned peaches in heavy syrup the sugar found naturally in the peaches and that added to sweeten the syrup are given together as one number so it is impossible to tell how much sugar has been added.

The ingredients list on food labels tells us the sources of carbohydrates The list of ingredients on a food label can provide information about the sources of carbohydrate in a food. For example, whole wheat bread lists whole wheat as the first ingredient whereas white bread lists wheat flour (see Off the Label: Finding Fiber). This list is also a source of information about sweeteners added to foods. Because ingredients are listed by prominence in terms of weight, a food with sweeteners early in the ingredient list contains a large proportion of added sweeteners. The only sweetener that can be called "sugar" is sucrose but sucrose may represent only one of many added sweeteners. Consumers need to increase their carbohydrate vocabulary to recognize all the sweeteners on the label (Off the Label: The Scoop on Sugars). Recognizing these sweeteners in the ingredient list will not tell you the number of grams of added sugar in your cereal or yogurt, but it will tell you if sugar has been added. Nutrient claims on food labels can also help you choose foods low in added sugars. The claim "no added sugar" or "without added sugar" on the label indicates that no sugars or foods composed mainly of sugars, such as fruit juices or apple sauce, have been added in processing (Table 4.4).

On the Side

If you go to Europe on vacation you will find that it is easier to tell how much sugar has been added to a food. This is because the labels in European countries not only list ingredients in order of prominence but also give the percent of each essential ingredient in the product. For example a label might tell you that your cereal is 15% sugar and 4% molasses by weight.

TABLE 4.4
Finding Low Sugar and High Fiber Foods[1]

What It Says	What It Means
Sugar free	Product contains no amount, or a trivial amount, of sugars (less than 0.5 gram per serving). Synonyms for "free" include "without," "no," and "zero."
Reduced sugar	Nutritionally altered product contains 25% less sugar than the regular or reference product.
Less sugar	Whether altered or not, a food contains 25% less sugar than the reference food. "Fewer" may be used as a synonym for "less."
No added sugars or without added sugars	No sugar or sugar-containing ingredient is added during processing.
High fiber	Food contains 20% or more of the Daily Value for fiber per serving. Synonyms for "high" include "rich in" and "excellent source of."
Good source of fiber	Food contains 10 to 19% of the Daily Value for fiber per serving. Synonyms for "good source of" include "contains" and "provides."
More fiber	Food contains 10% or more of the Daily Value for fiber per serving than an appropriate reference food. Synonyms for "more" include "added" (or "fortified" and "enriched"), "extra," or "plus."

[1]If a food is not low in total fat, the label must state total fat in conjunction with any fiber claim such as "More Fiber."

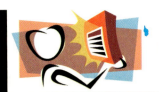

Off the Label: The Scoop on Sugar

Americans consume about 158 pounds of sweeteners per person per year.[1] This is more than is recommended. There are some easy ways to cut down on sugar—use less sugar in your coffee, sprinkle less on your cereal, drink fewer sweetened soft drinks, eat less candy. But finding and eliminating less obvious sources of added refined sugar in the diet isn't always easy. Knowing how to find sweeteners on food labels can help to sort out your sugar sources.

The sweeteners added to foods can be found in the ingredient list on food labels; they are listed in order of their prevalence by weight. Common sweeteners include sucrose, fructose, high-fructose corn syrup, honey, and molasses. Of these only sucrose, which is table sugar, can be listed as sugar. This could be brown sugar, powdered sugar, granulated sugar, or raw sugar. Fructose can be found in the ingredient list as fructose or as high-fructose corn syrup. It is sweeter and less expensive than sucrose and therefore has become the most commonly used added sweetener.[2] High-fructose corn syrup is produced by modifying starch extracted from corn to produce a syrup that is approximately half glucose and half fructose. It is used in snack foods, desserts, and sweetened beverages such as soft drinks. Because fructose does not cause as great a rise in blood glucose, it is sometimes used as an alternative to sucrose in products for people with diabetes. However, because fructose causes an increase in blood lipids, its use should be limited. Fructose consumed in fruits or juices can also cause diarrhea in children.

Less-refined sugars such as honey and blackstrap molasses are also added to sweeten food. These have been promoted as healthy alternatives to sucrose because they contain some nutrients that have been processed out of pure white table sugar. Although these sweeteners do have more micronutrients than table sugar, the amounts in most are too small to add much to the diet. Honey is derived from the nectar of flowering plants. Bees collect the nectar and convert some of the sucrose into fructose and glucose. The color, flavor, and proportions of the sugars in honey vary with the source of the nectar. Honey is somewhat sweeter than sucrose, so smaller amounts may be used for the same level of sweetness. Blackstrap molasses is a by-product of the refining of sucrose from sugar cane or sugar beets. It is a thick brown syrup that remains after the sucrose has crystallized. Refining of blackstrap molasses produces light and medium molasses. Unlike any other concentrated nutritive sweetener, molasses does contain significant amounts of some minerals; a tablespoon has over 100 mg of calcium and 2.4 mg of iron, both of which are often deficient in the American diet.

Other sweeteners such as brown sugar, maple syrup, and fruit juices are also sometimes thought of as healthier than sucrose. In fact, most are not significantly different from sucrose. Most brown sugar is simply refined white sugar containing some molasses to color it brown. Maple syrup is formed by boiling down the sap of maple trees. It is composed primarily of sucrose, which has been browned by the heat involved in processing. Fruit juices used as sweeteners may add small amounts of micronutrients but contribute primarily the sugar fructose to the product.

So, to cut down on added sugars use labels to find out which foods have sweeteners added to them. You might be surprised at how many products contain added sweeteners.

References
1. Coulston, A. M., and Johnson, R. K. Sugar and sugars: Myths and realities. *J. Am. Diet. Assoc.* 102:351–353, 2002.
2. American Diabetes Association. American Diabetes Association Position Statement: Evidence-based nutrition principles and recommendations for the treatment and prevention of diabetes and related complications. *J. Am. Diet. Assoc.* 102:109–118, 2002.

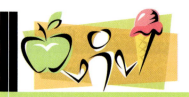

So, What Should I Eat?

Choose more unrefined carbohydrates
- Pass on the white bread and have your sandwich on a whole grain bread like whole wheat, oat bran, rye, or pumpernickel
- Have your stir fry over brown rice or try some new rice varieties
- Fill your cereal bowl with oatmeal
- Substitute whole grain flour for one-fourth to one-half of the white flour called for in recipes
- Satisfy your sweet tooth with a fresh fruit salad

Increase your fiber even more
- Put extra crunch in your salad by sprinkling on some almonds or sunflower seeds
- Add an extra vegetable at dinner—if you eat none have one, if you eat one have two
- Don't forget the beans—kidney beans, chick peas, black beans, and others have more fiber and resistant starch than any other veggies
- Eat eggplant for dinner
- Add berries and bananas to your cereal
- Add oats to cookies or other desserts
- Pop some corn
- Add some pearl barley or wild or brown rice to your favorite soup, stew, or casserole

Limit added sugars
- Next time you go to grab a soft drink choose a 12 ounce can instead of a 20 ounce bottle, or better yet, have a glass of milk
- Use one quarter less sugar in your recipe next time you bake
- Grab grapes instead of a candy bar
- Switch to an unsweetened breakfast cereal
- Snack on prunes and other dried fruits

On the next level of the Pyramid, the Milk, Yogurt, & Cheese Group provides unrefined simple carbohydrate in the form of lactose. Limit choices such as ice cream that are high in added sugars. Many of the choices in the Meat, Poultry, Fish, Dry Beans, Eggs, & Nuts Group contain no carbohydrate. Choosing dry beans from this group will provide a good source of unrefined complex carbohydrates and fiber that is also rich in protein.

The tip of the Pyramid also concerns carbohydrates. The carbohydrates in the tip are refined sweeteners, such as table sugar, honey, and syrup, and foods such as soda, jam, and candy that are almost pure refined sugar. These should be used sparingly. The relative amounts of these added sugars in each of the food groups are indicated in the Food Guide Pyramid by an upside-down triangle symbol (∇). The food groups that contain a higher proportion of foods with added sugar have more of these symbols. The tip of the Pyramid has the highest concentration of these symbols; the grain group, which includes sweetened bakery products like cakes and cookies, has a moderate concentration of symbols; and the Vegetable Group, which includes almost no foods with added sugar, has no symbols (see Figure 2.3).

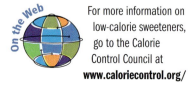

For more information on low-calorie sweeteners, go to the Calorie Control Council at **www.caloriecontrol.org/**

Alternative sweeteners can reduce the amount of sugar added to foods

America's love of sweets and the bad press surrounding sugar have promoted the development of an increasing number of alternative and non-nutritive sweeteners (Figure 4.23). These sugar substitutes, which provide little or no energy, are added to a host of sugar-free, low-calorie, and "light" foods such as yogurts, ice creams, and soft drinks. Although many sugar substitutes are technically not carbohydrates, they were developed to replace simple sugars in food products or as an alternative for table sugar at home. Alternative sweeteners are generally safe for healthy people;[27] however, to assure that they are not misused, the FDA has defined acceptable daily intakes (ADIs)—levels that should not be exceeded when using these products. The ADI is an estimate of the amount per kilogram of body weight that an individual can safely consume every day over a lifetime without risk.

Sugar substitutes are not the key to a healthy diet The average American eats about 20 teaspoons of added sweeteners per day.[28] Replacing some foods high in added sugars with sugar-free ones will cut down on calories and decrease sugar intake, but because foods that are high in added sugar tend to be nutrient-poor choices, replacing them with artificially sweetened alternatives does not necessarily make a diet healthy. If, however, sugar substitutes and foods containing them are used in moderation as part of a diet that is based on whole grains, vegetables, and fruits, these products can be part of a healthy diet.

Alternative sweeteners have been shown to reduce the incidence of dental caries and can be helpful for managing blood sugar levels in diabetes, but their usefulness for weight loss is debatable. If individuals trying to lose weight replace sugar and high-sugar foods with artificially sweetened products, they will reduce their energy intake. When used as part of a weight control program, alternative sweeteners may facilitate weight loss and long-term weight maintenance.[29] However, despite the variety of alternative sweeteners available, obesity has continued to increase in the American population. Clearly, these sugar substitutes are not the solution to the obesity epidemic.

There are a number of sugar substitutes to choose from
The main competitors in the artificial sweetener market in the United States today are saccharine, aspartame, acesulfame K (acesulfame potassium), and sucralose. Stevia is a sugar substitute that is sold as a dietary supplement. Though it is used extensively in Japan, it cannot be sold as a sweetener in the United States because the FDA considers it an unapproved food additive. Cyclamate, an artificial sweetener that was popular in the 1960s, was banned by the FDA in 1969. It is still sold in Canada and some 50 other countries. Sugar alcohols are also used as sweeteners.

Saccharine was once almost banned, but is now considered safe In 1977, after large doses of saccharine were found to increase the incidence of bladder cancer in rats, the FDA proposed banning saccharine. However, the public and industry protested. In response to the outcry, a moratorium was imposed on the banning of saccharine, and all products containing saccharine were required to display a warning on the label informing the public that it may cause cancer. In May 2000, saccharine was dropped from the government's list of cancer-causing substances so products containing saccharine no longer need to carry a warning. Saccharine intakes in the United States are estimated to be about 50 mg per person per day.[27] The ADI is 5 mg per kg of body weight or 350 mg for a 154 pound (70 kg) person. A 12-ounce diet beverage sweetened with saccharine can contain no more than 144 mg of saccharine and a packet of sweetener can contain no more than 20 mg. A 154 pound-person would have to consume 3 12-ounce saccharine-sweetened sodas or 18 packets of sweetener, such as Sweet'n Low, to exceed the ADI.

Aspartame is made from two amino acids In 1965, James Schlatter, at the pharmaceutical company G. D. Searle, was working with a chemical made up of two amino acids when he spilled some of the chemical on his fingers. Shortly afterward, he licked his finger to pick up a piece of paper and discovered an intensely sweet taste. This accidental discovery led to the development of the artificial

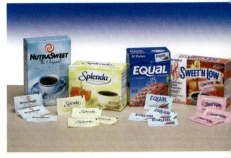

FIGURE 4.23

There are a variety of sugar substitutes on the market. Consumers often recognize their favorite by the color of the packaging. (© Andy Washnik)

sweetener aspartame. Since aspartame is made of two amino acids, the building blocks of protein, it is not a carbohydrate. It is about 200 times sweeter than sucrose. Because aspartame breaks down when heated, it works best in products that are not cooked, such as chewing gum, breakfast cereals, fruit spreads, yogurt, and beverages.

As with other alternative sweeteners, safety concerns have been raised about aspartame. It contains the amino acid phenylalanine and, therefore, can be dangerous to individuals with a genetic disorder called phenylketonuria (PKU). These individuals have an abnormality that affects the metabolism of phenylalanine. They must restrict their intake of this amino acid to prevent brain damage (see Chapter 6). There is also a concern that consuming aspartame might cause dangerously high blood phenylalanine levels in the general public. Phenylalanine occurs naturally in protein. A 4-ounce hamburger has 12 times more phenylalanine than a 12-ounce aspartame-sweetened soft drink. However, when phenylalanine is ingested without the other amino acids found in high-protein foods, blood and brain levels increase to a greater extent. There have been reports of headaches, dizziness, seizures, nausea, allergic reactions, and other side effects following ingestion of aspartame; however, double-blind placebo-controlled studies have not been able to reproduce these symptoms.[27] There has also been concern that the use of aspartame might be associated with an increased risk of brain cancer in children, but controlled studies found no evidence that aspartame is a carcinogen or that there was a correlation between aspartame use and brain cancer incidence.[30]

Overall, the consensus of the scientific community is that aspartame is safe for most people. The ADI is 50 mg per kg of body weight. To exceed this a 154-pound person would have to consume 95 packets of sweetener, such as Equal or NutraSweet, or 16 12-ounce sodas in a day.

Acesulfame K can be used in baked goods

Acesulfame K is a sweetener that is 200 times sweeter then sucrose. The K stands for potassium. It was approved for use in 1988 and is found in chewing gum, powdered drink mixes, gelatins, puddings, soft drinks, baked goods, and nondairy creamers. Sold under the brand names Sweet One and Sunett, it is heat stable, so it can be used in baking. Estimated intakes of this sweetener are well below the ADI of 15 mg per kg of body weight.

Sucralose is a derivative of sucrose

Sucralose (trichlorogalactosucrose) was discovered in 1976 and is the only noncaloric sweetener made from sugar. To make it, sucrose molecules are modified so they cannot be digested and pass through the digestive tract unchanged. It was approved for use in the United States in 1998. It is sold as Splenda and can be used as a tabletop sweetener that is added directly to foods. Since it is heat stable, it can be used in baked goods.[27] It is used in beverages, chewing gum, frozen desserts, puddings, jams and jellies, syrups, and many other products. It has been extensively tested for safety and found to be safe even for children and pregnant and lactating women.[31]

Sugar alcohols do not promote tooth decay

Because sugar alcohols are not digested, absorbed, or metabolized to the same extent as monosaccharides and disaccharides, they generally provide less energy than sucrose. Sugar alcohols can be used in products labeled "sugar free." Sugar-free products such as chewing gums, candies, ice creams, and baked goods sweetened with sugar alcohols may carry the health claim statement that they do not promote tooth decay. They are less likely to promote tooth decay because the bacteria in the mouth cannot metabolize sugar alcohols as rapidly as sucrose. Consumption of large amounts of sugar alcohols can cause diarrhea.

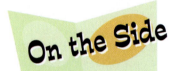

On the Side

Neotame is a new sugar substitute that is 8000 times sweeter than sucrose. Like aspartame it is made from the amino acids aspartic acid and phenylalanine, but the bond between the amino acids is harder to break than the bond in aspartame so it is more stable. Since it can't be broken down into phenylalanine it is not a problem for people with phenylketonuria. Although approved by the FDA it is too new to have appeared in many foods.

THINKING FOR YOURSELF

1. How much carbohydrate do you eat?
   a. Use the three-day diet record you kept in Chapter 2 to calculate your average carbohydrate and energy intake.
   b. What is the percent of energy from carbohydrate in your diet?
   c. How does your percent carbohydrate compare with the recommended 45 to 65% of energy from carbohydrate?

2. Are most of your carbohydrate choices from whole, minimally refined, or refined sources?
   a. Suggest some changes that would increase your intake of less refined carbohydrates.
   b. List some foods in your diet that are high in added refined sugars.

   c. Suggest some changes that would reduce the amount of added sugar in your diet.

3. How much fiber is in your diet?
   a. Calculate the grams of fiber in your original diet using the companion booklet, *Nutrition Composition of Foods*, a computer software program, or the exchanges in Table 4.3.
   b. Does it meet the AI for fiber for someone of your age and gender?
   c. How do the changes you suggested in question 2 affect the fiber content of your diet? If your modified diet still does not meet fiber recommendations, how might you further increase your intake?

SUMMARY

1. High-carbohydrate foods are the basis of the diet for most of the world. Unrefined foods, such as whole grains, fruits, and vegetables provide good sources of fiber and micronutrients. When these foods are refined, nutrients and fiber are lost. Added refined sugars contain few other nutrients, so foods high in added sugar are low in nutrient density.

2. Carbohydrates are chemical compounds that contain carbon, hydrogen, and oxygen. In food, they include sugar, starch, and fiber. Simple carbohydrates include monosaccharides and disaccharides and are found in foods such as table sugar, honey, milk, and fruit. Complex carbohydrates are oligosaccharides and polysaccharides. Polysaccharides include glycogen in animals and starch and fiber in plants. Sources of starch and fiber in the diet include whole grains, legumes, vegetables, and fruits.

3. Fiber cannot be digested by enzymes in the human stomach or small intestine and therefore is not absorbed into the body. Fiber benefits gastrointestinal function by increasing the amount of water and bulk in the intestine, which increases the ease and rate at which material moves through the gastrointestinal tract.

4. In the body, carbohydrate, primarily as glucose, provides a source of energy. Several tissues, including the brain and red blood cells, require glucose as an energy source. Glucose is metabolized through glycolysis, which breaks glucose molecules (6 carbons) into two 3-carbon pyruvate molecules, producing ATP. The complete breakdown of glucose through aerobic metabolism to form carbon dioxide and water produces a great deal more ATP.

5. The bloodstream delivers glucose to body cells. Blood glucose levels are maintained by the hormones insulin and glucagon. When blood glucose rises, insulin is released from the pancreas to allow body cells to take up the glucose. When blood glucose falls, glucagon is released. It increases blood glucose by causing the breakdown of glycogen and the synthesis of new glucose molecules.

6. Diabetes is characterized by high blood glucose. It damages tissues and causes complications including heart disease, kidney failure, blindness, and infections leading to amputations. This occurs either because insufficient insulin is produced or because there is a decrease in the sensitivity of body cells to insulin. Treatment to maintain glucose in the normal range includes diet, exercise, and medication.

7. Hypoglycemia is a condition in which blood glucose falls to abnormally low levels, causing symptoms such as sweating, headaches, and rapid heartbeat.

8. Diets high in carbohydrate, particularly added sugars, increase the risk of dental caries. Diets high in complex carbohydrates from whole grains, vegetables, fruits, and legumes may reduce the risk of chronic bowel disorders, colon cancer, diabetes, and heart disease.

9. Guidelines for healthy diets recommend 45 to 65% of energy from carbohydrates. Most choices should be whole grains, legumes, fruits, and vegetables. Foods high in added refined sugars should be consumed in moderation.

10. Alternative sweeteners or sugar substitutes are used to replace energy-containing sweeteners. They do not contribute to tooth decay.

REVIEW QUESTIONS

1. Why are foods high in added refined sugar said to contain empty calories?
2. How does the nutrient content of whole wheat bread compare to that of white bread?
3. What is a simple carbohydrate?
4. What is a complex carbohydrate?
5. What happens to carbohydrates that cannot be digested?
6. What is the main function of glucose in the body?
7. Why do we say that fiber does not provide energy?
8. Why is carbohydrate said to spare protein?
9. Why is it important to keep blood sugar levels in the normal range?
10. What is diabetes?
11. What is the difference between type 1 and type 2 diabetes?
12. What health benefits are associated with a diet high in unrefined carbohydrates?
13. How can you use the information on food labels to help you identify foods that are high in added sugars? In fiber?
14. How do the typical intakes of carbohydrates in the United States compare to recommendations?
15. What is wrong with consuming more than 25% of your calories from added sugar?
16. List the risks and benefits of alternative sweeteners?

REFERENCES

1. Institute of Medicine, Food and Nutrition Board. *Dietary Reference Intakes for Energy, Carbohydrates, Fiber, Fat, Protein and Amino Acids.* Washington, D.C.: National Academy Press, 2002.
2. American Dietetic Association. Position of the American Dietetic Association: Health implications of dietary fiber. *J. Am. Diet. Assoc.* 102:993–1000, 2003.
3. Lee, M. F., and Krasinski, S. D. Human adult-onset lactose decline: An update. *Nutr. Rev.* 56:1–8, 1998.
4. NIDDK Lactose Intolerance NIH Publication No. 98-2751, April 1994 e-text updated: November 1998. Available online at www.niddk.nih.gov/health/digest/pubs/lactose/lactose.htm/Accessed March 17, 2002.
5. USDA ARS Data Tables: Results from CSFII, 1996 ARS Food Surveys Research Group. Available online at www.barc.usda.bhnrc/foodsurveys/homt.htm/Accessed March 6, 2004.
6. Miller, D. L., Miller, P. F., and Dekker, J. J. Small bowel obstruction from bran cereal. *J.A.M.A.* 263:813–815, 1990.
7. National Diabetes Statistics. National Institute of Diabetes, and Digestive and Kidney Diseases. Available online at www.diabetes.niddk.nih.gov/ Accessed November 19, 2003.
8. American Diabetes Association. American Diabetes Association Position Statement: Evidence-based nutrition principles and recommendations for the treatment and prevention of diabetes and related complications. *J. Am. Diet. Assoc.* 102:109–118, 2002.
9. National Diabetes Education Program, Seven Steps to Controlling Diabetes. Available online at www.ndep.nih.gov/diabetes/control/principles.htm/Accessed November 19, 2003.
10. Willett, W. C. The dietary pyramid: Does the foundation need repair? *Am. J. Clin. Nutr.* 68:218–219, 1998.
11. U.S. Department of Health and Human Services. U.S. Public Health Service. Oral health in America: A report of the surgeon general. Rockville, MD: National Institutes of Health, 2000.
12. Wolraich, M. L., Wilson, D. B., and White, J. W. The effect of sugar on behavior or cognition in children: A meta analysis. *J.A.M.A.* 274:1617–1618, 1995.
13. Foster, G.D., Wyatt, H.R., Hill, J.O., et al., A randomized trial of a low-carbohydrate diet for obesity. *N. Engl. J. Med.* 348:2082–2090, 2003.
14. Wurtman, R. J., and Wurtman, J. J. Brain serotonin, carbohydrate craving, obesity and depression. *Obes. Res.* 4:477S–480S, 1995.
15. Kurzer, M. S. Women, food, and mood. *Nutr. Rev.* 55:268–276, 1997.
16. Fried, S. K., and Rao, S. P. Sugars, hypertriglyceridemia, and cardiovascular disease. *Am. J. Clin. Nutr.* 78:873S–880S, 2003.
17. Jacobs, D. R., Meyer, K. A., Kushi, L. H., and Folsom, A. R. Whole-grain intake may reduce the risk of ischemic heart disease death in postmenopausal women: The Iowa Women's Health Study. *Am. J. Clin. Nutr.* 68:248–257, 1998.
18. Kushi, L. H., Meyer, K. A., and Jacobs, D. R. Jr. Cereals, legumes, and chronic disease risk reduction: Evidence from epidemiologic studies. *Am. J. Clin. Nutr.* 70(Suppl):451S–458S, 1999.
19. Food and Nutrition Board, Institute of Medicine. A Report of the Panel on the Definition of Dietary Fiber and the Standing Committee on the Scientific Evaluation of Dietary Reference Intakes Food and Nutrition Board, *Proposed Definition of Dietary Fiber.* Washington, D.C.: National Academy Press, 2002.
20. Marlett, J. A. Sites and mechanisms for the hypocholesterolemic actions of soluble dietary fiber sources. In Kritevsky, D., and Bonfield, C., eds. *Fiber in Human Health and Disease.* New York: Plenum Press, 1997, 109–121.
21. Willett, W., Manson, J., and Liu, S. Glycemic index, glycemic load, and risk of type 2 diabetes. *Am. J. Clin. Nutr.* 76:274S–280S, 2002.
22. Peters, U., Sinha, R., Chatterjee, N., et. al. Dietary fibre and colorectal adenoma in a colorectal cancer early detection programme. *Lancet* 361:1491–1495, 2003.
23. Bingham, S. A., Day, N. E., Luben, R., et al. Dietary fibre in food and protection against colorectal cancer in the European Prospective Investigation into Cancer and Nutrition (EPIC): An observational study. *Lancet* 361:1496–1501, 2003.
24. Alberts, D. S., Martinez, M. E., Roe, D. J., et al. Lack of effect of a high-fiber cereal supplement on the occurrence of colorectal adenomias. *N. Engl. J. Med.* 342:1149–1155, 2000.
25. Schatzkin, A., Lanza, E., Corle, D., et al. Lack of effect of a low-fat, high-fiber diet on the recurrence of colorectal adenomias. *N. Engl. J. Med.* 342:1149–1155, 2000.
26. Krebs-Smith, S. M. Choose beverages and foods to moderate your intake of sugars: Measurement requires quantification. *J. Nutr.* 131:527S–535S, 2001.
27. American Dietetic Association. Position of the American Dietetic Association: Use of nutritive and non-nutritive sweeteners. *J. Am. Diet. Assoc.* 104:255–275, 2004.

28. Coulston, A. M., and Johnson, R. K. Sugar and sugars: Myths and realities. *J. Am. Diet. Assoc.* 102:351–353, 2002.

29. Blackburn, G. L., Kanders, B. S., Lavin, P. T., et al. The effect of aspartame as part of a multidisciplinary weight-control program on short- and long-term control of body weight. *Am. J. Clin. Nutr.* 65:409–418, 1997.

30. Gurney, J. G., Pogoda, J. M., Holly, E. A., et al. Aspartame consumption in relation to childhood brain tumor risk: Results from a case-control study. *J. Nat. Cancer Inst.* 89:1072–1074, 1997.

31. Calorie Control Council. Low calorie sweeteners: sucralose. Available online at www.caloriecontrol.org/sucralos.thml Accessed June 2, 2004.

Fats Add Flavor and Affect Your Health

⚠ **Lipids** A group of organic molecules, most of which do not dissolve in water.

It's the high fat content that gives ice cream its smooth texture and rich taste. In fact, **lipids**, or what we commonly call fats, contribute to the texture, flavor, and aroma of many of our foods. Olive oil imparts a unique flavor to salads and many traditional Italian and Greek dishes. Sesame oil gives egg rolls and other Chinese foods their distinctive aroma. The fats in our foods contribute to their appeal but also add to their caloric content and can affect our health.

Some fats are obvious and others are hidden

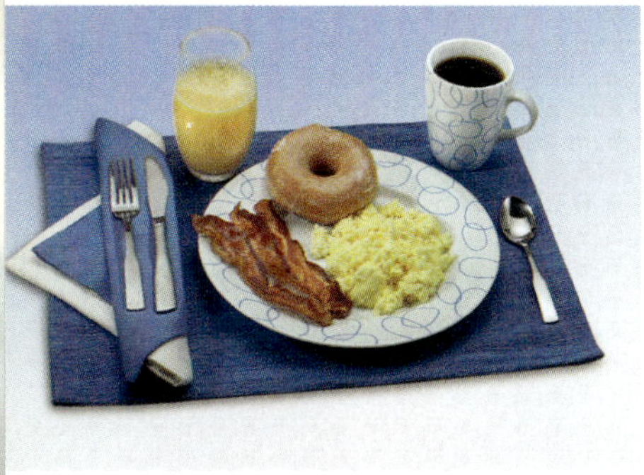

You can see the layer of fat around the outside of a steak and the stripes of fat in a slice of bacon sizzling on the stove. Other obvious sources of fat in our diets are the fats we add to foods at the table—the pat of butter melting on your hot baked potato, the cheese sauce you add to your broccoli, or the thick layer of cream cheese you spread on a bagel. We are also adding fat when we fry foods; french fries start as potatoes, which are low in fat, but when they are immersed in hot oil for frying they soak up fat. Other sources of fat in our diet are less obvious: dairy products, particularly cheese, ice cream, and whole milk, are high in fat. Crackers, doughnuts, cakes, cookies, pies, and muffins are also quite high in fat (Figure 5.1).

FIGURE 5.1

The fat in food is not always obvious. The three strips of bacon in this breakfast have 9 grams of fat, but the doughnut has 22 grams. (Andy Washnik)

Just cutting fat doesn't make your diet healthy

Fat has a bad reputation. Too much fat makes us fat, increases our risk of heart disease, and maybe even increases our chances of getting cancer. In response to messages that fat is bad, Americans responded by switching to low-fat milk, eating more chicken and fewer eggs, and gobbling up fat-free cookies, cakes, and ice cream. The food industry helped us by stocking the shelves with over 15,000 reduced-fat products. But we didn't get thinner, and heart disease and cancer are still major public health threats. Switching to fat-free cookies without paying attention to calories didn't promote weight loss. Limiting total fat without considering the type of fat and other components of the diet such as whole grains, fruits, and vegetables didn't reduce the incidence of obesity and other chronic diseases. A healthy diet requires eating the right kinds of fats and making healthy choices from all of the food groups.

Several Types of Lipids Are Important in Nutrition

⚠ **Triglycerides** The major form of lipid in food and in the body. These consist of three fatty acids attached to a glycerol molecule.

⚠ **Fatty acids** Organic molecules made up of a chain of carbons linked to hydrogens, with an acid group at one end.

⚠ **Phospholipids** Lipids composed of a glycerol molecule with two fatty acids and a phosphate group attached.

⚠ **Sterols** Lipids with a multiple ring structure.

What we usually think of as fat is a type of lipid called a **triglyceride**. Most of the fat in our food and in our bodies is triglycerides. Each triglyceride includes three **fatty acids**. Fatty acids are what we are really talking about when we say *trans* fat or saturated fat—they are really *trans* fatty acids and saturated fatty acids. **Phospholipids** and **sterols** are two other types of fat that are important in nutrition. The different structures of these lipids affect their function in the body and the properties they give to food.

Triglycerides are made of fatty acids

Triglycerides include a backbone of the 3-carbon molecule glycerol with three fatty acids attached (Figure 5.2). Each fatty acid is a chain of carbon atoms with an acid group at one end. The carbon chains of fatty acids vary in length from a few to 20 or more carbons. Most fatty acids in plants and animals, including humans, contain between 14 and 22 carbons.

Each carbon atom in the carbon chain of a fatty acid is attached to up to four other atoms. At one end of the carbon chain, there are three hydrogen atoms (CH_3) attached to the carbon; this is called the omega end of the fatty acid. At the other end of

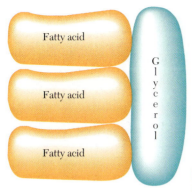

Triglyceride

FIGURE 5.2

A triglyceride is three fatty acids attached to a molecule of glycerol.

the chain, an acid group (COOH) is attached to the carbon. Each of the carbons in between is attached to the two carbons on either side and up to two hydrogens. If there is only one hydrogen attached to a carbon, a double bond forms between the two adjacent carbon atoms (Figure 5.3). The number and placement of double bonds affects the function of the fatty acid in food and in the body.

Saturated fatty acids are saturated with hydrogens
A **saturated fatty acid** is one in which all the carbons in the fatty acid chain are saturated with hydrogen atoms (see Figure 5.3). In other words, each carbon within the chain is bound to two other carbons and two hydrogens. Saturated fatty acids are more plentiful in animal foods such as meat and dairy products. Plant oils are generally low in saturated fatty acids. Exceptions include palm oil, palm kernel oil, and coconut oil, which are saturated plant oils. These are often called **tropical oils** because they are found in plants common in tropical climates. Because of their chemical structure, triglycerides that are high in saturated fatty acids are more solid at room temperature than triglycerides with unsaturated fatty acids of the same size.

Unsaturated fatty acids contain double bonds
An **unsaturated fatty acid** contains some carbons that are not saturated with hydrogens. The carbon chain therefore contains double bonds formed between carbons that are bound to only one hydrogen (see Figure 5.3). Unsaturated fats tend to be liquid oils at room

Saturated fatty acid A fatty acid in which the carbon atoms are bound to as many hydrogens as possible and therefore contains no carbon-carbon double bonds.

Tropical oils A term used in the media to refer to the saturated oils—coconut, palm, and palm kernel oil—that are derived from plants grown in the tropics.

Unsaturated fatty acid A fatty acid that contains one or more carbon-carbon double bonds.

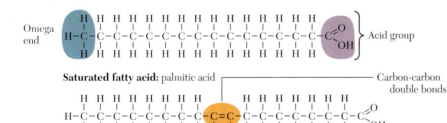

FIGURE 5.3

The structure of common saturated, monounsaturated, and polyunsaturated fatty acids.

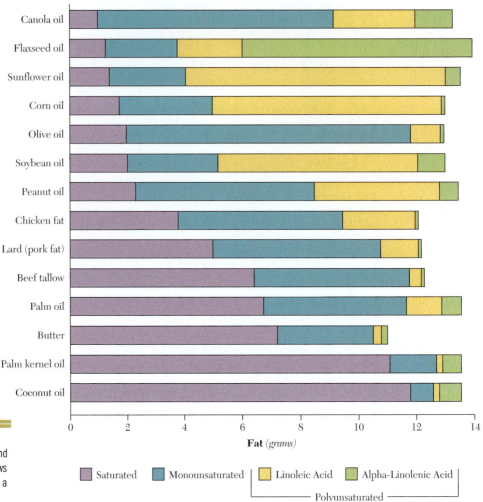

FIGURE 5.4

The fats and oils in foods contain varying amounts of saturated, monounsaturated, and polyunsaturated fatty acids. This graph shows the amounts of these types of fatty acids in a tablespoon of different types of fat.

⚠ **Monounsaturated fatty acid** A fatty acid that contains one carbon-carbon double bond.

⚠ **Polyunsaturated fatty acid** A fatty acid that contains two or more carbon-carbon double bonds.

⚠ **Omega-3 (ω-3) fatty acid** A fatty acid containing a carbon-carbon double bond between the third and fourth carbons from the omega end.

⚠ **Omega-6 (ω-6) fatty acid** A fatty acid containing a carbon-carbon double bond between the sixth and seventh carbons from the omega end.

temperature. A fatty acid containing one double bond in its carbon chain is called a **monounsaturated fatty acid**. In our diets, olive, canola, and peanut oils are high in monounsaturated fatty acids. A fatty acid with more than one double bond in its carbon chain is a **polyunsaturated fatty acid**. The most common polyunsaturated fatty acid is linoleic acid, found in corn, safflower, and soybean oils. The fats and oils in our diets contain combinations of saturated, monounsaturated, and polyunsaturated fatty acids (Figure 5.4).

The number and type of bonds in fatty acids determine their health effects
The way different fatty acids affect our health is determined by the number and location of the double bonds. A fatty acid with no double bonds is a saturated fatty acid. Diets high in saturated fats are associated with an increased risk of heart disease. A fatty acid with one double bond is a monounsaturated fatty acid; these tend to reduce heart disease risk. When a fatty acid contains many double bonds, the location of the double bonds affects its properties and function. When the first double bond occurs between the third and fourth carbons, counting from the omega end of the chain (see Figure 5.3), the fatty acid is said to be an **omega-3 (ω-3) fatty acid**. These fatty acids are found in flaxseed, soybean, and canola oils; nuts; and fatty fish, such as salmon, tuna, and trout. Diets high in these may reduce heart disease risk. If the first double bond occurs between the sixth and seventh carbons (from the omega end), the fatty acid is called an **omega-6 (ω-6) fatty acid**. They are found in nuts and corn, safflower, and sunflower oils.

The position of the hydrogen atoms around a double bond also affects the properties of unsaturated fatty acids. Most unsaturated fatty acids found in nature have both hydrogen atoms on the same side of the double bond, called the *cis* configuration

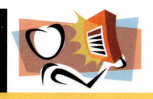

Off the Label: What Is Hydrogenated Fat?

Did you ever wonder what partially hydrogenated vegetable oil means on a food label? It's in the ingredients list, but what is it and where does it come from? Why is it in so many foods? Should you be concerned about it?

Hydrogenation is a process that bubbles hydrogen gas into liquid oil. The hydrogen atoms are accepted by some of the double bonds in the oil, making it more saturated and as a result more solid at room temperature. Hydrogenated or partially hydrogenated vegetable oils are a primary ingredient in margarine and vegetable shortening. In addition to making these products more solid, hydrogenation also makes the oils more stable and less likely to become rancid. Hydrogenated oils are therefore used in breakfast cereals and other processed foods such as cookies, crackers, and potato chips to protect against rancidity and thus preserve freshness and extend shelf life. For similar reasons, hydrogenated vegetable oil is often chosen for deep-fat frying. These oils keep longer than polyunsaturated fats and are cheaper to use than saturated fats.

Although good for food manufacturing, the use of hydrogenated vegetable oils has created some health concerns. During hydrogenation, only some of the bonds become saturated. Some of those that remain unsaturated are altered, converting them from the *cis* to the *trans* configuration. The resulting product therefore contains more *trans* fatty acids than the original oil. *Trans* fats raise

LDL cholesterol levels and increase the risk of heart disease. Because of the health risks associated with these, by January 2006 all Nutrition Facts labels will provide the number of grams of *trans* fat in a serving.

Trans fatty acids are found in small amounts in nature, but most of the *trans* fat we eat comes from hydrogenated fats (see Figure). So, limit your *trans* fats by keeping your eye on the label. When you see hydrogenated or partially hydrogenated vegetable oils in the ingredient list, you may want to consider choosing a different food.

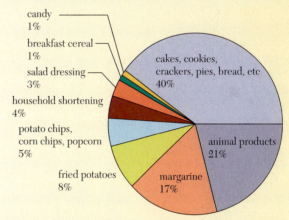

On average, adults in the United States consume 2.6% of their calories (5.8 grams) from *trans* fat. The major source is bakery products.

(Figure 5.5). When the hydrogens are on opposite sides of the double bond, called the *trans* configuration, the fatty acid is a **trans fatty acid**. Small amounts of *trans* fatty acids are present naturally in animal fats, but most of the *trans* fatty acids in our diets come from products that have undergone **hydrogenation** such as hard margarine and shortening. Diets high in *trans* fatty acids increase the risk of heart disease.[2]

The types of fatty acids in triglycerides determine their properties
Triglycerides may contain any combination of fatty acids: long, medium, or short chain, saturated or unsaturated. The types of fatty acids in triglycerides determine their texture, taste, and physical characteristics. For example, the amounts and types of fatty acids in the triglycerides in chocolate allow it to remain brittle at room temperature, snap when bitten into, and then melt quickly and smoothly in the mouth. The triglycerides in red meat contain predominantly long-chain, saturated fatty acids, so the fat on a piece of steak is solid at room temperature. The triglycerides in olive oil contain predominantly monounsaturated fatty acids, whereas those in corn oil are mostly polyunsaturated. These fats are liquid at room temperature. In our bodies, the triglycerides in adipose tissue provide a source of energy, help to cushion our internal organs, and insulate us from changes in temperature. The fatty acid composition of your adipose tissue varies, depending on the fatty acid composition of the triglycerides you consume in your diet.

Trans fatty acid An unsaturated fatty acid in which the hydrogens are on opposite sides of the carbon-carbon double bond.

Hydrogenation The process whereby hydrogens are added to the carbon-carbon double bonds of unsaturated fatty acids to increase their stability and shelf life.

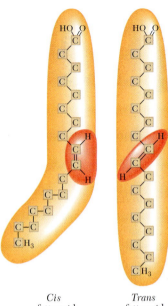

FIGURE 5.5

The orientation of hydrogens around the double bond distinguishes *cis* and *trans* fatty acids. In *cis* fatty acids, the hydrogens are on the same side of the double bond and cause a bend in the carbon chain. In *trans* fatty acids, the hydrogens are on opposite sides of the double bond and the carbon chain is straighter.

Cis fatty acid   *Trans* fatty acid

Ever wonder why the fat in beef stew forms solid clumps when you put the leftovers in the refrigerator, but the fat in your half and half stays liquid even in the refrigerator? Both contain saturated fats, but the fatty acids differ in chain length. The half and half contains more short-chain and medium-chain fatty acids, whereas beef fat has more long-chain fatty acids.

⚠ **Emulsifiers** Substances that allow water and fat to mix.

⚠ **Lecithin** A phospholipid that contains choline. It is found in eggs and is often added to foods as an emulsifier.

⚠ **Cholesterol** A lipid that consists of multiple chemical rings and is found only in animal foods.

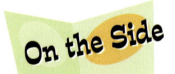

The drugs known as anabolic steroids are sterols. They are used by some athletes trying to increase muscle strength and muscle mass; however, their use is illegal and can cause liver damage and other devastating long-term health effects (see Chapter 11).

Phospholipids dissolve in both fat and water

Phospholipids are important in food and in the body because they allow water and fat to mix. It is the phospholipids in the egg yolks that allow the oil and water to mix in cake batter. Phospholipids can do this because one side of the molecule dissolves in water and the other side dissolves in fat. Like triglycerides, most phospholipids have a backbone of glycerol, but instead of three fatty acids, they contain only two. Instead of the third fatty acid, phospholipids have a chemical group containing phosphorus, called a phosphate group. The fatty acids in a phospholipid molecule are soluble in fat, but the phosphate is soluble in water. Because of this, phospholipids act as **emulsifiers**, a kind of chemical liaison that allows fat and water to mix.

In the body, cell membranes contain phospholipids that form a double layer called the lipid bilayer; this allows an aqueous (water) environment both inside and outside the cell with a lipid environment sandwiched between them. One of the best-known phospholipids is **lecithin**. In the body, lecithin is a major constituent of cell membranes. It is also used to synthesize the neurotransmitter acetylcholine, which is important in the memory center of the brain. Eggs and soybeans are natural sources of lecithin. Lecithin is also used by the food industry as an emulsifier in margarine, salad dressings, chocolate, frozen desserts, and baked goods to keep the oil from separating from the other ingredients.

Cholesterol is a sterol found only in animals

Sterols look very different from other lipids because they are made of interconnected rings of carbon atoms (Figure 5.6). **Cholesterol** is probably the best-known sterol. Cholesterol is needed in the body, but because it is manufactured by the liver, it is not essential in the diet. More than 90% of the cholesterol in the body is found in cell membranes. It is also part of myelin, the coating on many nerve cells. Cholesterol is the raw material for many other sterol molecules. It is needed to synthesize vitamin D in the skin; bile acids, which are emulsifiers in bile; some hormones, such as testosterone and estrogen, which promote growth and the development of sex characteristics; and cortisol, which promotes glucose synthesis in the liver.

In the diet, cholesterol is found only in foods from animal sources. Egg yolks and organ meats such as liver and kidney are high in cholesterol. One egg yolk contains about 212 mg of cholesterol. Organ meats contain about 300 mg per 3-ounce serving. Lean red meats and skinless chicken contain about 90 mg, whereas fish contains 50 mg in 3 ounces. Plant foods do not contain cholesterol unless it has been added in cooking

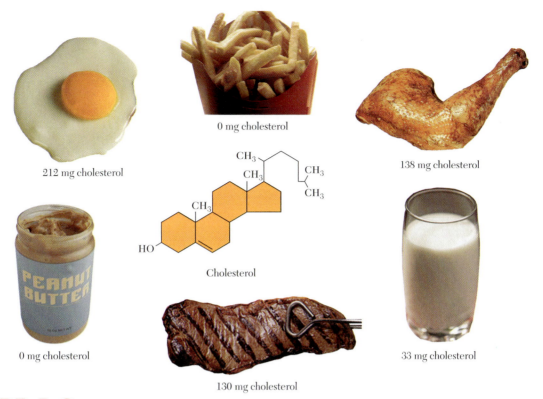

212 mg cholesterol

0 mg cholesterol

138 mg cholesterol

Cholesterol

0 mg cholesterol

130 mg cholesterol

33 mg cholesterol

FIGURE 5.6

Cholesterol is found only in animal foods. The ring structure is different from other lipids but common to all sterols. (*fries*: Corbis Images; *steak*: Jan Oswald/Foodpix/
PictureArts Corp.; *chicken*: Corbis Images; *milk*: Corbis Images; *peanut butter*: C Squared Studios/PhotoDisc, Inc./Getty Images; *egg*: Corbis Images)

or processing. Plants do contain other sterols. They have a role in plants similar to that
of cholesterol in animals; they help form plant cell membranes. When consumed in the
diet they help reduce cholesterol levels in the body.

Lipids Need Help to Move into and Through the Body

In a jar of salad dressing, the oil floats to the top. The fact that oil and water do not
mix poses a problem when transporting lipids throughout the body (Figure 5.7). Absorbing lipids from your intestines and transporting them in your blood requires special treatment in order to keep water and fat mixed together.

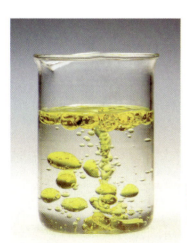

FIGURE 5.7

The oil droplets in this liquid are floating to the top. If this happened
to the fats in your bloodstream, it would be impossible for them to be
transported to your cells. (Charles D. Winters/Photo Researchers)

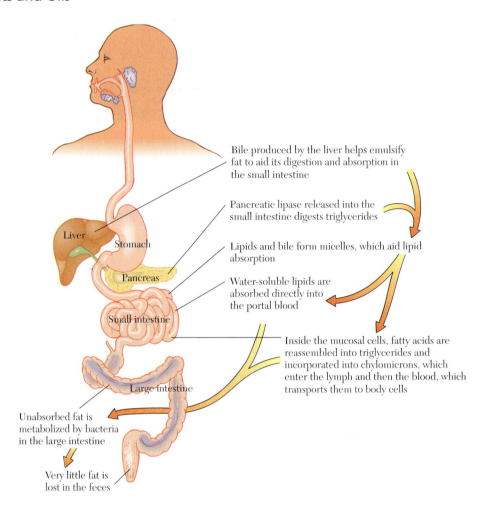

Bile produced by the liver helps emulsify fat to aid its digestion and absorption in the small intestine

Pancreatic lipase released into the small intestine digests triglycerides

Lipids and bile form micelles, which aid lipid absorption

Water-soluble lipids are absorbed directly into the portal blood

Inside the mucosal cells, fatty acids are reassembled into triglycerides and incorporated into chylomicrons, which enter the lymph and then the blood, which transports them to body cells

Liver

Stomach

Pancreas

Small intestine

Large intestine

Unabsorbed fat is metabolized by bacteria in the large intestine

Very little fat is lost in the feces

FIGURE 5.8

An overview of lipid digestion and absorption.

Bile is an emulsifier that helps digest and absorb fats

Fat must be digested to be absorbed. In healthy adults, most fat digestion occurs in the small intestine (Figure 5.8). Here, **bile** secreted by the gallbladder aids this process by breaking large fat drops into small globules, which can then be broken down by fat-digesting enzymes from the pancreas. The mixture of fatty acids, partially digested triglycerides, and bile forms smaller droplets called **micelles** (Figure 5.9), which facilitate absorption. Once absorbed, the triglycerides are reassembled and most of the bile acids are returned to the liver to be reused.

Bile A substance that aids in fat digestion and absorption. It is made in the liver and stored in the gallbladder.

Micelles Particles formed in the small intestine when droplets of lipid are surrounded by bile.

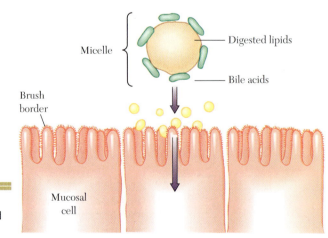

Micelle

Digested lipids

Bile acids

Brush border

Mucosal cell

FIGURE 5.9

Bile mixes with fats to form small droplets called micelles. When micelles come in contact with the microvilli that line the wall of the small intestine, the fatty acids and partially digested triglycerides diffuse into the mucosal cells.

These processes, necessary for fat digestion and absorption, are also necessary for the absorption of the fat-soluble vitamins (vitamins A, D, E, and K). These vitamins must be incorporated into micelles to be absorbed, and therefore absorption can be reduced if dietary fat is very low or if disease, medications, or other dietary components interfere with fat absorption.

Lipoproteins help transport lipids through the blood

Lipids that do not dissolve in water require special packaging to travel in the bloodstream. They are covered with a water-soluble envelope of phospholipid and protein to form particles called **lipoproteins**. Different types of lipoproteins transport dietary lipids from the small intestine and stored or newly synthesized lipids from the liver.

Chylomicrons carry lipids from the small intestine to body cells
After you eat, the lipids from the meal are absorbed into the intestinal mucosal cells. Shorter-chain fatty acids, which are soluble in water, are then absorbed into the blood and travel to the liver for further processing. Water-insoluble lipids, such as long-chain fatty acids, cholesterol, and fat-soluble vitamins, cannot enter the bloodstream directly. First, long-chain fatty acids are reassembled into triglycerides. These triglycerides, along with cholesterol, and fat-soluble vitamins are surrounded by a coat of phospholipids and a small amount of protein to form lipoproteins called **chylomicrons**. Chylomicrons are absorbed from the intestinal mucosa into the lymph and enter the bloodstream without first passing through the liver. They circulate in the blood, delivering triglycerides to body cells. Delivery is aided by an enzyme called **lipoprotein lipase**, present on the surface of the cells lining the blood vessels. Lipoprotein lipase breaks the triglycerides in chylomicrons into fatty acids and glycerol, which enter the surrounding cells. Once in the cells, fatty acids can be either broken down as fuel or reassembled into triglycerides for storage. What remains of the chylomicron is mostly cholesterol and protein and goes to the liver to be disassembled (Figure 5.10).

VLDLs transport lipids from the liver to body cells
Lipids are transported from the liver in **very-low-density lipoproteins (VLDLs)**. These lipoproteins contain proportionately less triglyceride than chylomicrons (Figure 5.11) but are similar to chylomicrons because both particles deliver triglycerides to body cells with the help of the enzyme lipoprotein lipase. As VLDLs circulate in the blood, lipoprotein lipase on the surface of blood vessels breaks down the triglycerides so that the fatty acids can be taken up by surrounding cells. Once the triglycerides are removed from the VLDLs, a denser, smaller particle remains. About two-thirds of these particles are returned to the liver, and the rest are transformed in the blood into **low-density lipoproteins (LDLs)**.

LDLs deliver cholesterol to cells
LDLs are the primary cholesterol delivery system for cells. They contain a higher proportion of cholesterol than chylomicrons or VLDLs (see Figure 5.11). High levels of LDLs in the blood have been associated with an increased risk for heart disease. For this reason they are sometimes referred to as "bad cholesterol." For LDLs to deliver cholesterol, a protein on the LDL particle must bind to a protein on the cell membrane called an **LDL receptor**. This binding allows the whole LDL particle to be removed from circulation and enter the cell, where the cholesterol and other components can be used (see Figure 5.10).

HDLs return cholesterol to the liver
Since most body cells have no system for breaking down cholesterol, it must be returned to the liver to be eliminated from the body. This reverse cholesterol transport is accomplished by the densest of the lipoprotein particles, called **high-density lipoproteins (HDLs)**. These particles circulate in the blood, picking up cholesterol from other lipoproteins and body cells. Some of the cholesterol in HDLs is taken directly to the liver for disposal, and some is transferred to organs that have a high requirement for cholesterol, such as those that synthesize steroid hormones. HDL cholesterol is often called "good cholesterol" because high levels of HDL in the blood are associated with a reduction in heart disease risk.

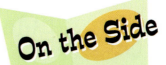
On the Side

People who have had their gallbladders removed can still digest fat because bile is only stored in the gallbladder. It is made in the liver. Without a gallbladder, bile is less concentrated and fat digestion may be less efficient.

Lipoproteins Particles containing a core of triglycerides and cholesterol surrounded by a shell of protein, phospholipid, and cholesterol that transport lipids in blood and lymph.

Chylomicrons Lipoproteins that transport lipids from the mucosal cells of the small intestine and deliver triglycerides to other body cells.

Lipoprotein lipase An enzyme attached to the outside of cells that line blood vessels. It breaks down triglycerides into fatty acids and glycerol that can enter cells.

Very-low-density lipoproteins (VLDLs) Lipoproteins assembled by the liver that carry lipid from the liver and deliver triglycerides to body cells.

Low-density lipoproteins (LDLs) Lipoproteins that transport cholesterol to cells. Elevated LDL cholesterol increases the risk of cardiovascular disease.

LDL receptor A protein on the surface of cells that binds to LDL particles and allows them to be taken up by the cell.

High-density lipoproteins (HDLs) Lipoproteins that pick up cholesterol from cells and transport it to the liver so that it can be eliminated from the body. High HDL levels reduce the risk of cardiovascular disease.

On the Side

The more fat you eat in a meal, the more chylomicrons appear in your blood. If you were to have a blood sample taken after eating a high-fat meal, your blood plasma would look white like milk because of the large number of chylomicrons floating around in it. After a few hours, the chylomicrons would clear from the blood and the plasma would be a clear yellowish color again.

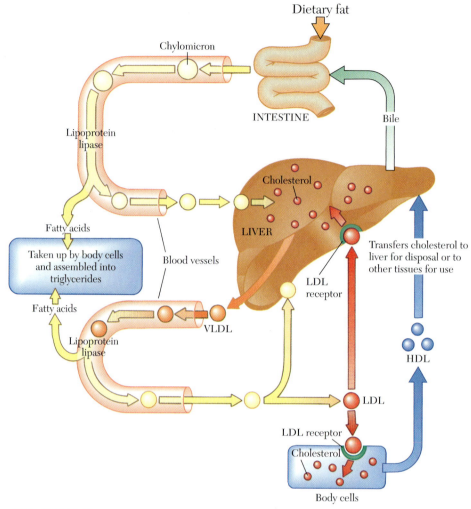

FIGURE 5.10

Chylomicrons carry lipids from the intestines and deliver triglycerides to body cells. VLDLs carry lipids from the liver and deliver triglycerides to body cells. LDLs are the primary cholesterol delivery system for body cells. HDLs carry cholesterol away from cells and return it to the liver.

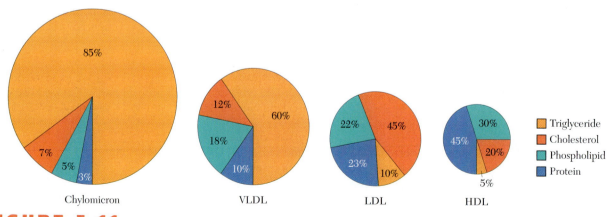

FIGURE 5.11

All lipoproteins consist of a shell of phospholipid, protein, and cholesterol and a center of triglycerides and cholesterol, but they vary in size and density. Particles with proportionately more triglyceride and less protein are larger and less dense. Chylomicrons are the largest, least-dense particles and contain the most triglyceride, whereas HDLs are the smallest, densest particles and have the greatest percentage of protein.

Lipids Provide Structure, Regulation, and Energy

We generally try to avoid too much fat—in our diets and in our bodies—but some fat is necessary to maintain health. Lipids provide structure and regulation and are a concentrated source of energy. Because each gram of fat provides 9 Calories, compared with only 4 Calories per gram from carbohydrate or protein, a large amount of energy can be stored in the body as fat without a great increase in size or weight. Even a lean man whose body fat is only about 10% of his weight stores over 50,000 Calories of energy as fat.

Lipids form structures and lubricate surfaces

Most lipids in the body are triglycerides stored in **adipose tissue**, which lies under the skin and around internal organs. The amount and location of our adipose tissue affects our body size and shape. In addition to providing stored energy, adipose tissue insulates the body from changes in temperature and provides a cushion to protect against shock. Lipids are also an important structural component of cells, particularly in the brain and nervous system. As components of all cell membranes, lipids protect the internal environment of cells. Lipids are also important for lubricating body surfaces. For example, the oils in your skin keep it soft and supple.

Lipids have important regulatory roles

Cholesterol and fatty acids are both used to synthesize regulatory molecules in the body. Cholesterol, either consumed in the diet or made in the liver, is used to make a number of hormones, including the sex hormones estrogen and testosterone and the stress hormone cortisol. Polyunsaturated fatty acids are also used to make hormone-like molecules that help regulate body functions.

Essential fatty acids must be consumed in the diet
The body is capable of synthesizing most of the fatty acids it needs from glucose or other sources of carbon, hydrogen, and oxygen. However, humans are not able to synthesize fatty acids that have double bonds in the omega-6 and omega-3 positions. Therefore, the fatty acids linoleic acid (omega-6) and α-linolenic acid (omega-3) are considered **essential fatty acids**; they must be consumed in the diet to make other omega-6 and omega-3 fatty acids.

Omega-6 fatty acids are important for growth, skin integrity, fertility, and maintaining red blood cell structure. Omega-3 fatty acids are important for the structure and function of cell membranes, particularly in the retina of the eye and the central nervous system. If the diet is low in linoleic acid or α-linolenic acid, other fatty acids synthesized from them become dietary essentials. For example, arachidonic acid is an omega-6 fatty acid found in both animal and vegetable fats. It is essential in the diet only when the diet is low in linoleic acid. Eicosapentaenoic acid (EPA) and docosahexaenoic acid (DHA) are omega-3 fatty acids synthesized from α-linolenic acid; in our diet they are found in fatty fish. Arachidonic acid and DHA are necessary for normal brain development in infants and young children.

If adequate amounts of linoleic and α-linolenic acid are not consumed, an **essential fatty acid deficiency** will result. Symptoms include scaly, dry skin, liver abnormalities, poor wound healing, impaired vision and hearing, and growth failure in infants. Essential fatty acid deficiency is rare because the requirement for essential fatty acids is well below the typical intake. However, deficiencies have occurred in infants and young children fed low-fat diets, in individuals who are unable to absorb lipids, and in adults consuming a weight-loss diet consisting of only skim milk.

You need a balance of both omega-6 and omega-3 fats
Both omega-6 and omega-3 fatty acids are used to make hormone-like molecules called **eicosanoids**. Eicosanoids help regulate blood clotting, blood pressure, immune function, and other body processes. The effect an eicosanoid has on these functions

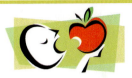

Carbohydrate, protein, and fat are all fattening if you eat more than you need, but gram for gram, fat provides the most calories. Cutting 20 grams of fat out of your diet will eliminate 180 Calories, but cutting out 20 grams of carbohydrate will reduce your intake by only 80 Calories.

Adipose tissue Tissue found under the skin and around body organs that is composed of fat-storing cells.

Essential fatty acids Fatty acids that must be consumed in the diet because they cannot be made by the body or cannot be made in sufficient quantities to meet needs.

Essential fatty acid deficiency A condition characterized by dry, scaly skin and poor growth that occurs when the diet does not supply sufficient amounts of the essential fatty acids.

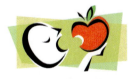

A diet with no fat at all will not support life. Some fatty acids are essential nutrients that must be supplied in the diet. In general a diet that provides at least 10% of calories from fat will provide sufficient essential fatty acids.

Eicosanoids Regulatory molecules that can be synthesized from omega-3 and omega-6 fatty acids.

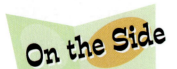

depends on the fatty acid from which it is made. For example, when the omega-6 fatty acid arachidonic acid is the starting material, the eicosanoid synthesized increases blood clotting; when the eicosanoid is made from the omega-3 fatty acid EPA, it decreases blood clotting. The ratio of dietary omega-6 to omega-3 essential fatty acids affects the balance of these fatty acids in the tissues and therefore the balance of the regulatory molecules made from omega-6 and omega-3 fats. In order to maintain a healthy balance in the body, a dietary ratio of linoleic to α-linolenic acid between 5:1 and 10:1 is recommended. To provide this ratio, a diet that contains 20 grams of linoleic acid would need to include 2 to 4 grams of α-linolenic acid. However, if the diet contains plenty of the fatty acids arachidonic acid, EPA, and DHA, which are made from linoleic and α-linolenic acid, the actual ratio of linoleic to α-linolenic is less of a concern.[2] The typical American diet contains plenty of omega-6 fatty acids, so to get a healthy mix of fatty acids, try to increase your intake of omega-3s by eating fish, flax seed, leafy green vegetables, and canola oils.[3]

Fat provides energy

Fat is an important source of energy in the body. Triglycerides consumed in the diet can either be used immediately to fuel the body or be stored in adipose tissue. Throughout the day, triglycerides are continuously stored and then broken down, depending on the immediate energy needs of the body. For example, after a meal some triglyceride will be stored; then, between meals some of the stored triglyceride will be broken down to provide energy. When the energy in the diet equals the body's energy requirements, the net amount of stored triglyceride in the body does not change.

Triglycerides can be used for fuel The triglycerides we eat in our meals are broken down to fatty acids and a small amount of glycerol. These can then be used to provide energy to fuel the body. This occurs by breaking the carbon chain of the fatty acids into two-carbon units, which can be further broken down to generate additional ATP (Figure 5.12). The glycerol molecules, which contain three carbons, can also be used to produce ATP or small amounts of glucose.

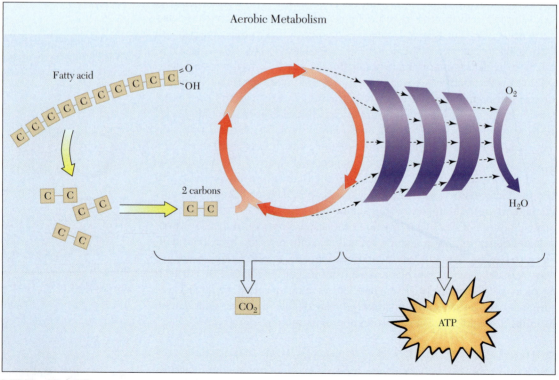

FIGURE 5.12

Fatty acids can be used to produce ATP. These are first broken into two-carbon units which can then be broken down by aerobic metabolism.

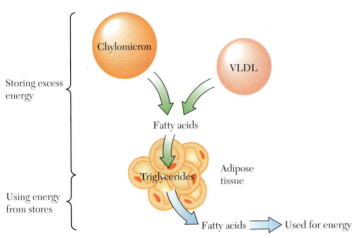

When we eat too much, excess calories are stored in adipose tissue as triglycerides. When we don't eat enough, triglycerides in adipose tissue are broken down, releasing fatty acids, which can be used for energy.

Triglycerides can be stored in adipose tissue If you eat more calories than you need, the excess can be converted into triglycerides and stored in adipose tissue. When your excess calories come from fat, no conversion is necessary; the fat is transported directly to the adipose tissue in chylomicrons. Excess calories consumed as carbohydrate and protein must first go to the liver, where they can be used to synthesize fatty acids, which are then assembled into triglycerides and transported in VLDLs to adipose tissue (Figure 5.13). The ability of the body to store excess triglycerides is theoretically limitless. Cells in your adipose tissue can increase in weight by about 50 times, and new fat cells can be made when existing cells reach their maximum size (see Chapter 7).

Stored triglycerides can be used for energy When you eat fewer calories than you use, your body takes energy from fat stores. In this situation, an enzyme inside the fat cells receives a signal to break down stored triglycerides. The fatty acids and glycerol that result are released directly into the blood and circulate throughout the body. They are taken up by cells and used to produce ATP. If there is not enough carbohydrate to allow the two carbon units from fatty acid breakdown to enter aerobic metabolism, they will be used to make ketones (see Chapter 4). Ketones can be used as an energy source by muscle and adipose tissue. During prolonged starvation or fasting, the brain can adapt to use ketones to meet about half of its energy needs. For the other half, it continues to require glucose. Fatty acids cannot be used to make glucose, and only a small amount of glucose can be made from the glycerol released from triglyceride breakdown.

On the Side

When the fattest man on record died in 1983 at age 42, he weighed 1397 pounds and 80% of his body weight was estimated to be from fat—that is over 4 million stored Calories.

The Type and Amount of Fat You Eat Affects Your Health

Your fat intake affects your health. Eating too little fat can cause an essential fatty acid deficiency and reduce the absorption of fat-soluble vitamins. Eating too much of the wrong types of fat can contribute to chronic diseases such as heart disease and cancer. The development of heart disease has been linked to diets high in cholesterol, saturated fat, and *trans* fat.[2] The risk of certain types of cancer, including that of the breast, colon, and prostate, may be increased with a high intake of saturated and *trans* fat or reduced with a higher intake of monounsaturated fat.[4,5] Consuming too much fat can add calories and contribute to weight gain. Excess body fat in turn is associated with an increased risk of diabetes, cardiovascular disease, and high blood pressure.

Fat affects the risk of heart disease

Over 64 million people in the United States suffer from some form of **cardiovascular disease**, which is any disease that affects the heart and blood vessels. It is the number one cause of death of both men and women in the United States.[6] **Atherosclerosis** is

Go to the American Heart Association for information on heart disease, its risk factors, incidence, prevention, and treatment:
www.americanheart.org/

⚠ **Cardiovascular disease** Any disease affecting the heart and blood vessels.

⚠ **Atherosclerosis** A type of cardiovascular disease that involves the buildup of fatty material in the artery walls.

the type of cardiovascular disease in which cholesterol is deposited in the artery walls, reducing their elasticity and eventually blocking the flow of blood.

Cholesterol accumulates in artery walls
Our current understanding of how atherosclerosis develops is based on the work of Michael Brown and Joseph Goldstein, who were awarded the Nobel Prize in 1985 for their discoveries. Their work identified LDL receptors on cells and demonstrated how they bind LDL particles in the blood. When LDL receptors bind LDL particles, cholesterol synthesis is shut off in the body. The LDL particles are taken up by the cells, reducing blood levels of LDL cholesterol. If the amount of LDL cholesterol in the blood exceeds the amount that can be taken up by cells—because of either too much LDL cholesterol or too few LDL receptors—the result is a high level of LDL cholesterol. High LDL cholesterol increases the risk of atherosclerosis because excess LDL cholesterol in the blood can lead to the deposition of cholesterol in the artery walls.

Atherosclerosis begins with damage to the artery walls
The exact events that cause the buildup of cholesterol in artery walls are still not fully understood. One theory is that an injury to the arterial wall—possibly caused by high blood pressure, high blood sugar levels, high cholesterol levels, infection, or some other factor—begins the process. Therefore, having diabetes, high blood pressure, or high blood cholesterol levels directly increases the risk of developing heart disease. Obesity also increases risks because it increases the amount of work required by the heart and also increases blood pressure, blood cholesterol levels, and the risk of diabetes.

LDL oxidation leads to cholesterol deposits
Once an artery wall has been injured, LDL particles, immune system cells, and blood cell fragments involved in blood clotting, called platelets, enter the wall of the artery. Inside the artery wall, LDL that comes in contact with highly reactive oxygen molecules is **oxidized**. Immune cells pick up this toxic oxidized LDL cholesterol and eventually burst open, depositing cholesterol in the artery wall. Platelets signal muscle cells to grow in the artery wall and secrete fibrous proteins. The result is a mass of cholesterol, muscle cells, and fibrous tissue called a **plaque**. Eventually, calcium also collects in the plaque and causes it to harden. Blood clots form around the plaque and it continues to enlarge, causing the artery to narrow and lose its elasticity (Figure 5.14). The buildup of material can become so large that it completely blocks the artery, or a blood clot can break loose and block a smaller artery elsewhere. When an artery is blocked, blood can no longer move through it to supply oxygen and nutrients to the cells, and they

On the Side

People with an inherited condition called familial hypercholesterolemia do not make LDL receptors normally. In these people cholesterol cannot be removed from the blood and levels can be so high that cholesterol deposits can accumulate in the tendons and skin. The risk of a fatal heart attack before 40 years of age is much higher in those with this condition than among the general population.

⚠ **Oxidized** Having undergone a chemical change involving the loss of electrons.

⚠ **Plaque** The cholesterol-rich material that is deposited in the blood vessels of individuals with atherosclerosis. It consists of cholesterol, muscle cells, fibrous tissue, and calcium.

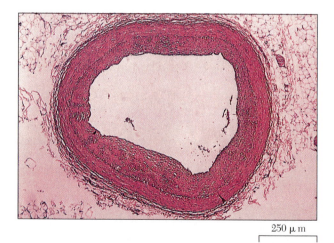
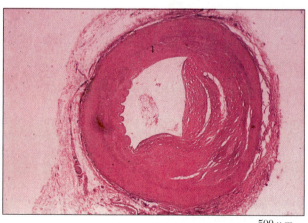

250 μm   500 μm

FIGURE 5.14

The photograph on the left shows a cross-section of a normal artery. The one on the right shows a cross-section of an artery partially blocked by atherosclerotic deposits. (*left*: Cabisco/Visuals Unlimited; *right*: Ober/Visuals Unlimited)

die quickly. If blood flow to the heart muscle is interrupted, heart cells die, resulting in a heart attack or myocardial infarction. If the blood flow to the brain is interrupted, a stroke results.

Blood cholesterol levels affect plaque formation High levels of LDL cholesterol increase the risk of developing atherosclerotic plaques. If you have your blood cholesterol measured, you will likely get results that show levels of total cholesterol as well as LDL and HDL. The desirable level for total blood cholesterol in adults is below 200 mg per 100 ml of blood. In healthy adults, LDL cholesterol level should be below 100 mg per 100 ml of blood. In those at high risk for a heart attack, LDL should be ≤70 mg per 100 ml. HDL cholesterol is protective against heart disease; an HDL level of <40 mg per 100 ml increases risks; a level of at least 60 mg per 100 ml of blood or above decreases risk (see Table 5.1 and Appendix C).[7] Comparing your LDL and HDL levels with these standards can help assess your risk of heart disease.

Genetics, health, and lifestyle affect your heart disease risk Your risk of developing atherosclerosis is affected by the genes you inherit from your parents, other health conditions you have, and your lifestyle (see Table 5.1). The risk of developing heart disease increases with age. Men and women are both at risk, but men are generally affected a decade earlier than women. This is due in part to the protective effect of the hormone estrogen in women. As women age, the effects of menopause—including the decline in estrogen level and gain in weight—increase heart disease risk.

Having diabetes, high blood pressure, elevated LDL cholesterol or triglycerides, low HDL cholesterol, or obesity increases your risk of developing atherosclerosis. Likewise, if your parents had heart disease, you are more likely to develop it. Scientists

On the Side

High LDL cholesterol increases your risk of heart disease, but researchers have found an even better marker of heart disease risk. It is a protein found in LDL and VLDL particles called **apolipoprotein B,** or **apo B.** High levels of apo B indicate an increased cholesterol-depositing capacity of the blood.

TABLE 5.1
Factors that Increase Your Heart Disease Risk

Age:
- Men, ≥ 45 years
- Women, ≥ 55 years

Family history:
- Male relative with heart disease before age 55 years
- Female with heart disease before age 65 years

Medical conditions:
- **Diabetes:** fasting blood sugar of ≥ 126 mg/100 ml
- **High blood pressure:** > 140/90 mm Hg
- **Obesity:** Body Mass Index > 27* and waist circumference > 35 inches for women or > 40 inches for men
- **Altered blood lipid level**
  LDL cholesterol > 100 mg/100 ml
  HDL cholesterol < 40 mg/100 ml
  Total cholesterol ≥ 200 mg/100 ml
  Triglycerides ≥ 150 mg/100 ml

Lifestyle:
- Cigarette smoking
- A sedentary lifestyle
- A diet high in saturated fat, *trans* fat, and cholesterol and low in fiber, fruits, and vegetables

*See Chapter 7 for information about Body Mass Index and how it can be calculated.

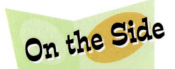

are making progress in identifying genetic factors that increase heart disease risk. African Americans have a higher risk of heart disease than the general population because they are more likely to have high blood pressure. Mexican Americans, Native Americans, Hawaiians, and some Asian Americans have higher risk, in part because of a higher incidence of diabetes and obesity in these groups.

Lifestyle factors that affect risk include activity level, smoking, and diet. A sedentary lifestyle increases the risk of heart disease, as does cigarette smoking. On the other hand, regular exercise decreases risk by promoting a healthy body weight, reducing the risk of diabetes, increasing HDL cholesterol, and reducing blood pressure. Some dietary factors, including high intakes of saturated and *trans* fat and cholesterol, increase risk. Other dietary factors, including adequate intakes of fiber, fruits and vegetables, unsaturated fats, and antioxidants, may offer a protective effect. You can't change your age, ethnicity, or genetic background, but you can control these lifestyle factors.

Dietary cholesterol, saturated fat, and *trans* fat increase heart disease risk

Cholesterol in the blood comes from cholesterol both consumed in the diet and made by the liver. Generally, about three to four times more cholesterol is made by the liver than is consumed in the diet. In some people an increase in dietary cholesterol causes liver cholesterol synthesis to decrease so that blood levels do not change. In others, however, liver synthesis does not decrease in response to an increase in dietary cholesterol, so blood cholesterol levels rise. In general, however, the effect of dietary cholesterol on blood cholesterol levels is low in comparison with other dietary factors such as the amount of saturated fat.[8]

Diets high in saturated fat increase LDL cholesterol in the blood, which in turn increases the risk of atherosclerosis. This occurs because a diet high in saturated fatty acids increases liver production of cholesterol-carrying lipoproteins and reduces the activity of LDL receptors in the liver, so that LDL cholesterol cannot be removed from the blood.[9] When the diet is low in saturated fat, lipoprotein production decreases and the number of LDL receptors increases, allowing more LDL cholesterol to be removed from the blood. Not all saturated fats increase LDL cholesterol levels. Some types, such as stearic acid found in chocolate and beef, do not increase blood cholesterol levels. However, these may contribute to heart disease by decreasing HDL cholesterol and affecting blood platelets and blood clotting, both of which are involved in plaque formation.[10]

Another type of dietary fat that increases the risk of heart disease is *trans* fatty acids. Some of the increase in risk is due to the effect of *trans* fatty acids on blood cholesterol levels. *Trans* fatty acids can raise LDL cholesterol, lower HDL cholesterol, or both. The overall effect of *trans* fats on blood lipids is worse than that of all other types of dietary fatty acids, including saturated fats.[11]

Dietary unsaturated fats protect against heart disease

When saturated fat in the diet is replaced by polyunsaturated fat, there is a beneficial decrease in LDL cholesterol.[12] However, a high intake of omega-6 fats, such as that in corn and sunflower oils, may also decrease HDL cholesterol, which increases heart disease risk. If instead your polyunsaturated fats are high in omega-3 fatty acids, such as those in fish oils, LDL cholesterol is decreased without a drop in HDL cholesterol. In addition to their effect on blood lipids, omega-3 fatty acids have other effects that also reduce heart disease risk. They prevent the growth of atherosclerotic plaque, reduce blood clotting and blood pressure, and affect immune function by decreasing inflammation.[13] Populations that consume a diet high in omega-3s, such as the Inuits in Greenland, have a low incidence of heart disease.[14] The traditional Inuit diet consists mainly of seals, whales, and fish. Although supplements of fish oil are marketed to reduce your risk of heart disease, factors in fish other than omega-3 fats may also protect against heart disease; the benefits are greater when the omega-3 fatty acids are consumed in fish, such as salmon and tuna, rather than in supplements.[15]

Monounsaturated fats also decrease heart disease risk. Populations with diets high in monounsaturated fats, such as those in Mediterranean countries where olive oil is

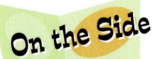

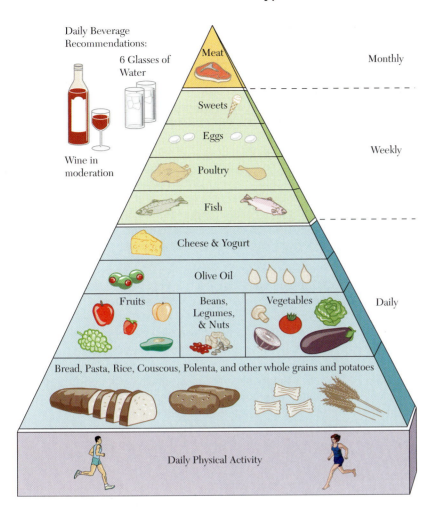

Daily Beverage Recommendations:
6 Glasses of Water

Wine in moderation

Meat — Monthly

Sweets

Eggs — Weekly

Poultry

Fish

Cheese & Yogurt

Olive Oil

Fruits   Beans, Legumes, & Nuts   Vegetables — Daily

Bread, Pasta, Rice, Couscous, Polenta, and other whole grains and potatoes

Daily Physical Activity

FIGURE 5.15

A Mediterranean Diet Pyramid has been developed, based on the eating patterns in Mediterranean countries. Like the USDA Food Guide Pyramid, it emphasizes eating plenty of grains, vegetables, and fruits. But it also differs from the Food Guide Pyramid in a number of ways. Most of the fat in the Mediterranean diet is from olive oil, which is placed in the middle of the pyramid rather than in the very tip. Instead, red meat, which is eaten infrequently in the Mediterranean diet and is a source of saturated fat and cholesterol, is in the small tip of the pyramid. Plant sources of protein, such as legumes and nuts, are lower down on the pyramid, between fruits and vegetables.

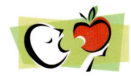

Dipping your bread in olive oil, Italian style, is the best bet because it is rich in monounsaturated fatty acids, which help protect you from heart disease. If you are choosing spreads, a trans*-free margarine is probably better than butter because it has less saturated fat.*

commonly used, have a mortality rate from heart disease that is half of that in the United States. This is true even when total fat intake provides 40% or more of energy intake.[16] Substituting monounsaturated fat for saturated fat reduces LDL cholesterol without decreasing HDL cholesterol.[17] However, the type of fat in the diet is unlikely to be the only factor responsible for the difference in the incidence of heart disease between the Mediterranean countries and the United States. The diet in olive-growing regions of the Mediterranean is higher in plant foods and lower in red meat than the American diet, and the lifestyle is more active and less stressful (Figure 5.15).

Fat is not the only dietary factor that affects heart disease risk The amount and type of fat are not the only dietary factors that affect your risk of developing heart disease. Adequate intakes of foods high in fiber, antioxidants, and B vitamins; moderate alcohol consumption; and a combination of diet and exercise that keeps your weight in the healthy range can reduce the risk of developing heart disease. On the other hand, too much salt and added sugar can increase your blood pressure and blood triglycerides, thereby increasing your heart disease risk.

Many of the dietary components that protect you from heart disease are found in plant foods. Fruits, vegetables, grains, and legumes are a good source of fiber, vitamins, minerals, and phytochemicals. Soluble fibers, such as those in oat bran, legumes, psyllium, pectin, and gums, have been show to reduce blood cholesterol levels and therefore reduce heart disease risk. The vitamins, minerals, and phytochemicals in plant foods protect against heart disease because many have antioxidant functions. Antioxidants decrease the oxidation of LDL cholesterol and therefore the development of plaque in artery walls.[17]

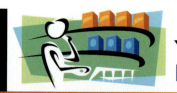

Your Choice: Cholesterol-Lowering Extras

Over 100 million American adults have blood cholesterol values that put them at risk for a heart attack.[1] Many of these people are taking medications to reduce their cholesterol and their risk. But in some cases prescription drugs may not be necessary. A recent study found that a dietary pattern that includes soluble (viscous) fiber, plant sterols, soy protein, and nuts can reduce blood cholesterol as much as medication.[2] So, if you are concerned about your cholesterol level and your risk of heart disease, you can help lower both by choosing from the following shopping list to create your own dietary portfolio of cholesterol-lowering foods.

Oats and Other Soluble Fibers

One of the easiest cholesterol-lowering foods to include in your diet is oatmeal. Oatmeal, as well as other products that contain oat bran, provides soluble or viscous fiber, which lowers total and LDL cholesterol in those with elevated levels.[3] The evidence of the cholesterol-lowering effect of foods such as oats, apples, beans, and barley, which contain viscous fiber, is substantial enough for the FDA to allow a health claim related to the cholesterol-lowering effects of foods containing sufficient amounts of this fiber. Ten grams per day of the viscous fiber psyllium, found in Metamucil, has also been shown to lower total and LDL cholesterol without affecting HDL cholesterol.[4] So to lower your cholesterol, have oatmeal for breakfast, apples with your lunch, and beans and barley in your stew, and add a tablespoon of psyllium to your orange juice in the morning.

Flaxseed

Another food that can lower LDL cholesterol without lowering HDL cholesterol is flaxseed. These small seeds, which can be ground up and sprinkled on your cereal or mixed into your yogurt, provide soluble fiber that helps lower cholesterol and protect against cardiovascular disease, but they are also high in omega-3 fatty acids. These fats offer additional protection against high blood lipids and heart disease. Flaxseed is also high in lignan, a phytochemical that may help to block the action of certain substances that can contribute to the development of cancer.

Soy

When soy protein replaces animal protein in the diet, it lowers LDL cholesterol and either increases or has no effect on HDL cholesterol.[5] This effect may be due to the amino acid composition of soy protein or it may be related to phytochemicals called phytoestrogens in soybeans.[6] When consumed in food, soy phytoestrogens lower cholesterol, though the same effect does not occur when phytoestrogens are consumed in supplements.[7] The American Heart Association recommends about 25 grams of soy protein daily to help lower cholesterol. You can get this amount by eating about 2 heaping tablespoons of soy protein powder or having 2 cups of low-fat soymilk and 4 ounces of firm tofu. Foods that are low in fat, saturated fat, and cholesterol and contain 6.25 grams or more of soy protein can display a health claim on their label stating that soy protein may help reduce the risk of coronary heart disease.

Plant Sterols and Stanols

Plant sterols and stanols are compounds found in plant cell membranes. They resemble cholesterol chemically, making it difficult for the digestive tract to distinguish them from cholesterol. They lower blood cholesterol by reducing cholesterol absorption.[8] Small quantities of these compounds are present naturally in many fruits, vegetables, nuts, seeds, cereals, legumes, vegetable oils, and other plant foods. Larger amounts have been added to margarines, salad dressings, and orange juice. These foods can include a health claim on their label about the relationship between plant sterols and reduced risk of heart disease.

Nuts

Epidemiologic studies have shown that diets rich in nuts are associated with a lower incidence of cardiovascular disease. Almonds have been studied more extensively than other nuts; studies have demonstrated that the addition of almonds to a typical diet reduces cholesterol levels.[9] This benefit may be due not only to the monounsaturated fat they contain but also to their protein, fiber, and high polyunsaturated fatty acid content. So, go nuts! Grab some for a snack, add them to breads and muffins, and sprinkle them in stir fries.

Fish

Fatty fish, such as mackerel, lake trout, herring, sardines, tuna, and salmon, can help reduce your risk of heart disease. Fatty fish are high in the omega-3 fatty acids EPA and DHA. Regular consumption of these lowers the risk of heart disease and protects against sudden cardiac death.[10] They do affect blood lipids but they have more important effects that protect against heart disease. These include stabilizing the heart electrically so irregular heart beats occur less often, decreasing the growth of atherosclerotic plaque, and lowering blood pressure. The American Heart Association recommends eating two servings of fatty fish a week.[11]

References
1. American Heart Association. Cholesterol statistics. Available at www.americanheart.org/presenter.jhtml?identifier=536/Accessed June 22, 2004.
2. Jenkins, D.J.A., Kendall, C.W.C., Marchie, A., et al. Effects of a dietary portfolio of cholesterol-lowering foods vs lovastatin on serum lipids and C-reactive protein. JAMA 290:502–510, 2003.

3. Brown, L., Rosner, B., Willett, W. W., and Sacks, F. M. Cholesterol-lowering effects of dietary fiber: a meta-analysis. *Am. J. Clin. Nutr.* 69(1):30–42, 1999.

4. Anderson, J. W., Allgood, L. D., Lawrence, A., et al. Cholesterol-lowering effects of psyllium intake adjunctive to diet therapy in men and women with hypercholesterolemia: Meta-analysis of 8 controlled trials. *Am. J. Clin. Nutr.* 71:472–479, 2000.

5. Anthony, M. S. Soy and cardiovascular disease: Cholesterol lowering and beyond. *J. Nutr.* 130:662S–663S, 2000.

6. Nicolosi, R. J., Wilson, T. A., Lawton, C., and Handelman, G. J. Dietary effects on cardiovascular disease risk factors: beyond saturated fatty acids and cholesterol. *J. Am. College Nutr.* 20:421S–427S, 2001.

7. Demonty, I., Lamarche, B., and Jones, P.J.H. Role of isoflavones in hypercholesterolemic effect of soy. *Nutr. Rev.* 61:189–203, 2003.

8. Law, M., Plant sterol and stanol margarines and health. *B.M.J.* 320:861–864, 2000.

9. Sabaté, J., Haddad, E., Tanzman, J.S., et al. Serum lipid response to the graduated enrichment of a Step I diet with almonds: a randomized feeding trial. *Am. J. Clin. Nutr.* 77:1379–1384, 2003.

10. Lee, K. W., and Lip, G.Y.H. The role of omega-3 fatty acids in the secondary prevention of cardiovascular disease. *Q. J. Med.* 96:465–480, 2003.

11. American Heart Association. *Fish and Omega-3 Fatty Acids: AHA Recommendations.* Available online at www.americanheart.org/presenter.jhtml?identifier=4632/ accessed June 22, 2004.

Adequate intakes of vitamin B_6, vitamin B_{12}, and folic acid can help protect against heart disease because they keep blood levels of the amino acid homocysteine low (see Chapter 8). Elevated homocysteine levels are associated with a higher incidence of heart disease.[18] Higher levels of B vitamins in the blood are related to lower levels of homocysteine. The American grain supply was recently fortified with folic acid resulting in a reduction in blood homocysteine levels in the population.[19] There is insufficient evidence on the relationship between intake of these vitamins and homocysteine levels to recommend supplements, but a diet high in grains, fruits, and vegetables is advised to ensure adequate intake. Another B vitamin that may affect heart disease risk is niacin, but the amount consumed in the diet will not have an impact. When consumed in extremely high doses, the nicotinic acid form of niacin can be used to lower blood cholesterol. Nicotinic acid is inexpensive and widely available without a prescription, but at the high doses needed to lower cholesterol it is really a drug, not a nutrient. Because of the potential side effects, an individual using nicotinic acid as a drug to lower cholesterol should be monitored by a physician.

Alcohol is a dangerous drug, but moderate alcohol consumption has been shown to reduce stress, to raise levels of HDL cholesterol, and to reduce blood clotting. These effects are protective against heart disease. Some of the protection may also be due to compounds in red wine known as phenols, which are antioxidants that protect against LDL oxidation, thereby preventing the development of atherosclerotic plaques.[20] The Dietary Guidelines for Americans recognize that in men over age 45 years and women over age 55 years, moderate drinking can lower the risk of heart disease. Moderate drinking means no more than one drink per day for women and two drinks per day for men. One drink is defined as 12 ounces of beer, 5 ounces of wine, or 1.5 ounces of 80-proof distilled spirits. Greater intake of alcohol increases the risk of accidental deaths, heart disease, cancer, birth defects, and drug interactions and should be avoided. Alcohol consumption is not recommended for children or adolescents, pregnant women, individuals who cannot restrict their drinking to a moderate amount, or individuals who plan to drive or perform other activities that require concentration.

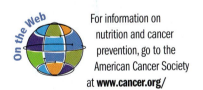

Just cutting the fat in your diet will not necessarily protect you from heart disease. A heart-healthy diet limits cholesterol, trans fat, and saturated fat, has just enough calories to maintain a healthy weight, and provides plenty of fiber, antioxidants, and B vitamins.

On the Web

For information on nutrition and cancer prevention, go to the American Cancer Society at **www.cancer.org/**

Cancer is linked to fat in the diet

Cancer is the second leading cause of death in the United States, and it is estimated that 30 to 40% of cancers are directly linked to dietary choices.[21] As with cardiovascular disease, there is epidemiologic evidence that diet and lifestyle affect cancer risk. Populations consuming diets high in fruits and vegetables tend to have a lower cancer risk. These foods provide more antioxidants such as vitamin C, vitamin E, and β-carotene. In contrast, populations who consume diets high in fat, particularly animal fats, have a higher cancer incidence.

The good news is that for the most part the same type of diet that protects you from cardiovascular disease will also protect you from certain forms of cancer. The incidence of breast cancer in Mediterranean women who rely on olive oil, which is high in monounsaturated fat, as a source of dietary fat is low despite a total fat intake similar to that in the United States.[5] *Trans* fatty acids, on the other hand, not only raise LDL cholesterol levels but also have been suggested to increase the risk of breast cancer.[22] Diets high in saturated fats from red meat are associated with a higher incidence of colon and prostate cancer.[4]

PIECE IT TOGETHER

Evaluating Heart Disease Risk

Michael's mother died of a heart attack at age 60. Michael is worried about his own heart disease risk, so he decides to attend a "healthy heart" class at the local hospital. During the first week of the class he fills out a questionnaire about his medical history and lifestyle and has blood drawn for lipid analysis. The table below summarizes the "risk report" he receives after all the analyses are completed.

Heart Disease Risk Report

Gender	Male
Age	35 years
Family history	Mother had heart attack at age 60
Height/weight	68 inches/160 pounds
Blood pressure	119/70 mm Hg
Cigarette smoker	Yes
Activity level	Sedentary
Blood values	
Total cholesterol	210 mg/100 ml
LDL cholesterol	160 mg/100 ml
HDL cholesterol	34 mg/100 ml
Triglycerides	120 mg/100 ml

Energy from	
Total fat	33%
Saturated fat	20%
Polyunsaturated fat	8%
Monounsaturated fat	6%
Trans fat	7%
Cholesterol	350 mg
Fiber	23 g
Number of servings from the Food Guide Pyramid groups:	
Bread, Cereals, Rice, & Pasta	11
Vegetables	2
Fruits	1
Milk, Yogurt, & Cheese	2
Meat, Poultry, Fish, Dry Beans, Eggs, & Nuts	4

WHAT RISK FACTORS DOES MICHAEL HAVE FOR DEVELOPING CARDIOVASCULAR DISEASE?

His mother died of a heart attack before the age of 65. He smokes cigarettes. He is sedentary. His LDL cholesterol and HDL cholesterol values both put him at high risk.

WHAT LIFESTYLE CHANGES COULD HE MAKE TO REDUCE HIS RISKS?

Your answer:

For his next class he keeps a 3-day record of his food intake and uses a computer program to analyze it. He also records the number of servings he gets from each group of the Food Guide Pyramid. Some of this information is given here.

HOW DOES MICHAEL'S DIET AFFECT HIS HEART DISEASE RISK?

Although his total fat intake is within the range recommended for a healthy diet, much of this fat is saturated, and his *trans* fat intake is well above the average intake of about 3% of energy. The recommendation for cholesterol intake is less than 300 mg, and he eats an average of 350 mg per day. High levels of dietary saturated fat, *trans* fat, and cholesterol all increase heart disease risk. His diet is also well below the recommended 38 grams of fiber per day and does not meet the recommended number of servings of fruits and vegetables.

WHY DO HIS LOW INTAKES OF FIBER AND FRUITS AND VEGETABLES INCREASE HIS RISK OF HEART DISEASE?

Your answer:

Fat doesn't make you fat; too many calories do

Fat has 9 Calories per gram. If you eat a high-fat diet, will it lead to obesity? There is little evidence that the amount of fat in the diet is related to body weight.[23] In fact, as the percentage of fat in the American diet decreased over the last 2 decades, the prevalence of obesity actually increased. This was most likely due to the fact that we increased our calorie intake by adding extra carbohydrates as we reduced our fat intake.[24]

Consuming more energy than is expended increases body fat, regardless of whether the extra energy comes from fat, carbohydrate, or protein. Excess body fat increases the risk of elevated blood cholesterol levels, high blood pressure, diabetes, and heart disease in general. A reduction in body weight has been shown to reduce blood cholesterol levels, blood pressure, and heart disease risk and to help control diabetes. Maintaining a healthy body weight throughout life can help you avoid these conditions.

Fat Is Part of a Healthy Diet

About 33% of the energy in the typical North American diet comes from fat.[24] This amount will easily meet the minimum requirements for essential fatty acids and is within the range of acceptable fat intakes for healthy adults. However, a healthy diet must also limit certain types of fat and include plenty of whole grains, legumes, vegetables, and fruits, which are high in fiber, micronutrients, and phytochemicals (Figure 5.16).

Healthy diets can include a wide range of fat intakes

Fat is needed in the diet to provide essential fatty acids, to allow the absorption of fat-soluble vitamins and phytochemicals, and to provide energy. The amounts needed for this are small, but a diet that provides only the minimum amount of fat would be very high in carbohydrate, not be very palatable, and not necessarily be any healthier than diets with more fat. Therefore, the DRIs recommend a total fat intake of 20 to 35% of calories for adults; this range allows for a variety of individual preferences in terms of food choices.

Small amounts of essential fatty acids are needed to support life The amounts of the essential fatty acids recommended by the DRIs are based on the amounts consumed by the healthy U.S. population. The AI for linoleic acid is 12 grams per day for women and 17 grams per day for men. This is the amount in a half cup of walnuts or 2 tablespoons of safflower oil. For α-linolenic acid, the AI is 1.1 grams per day for women and 1.6 grams per day for men. This is the amount in a quarter cup of walnuts or a tablespoon of canola oil or ground flax seeds. Rather than a UL, AMDRs of 5 to 10% of energy for linoleic acid and 0.6 to 1.2% of energy for α-linolenic acid (with 10% or less of this as EPA and DHA) have been set.[2]

Intakes of saturated fat, cholesterol, and *trans* fat should be limited The DRIs have not set specific guidelines for cholesterol, saturated fat, or *trans* fat, but they recommend that intake of these be kept to a minimum because the risk of heart disease increases with higher intake. The Daily Values on food labels give more specific recommendations: less than 30% of energy as fat, no more than 300 mg of cholesterol per day, and no more than 10% of energy as saturated fat. No Daily Value has been established for *trans* fat, but it is recommended that our intake of *trans* fat should not increase above current average levels of 5.8 grams daily or 2.6% of calorie intake.[25]

Children and teens need more total fat The acceptable ranges of fat intake are higher for children than for adults: 30 to 40% of energy for ages 1 to 3 years and 25 to 35% of energy for ages 3 to 18 years. These levels are higher than for adults because fat provides a concentrated energy source and a higher-fat diet can more easily meet energy needs, especially for young children, who can consume only small amounts of food. These recommendations meet the needs for growth and are unlikely to increase the risk of chronic disease. Specific recommendations for each of the life stage groups in children are given on the inside cover. As with adults, a healthy diet that meets these needs should be based on whole grain products, fruits, vegetables, low-fat dairy products, legumes, and lean meats. The American Academy of Pediatrics specifies a lower limit of 20% of energy from total fat for children and adolescents.[26]

The acceptable ranges of fat intake are not increased during pregnancy or lactation, but the AIs for essential fatty acids are slightly higher than those for non-pregnant women. Recommendations are not different for older adults. In this population, fat intake must be carefully balanced with other nutrients to reduce the risk of malnutrition (see Chapter 13).

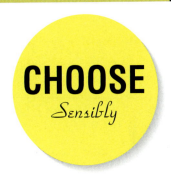

CHOOSE *Sensibly*

- Choose a diet that is low in saturated fat and cholesterol and moderate in total fat.

FIGURE 5.16

The Dietary Guidelines for Americans recommend a diet low in saturated fat and cholesterol and moderate in total fat. (USDA, DHHS, 2000)

On the Side

The traditional Japanese diet provides only about 10% of calories from fat. People living on the Mediterranean island of Crete eat 35% or more of their calories as fat, and the traditional Inuit diet may have provided as much as 60% of calories from fat. Yet, the incidence of heart disease is low in all of these cultures.

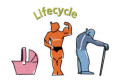

Lifecycle

TABLE 5.2
Diet Tips to Reduce Your Cancer Risk

- Choose a diet rich in a variety of plant-based foods.
- Eat plenty of vegetables and fruits.
- Maintain a healthy weight and be physically active.
- Drink alcohol only in moderation, if at all.
- Select foods low in fat and salt.
- Prepare and store foods safely.
- And always remember: do not use tobacco in any form.

Adapted from AICR Guidelines for reducing cancer risk, available online at www.aicr.org.

Guidelines for prevention of specific diseases are more restrictive In addition to these general recommendations for fat intake, some dietary recommendations target populations at risk for specific diseases. Recommendations for a diet to reduce cancer risk are included in Table 5.2. The American Heart Association (Appendix G) and the National Cholesterol Education Program (NCEP) have developed recommendations to lower heart disease risk.[7] The NCEP recommends that people with heart disease and those with risk factors for heart disease, including diabetes (see Table 5.1), change their diet and lifestyle to reduce their risk (Table 5.3). The NCEP also recommends drug therapy for individuals with extremely high cholesterol levels or for those for whom lifestyle changes are not effective. The drugs most commonly used to treat elevated cholesterol are the statins; these work by blocking cholesterol synthesis in the liver and by increasing the capacity of the liver to remove cholesterol from the blood. Other cholesterol-lowering drugs act in the gastrointestinal tract by preventing cholesterol and bile absorption.

Does your diet meet recommendations for fat intake?

How does your fat intake compare with recommendations? Most of the recommendations for fat intake are based on the percentage of fat calories in your diet. To calculate fat intake as a percentage of calories, you need to know the number of grams of fat in

For more information about coronary heart disease and how to lower your blood cholesterol, go to the National Heart, Lung, and Blood Institute site at **www.nhlbi.nih.gov/guidelines/**

TABLE 5.3
Reduce Your Heart Disease Risk

How Much is Recommended	
Saturated fat	Less than 7% of calories
Polyunsaturated fat	Up to 10% of calories
Monounsaturated fat	Up to 20% of calories
Cholesterol	Less than 200 mg/day
Total fat	25 to 35% of calories
Protein	Approximately 15% of calories
Carbohydrate	50–60% of total calories
Soluble fiber	10–25 g/day
Plant stanols	2 g/day
Sodium	2400 mg/day or less
Total energy (calories)	Balance to maintain a desirable body weight
Exercise	Equivalent to 200 Calories per day

Source: Adapted from the National Cholesterol Education Program.

TABLE 5.4
How Much Fat DO You Eat?

If you want to know the number of calories you eat from fat:
- Determine the number of grams of fat in a food or diet
- Multiply the grams of fat by 9 Calories per gram
  Example: For a diet that contains 75 grams of fat,

75 grams × 9 Calories per gram = 675 Calories from fat

If you want to know the percentage of calories from fat:
- Determine the total Calories in the food or diet
- Divide Calories from fat by total Calories, and multiply by 100 to express as a percentage
  Example: For a diet that contains 2000 total Calories and 675 Calories of fat,

675 Calories ÷ 2000 Calories = 0.34 × 100 = 34% calories from fat

the diet and the number of calories consumed (Table 5.4). This same calculation can be used to determine the percentage of fat in individual foods. Exchange lists can also be used to calculate the amount of fat in your diet. These calculations, however, don't tell you where your fats are coming from. To get this type of information, food composition tables and food labels can be used.

Use Exchange lists to estimate fat content The Exchange Lists can be used to give a quick estimate of the total amount of fat in a food or in a diet (Table 5.5; Appendix I). An exchange of fruits, vegetables, or breads contains 1 gram of fat or less. An exchange of dairy products provides 0 to 8 grams, depending

TABLE 5.5
Use Exchange Lists to Estimate the Fat in Foods

Exchange Groups/Lists	Foods	Serving Size	Fat (g)
Carbohydrate group			
Starch	Rice, cereal, potatoes	1/2 cup	0–1
	Bread	1 slice	
Fruit	Apple, peach, pear	1 small	0
	Banana	1/2 medium	
	Canned fruit	1/2 cup	
Milk	Milk or yogurt	1 cup	
Fat-free or low-fat			0–3
Reduced-fat			5
Whole			8
Vegetables	Cooked vegetables	1/2 cup	0
	Raw vegetables	1 cup	
Meat group	Meat	1 ounce	
Very Lean			0–1
Lean			3
Medium fat			5
High fat			8
Fat group	Butter, oil, margarine	1 tsp	5

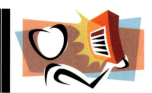

Off the Label: Choosing Lean Meat

Looking for some lean meat? Although fresh meats are not required to carry a Nutrition Facts label, they often do carry information about the fat content of the meat. Understanding this can help you choose meats that will fit into your diet plan.

The terms "lean" and "extra lean" are used to describe the fat content of packaged meats, such as hot dogs and lunch meat, and fresh meats, such as pork chops and steaks. "Lean" means that the meat contains less than 10% fat by weight, and "extra lean" means that it contains no more than 5% fat by weight (see Table 5.6 in text). Ground beef, which accounts for almost half of the beef sold in the United States, is an exception to these labeling rules. The USDA allows ground beef to be labeled "lean" even if it has as much as 22.5% of its weight as fat. Since there is no specific definition for lean ground beef, the amounts of fat in ground beef labeled lean and extra lean can vary from store to store. Despite this, you can still figure out how much fat is in your lean ground beef because ground meats labeled "lean" or "extra lean" must indicate the actual percentage of fat versus lean. This is done by stating that it is a certain "percent lean" (see Figure). But "% lean" claims can be confusing. A food that is 80% lean has only 20% fat—this doesn't sound like much but the "% lean" refers to the weight of the meat that is lean, not the percent of calories

that is from lean. So when the label says it is 80% lean, it means that 20% of the weight of the meat is fat, or that there are 20 grams of fat in 100 grams (3.5 ounces) of raw hamburger. This works out to about 50% of calories as fat.

So, if even lean ground beef is high in fat, should we cut it out of our diets? Not necessarily. The label-savvy consumer can purchase lean ground meats by choosing those labeled as 90% lean or greater. If you choose a lower percent lean ground beef for your burgers, tacos, meatloaf, or lasagna, balance this with lower-fat choices throughout the day.

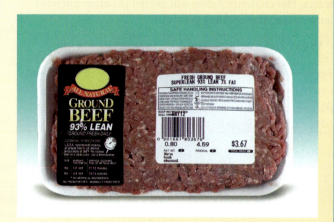

(Andy Washnik)

and the number of milligrams of cholesterol in a serving.[25] With the exception of *trans* fat, these are also presented as a percentage of the Daily Value. This information allows consumers to tell at a glance how one food will fit into the recommendations for fat intake for the day. For example, if a serving provides 50% of the Daily Value for fat—that is, half the recommended maximum daily intake for a 2000-Calorie diet—the rest of the day's foods will have to be carefully selected to not exceed the recommended maximum. To choose foods low in saturated fat and cholesterol, use the general rule that 5% of the Daily Value or less is low and 20% or more is high.

The amount of monounsaturated and polyunsaturated fat is voluntarily included on the labels of some products. For example, in addition to listing the 2 grams of saturated fat, the label on a bottle of olive oil may indicate that it contains 2 grams of polyunsaturated fat and 10 grams of monounsaturated fat per tablespoon. There are no Daily Values for polyunsaturated and monounsaturated fat.

If you want to know the source of fat, you can check the ingredient list. This will show you, for example, if a food contains corn oil, soybean oil, coconut oil, or partially hydrogenated vegetable oil. Labels may also include terms such as "low fat," "fat free," and "low cholesterol" that describe their fat content. Food labeling regulations have developed standard definitions for these terms, and they can be used only in ways that do not confuse consumers (Table 5.6). For instance, a food that is low in cholesterol but high in saturated fat, such as crackers containing coconut oil,

TABLE 5.6
Using Food Labels to Find Low-Fat, Low-Cholesterol Foods

What the Label Says	What It Means
Fat-free	Contains < 0.5 gram of fat per serving
Low-fat	Contains ≤ 3 grams of fat per serving
Percent fat-free	May be used only to describe foods that meet the definition of fat-free or low-fat
Reduced or less fat	Contains at least 25% less fat per serving than the regular or reference product
Saturated fat-free	Contains < 0.5 gram of saturated fat per serving and < 0.5 gram *trans* fatty acids per serving
Low saturated fat	Contains ≤ 1 gram of saturated fat and not more than 15% of calories from saturated fat per serving
Reduced or less saturated fat	Contains at least 25% less saturated fat than the regular or reference product
Cholesterol-free	Contains < 2 mg of cholesterol and ≤ 2 grams of saturated fat per serving
Low cholesterol	Contains ≤ 20 mg of cholesterol and ≤ 2 grams of saturated fat per serving
Reduced or less cholesterol	Contains at least 25% less cholesterol than the regular or reference product and ≤ 2 grams of saturated fat per serving
Lean	Contains < 10 grams of fat, ≤ 4.5 grams of saturated fat, and < 95 mg of cholesterol per serving and per 100 grams
Extra lean	Contains < 5 grams of fat, < 2 grams of saturated fat, and < 95 mg of cholesterol per serving and per 100 grams

FDA, Center for Food Safety and Applied Nutrition, available at www.cfsan.fda.gov/.

cannot be labeled "low cholesterol" because saturated fat in the diet raises blood cholesterol. Food labels may also include health claims related to their fat content. For example, a food low in saturated fat may claim to reduce the risk of heart disease (see Appendix D).

Healthy fat choices are one part of a healthy diet

A healthy diet must meet nutrient needs, balance energy intake from carbohydrate, protein, and fat, and at the same time limit *trans* fat, saturated fat, and cholesterol. Following the recommendations of the Dietary Guidelines for Americans and the Food Guide Pyramid can help you plan such a diet.

Both of these guidelines propose a diet that is high in whole grains, fruits, and vegetables. These foods, shown at the base of the Pyramid, are naturally low in fat (Figure 5.17). However, choices from these groups need to be made with care to avoid fats that are added in processing or preparation. For example, within the grain group,

SUMMARY

1. Lipids in our diet contribute energy, texture, flavor, and aroma. Some of the fat in our food is clearly visible, but other foods are less obvious sources of fat. The amount and type of fat in a diet are only two of many factors that determine the overall healthfulness of the diet.

2. There are many different types of lipids. Most of the lipids in our diets and in our bodies are triglycerides, commonly called fat. Triglycerides are made by linking three fatty acids to a molecule of glycerol. Fatty acids consist of a carbon chain with an acid group at one end. Saturated fatty acids are saturated with hydrogens and tend to be solid at room temperature. Larger amounts are found in animal foods. Unsaturated fatty acids are found in vegetable oils; they tend to be liquid at room temperature. *Trans* fatty acids are unsaturated, but the orientation of the hydrogen atoms around the double bond gives them properties more similar to saturated fats.

3. Phospholipids are a type of lipid that allows oil and water to mix; this property is important in the body and in food. Phospholipids consist of a backbone of glycerol, two fatty acids, and a phosphate group.

4. Sterols, of which cholesterol is the best known, are made up of multiple chemical rings. Cholesterol is made by the body and consumed in animal foods in the diet. In the body, it is a component of cell membranes and is used to synthesize vitamin D, bile acids, and a number of hormones.

5. Most fat digestion takes place in the small intestine. Bile from the gallbladder helps break large fat globules into small droplets. This allows enzymes to access these fats for digestion. The products of fat digestion combine with bile to form micelles, which facilitate the absorption of these materials into the cells of the small intestine.

6. Water-insoluble lipids are transported in the blood in lipoproteins. Lipids absorbed from the intestine are packaged with protein to form lipoproteins called chylomicrons, which transport triglycerides from the intestine to body cells. Very-low-density lipoproteins (VLDLs) are synthesized by the liver; they take triglycerides from the liver to body cells. Once the triglycerides have been removed from VLDLs, some are transformed into low-density lipoproteins (LDLs). LDLs deliver cholesterol to tissues by binding to LDL receptors on the cell surface. High levels of LDL are associated with an increased risk of heart disease. High-density lipoproteins (HDLs) are lipoproteins that help remove cholesterol from cells for disposal. High levels protect against cardiovascular disease.

7. In the body, lipids provide lubrication, insulate against shock, and help regulate body temperature. They are a structural component of cell membranes and are used to synthesize hormones and regulatory molecules called eicosinoids. Small amounts of both omega-3 and omega-6 fatty acids are essential in the diet.

8. Lipids provide a concentrated source of energy. Some triglycerides are used immediately for energy and others are stored for future use. During fasting, triglycerides stored in adipose tissue are broken down and the fatty acids and glycerol are released into the blood.

9. Atherosclerosis occurs when a blood vessel is damaged and LDL cholesterol, immune system cells, and platelets enter the artery wall. Oxidation of LDL cholesterol leads to deposits called plaque, which stiffen the artery and block blood flow. The risk of heart disease is affected by age, gender, and family history as well as by other health conditions such as diabetes, high blood pressure, obesity, and high levels of LDL blood cholesterol. High levels of HDL cholesterol in the blood are associated with a reduced risk.

10. Diets high in saturated fat, *trans* fatty acids, and cholesterol increase the risk of heart disease. Diets high in omega-6 and omega-3 polyunsaturated fatty acids, monounsaturated fatty acids, certain B vitamins, and plant foods containing fiber, antioxidants, and phytochemicals reduce the risk of heart disease. Total dietary and lifestyle pattern is more important than any individual dietary factor in reducing heart disease risk.

11. Diets high in certain types of fat correlate with an increased incidence of some cancers, but as with heart disease, fat intake is only one dietary factor that affects cancer risk.

12. The acceptable range of fat intake for adults is 20 to 35% of energy. Acceptable ranges of intake and AIs have been established for the essential fatty acids linoleic acid (omega-6) and α-linolenic acid (omega-3). The DRIs suggest that intakes of cholesterol, *trans* fatty acids, and saturated fatty acids should be minimized. The Daily Values recommend that total fat account for no more than 30% of energy, that saturated fat account for no more than 10% of energy, and that dietary cholesterol be no more than 300 mg per day.

13. Total fat intake can be estimated using the Exchange Lists. Food labels provide information on the amounts of different types of fat in packaged foods.

14. The Dietary Guidelines for Americans and the Food Guide Pyramid are designed to help you choose a diet that meets the recommendations for fat intake. Reducing saturated fat, *trans* fat, and cholesterol intake requires decreasing your intake of animal fats and processed convenience foods that contain partially hydrogenated vegetable oil. To increase your intake of mono- and polyunsaturated fats, use olive, canola, and peanut oil as well as a variety of other vegetable oils and choose nuts and fish often. The total dietary pattern, not just fat intake, determines the healthfulness of your intake.

15. Artificial fats are used to create reduced-fat products with taste and texture similar to the originals. A healthy diet does not need to include artificial fats, but if used wisely they can be part of a healthy diet.

REVIEW QUESTIONS

1. What is a lipid?
2. What type of lipid is most plentiful in our body and our food?
3. Why are phospholipids important?
4. What distinguishes a saturated fat from a monounsaturated fat? From a polyunsaturated fat?
5. Name two functions of fat in foods.
6. What types of foods contain cholesterol?
7. What is hydrogenation and how is it related to *trans* fatty acids?
8. What is the function of bile in fat digestion?
9. List three functions of fat in the body.
10. Why is it important to have a balance of omega-6 and omega-3 fatty acids in your diet?
11. What is the advantage of storing energy in the body as fat rather than as carbohydrate?
12. What is the first step in the development of atherosclerosis?
13. How is oxidation related to the development of atherosclerosis?
14. How are blood levels of LDLs and HDLs related to the risk of cardiovascular disease?
15. How much fat can be included in a healthy diet?
16. Do you think essential fatty acid deficiency is common in developed countries? Why or why not?
17. High intakes of what types of dietary fats increase the risk of heart disease?
18. What dietary components help reduce the risk of heart disease?

REFERENCES

1. Carroll, J., and Leung, S. U.S. consumption of french fries is sliding as diners opt for healthy. February 20, 2002. Available online at www.gsu.edu/~ecojxm/micro/articles/w0220021.htm accessed June 28, 2004.
2. Institute of Medicine, Food and Nutrition Board. *Dietary Reference Intakes for Energy, Carbohydrates, Fiber, Fat, Protein, and Amino Acids.* Washington, DC: National Academy Press, 2002.
3. Kris-Etherton, P. M., Harris, W. S., and Appel, L. J. Fish consumption, fish oil, omega-3 fatty acids, and cardiovascular disease. *Circulation* 106:2747–2752, 2002.
4. Kushi, L., and Giovannucci, E. Dietary fat and cancer. *Am. J. Med.* 113 (Suppl 9B): 63S–70S, 2002.
5. Alarcon de la Lastra, C., Barranco, M. D., Motilva, V., and Herrerias, J. M. Mediterranian diet and health. *Curr. Pharm. Des.* 7: 933–950, 2001.
6. American Heart Association. Heart Disease and Stroke Statistics: 2004 Update. Available online at www.americanheart.org/presenter.jhtml?identifier=3000333 accessed June 17, 2004.
7. National Cholesterol Education Program *Adult Treatment Panel III Report, 2001, 2004.* Available online at www.nhlbi.nih.gov/guidelines/cholesterol/atp3upd04.htm/accessed July 30, 2004.
8. Huff, M. W., Dietary cholesterol, cholesterol absorption, postprandial lipemia and atherosclerosis. *Can. J. Clin. Pharmacol.* 10 (Suppl A):26A–32A, 2003.
9. Ginsberg, H. N., and Karmally, W. Nutrition, lipids, and cardiovascular disease. In *Biochemical and Physiological Aspects of Human Nutrition.* M. H. Stipanuk, ed. Philadelphia: WB Saunders, 2000, 917–944.
10. Connor, W. E. Harbingers of coronary heart disease: dietary saturated fatty acids and cholesterol. Is chocolate benign because of its stearic acid content? *Am. J. Clin. Nutr.* 70:951–952, 1999.
11. Sacks, F. M., and Katan, M. Randomized clinical trials on the effects of dietary fat and carbohydrate on plasma lipoproteins and cardiovascular disease. *Am. J. Med.* 113:13S–24S, 2002.
12. Dietschy, J. M. Dietary fatty acids and the regulation of plasma low density lipoprotein cholesterol concentrations. *J. Nutr.* 128:444S–448S, 1998.
13. Lee, K. W., and Lip, G. Y. The role of omega-3 fatty acids in the secondary prevention of cardiovascular disease. *Q.J.M.* 96:465–480, 2003.
14. Ascherio, A., Rimm, E. B., Stampfer, M. J., et al. Marine ω-3 fatty acids, fish intake, and the risk of coronary disease among men. *N. Engl. J. Med.* 332:977–982, 1995.
15. Schoene, N. W., and Fitzgerald, G. A. Thrombogenic potential of dietary long-chain polyunsaturated fatty acids: session summary. *Am. J. Clin. Nutr.* 56(suppl):825S–826S, 1992.
16. Willett, W. C., Sacks, F., Trichopouluo, A., et al. Mediterranean diet pyramid: A cultural model for healthy eating. *Am. J. Clin. Nutr.* 61(suppl):1402S–1406S, 1995.
17. Kwiterovich, P. O. The effect of dietary fat, antioxidants and pro-oxidants on blood lipids, lipoproteins and atherosclerosis. *J. Am. Diet. Assoc.* 97(suppl): S231–S241, 1997.
18. American Heart Association. Homocysteine, Folic Acid and Cardiovascular Disease. Available online at 216.185.112.5/presenter.jhtml?identifier54677/accessed April 4, 2004.
19. Selhub, J., Jacques, P. F., Bostom A. G., et al. Relationship between plasma homocysteine and vitamin status in the Framingham study population. Impact of folic acid fortification. *Public Health Rev.* 28:117–1145, 2000.
20. Waterhouse, A. L., German, B. L., Walzem, R. L., et al. Is it time for a wine trial? *Am. J. Clin. Nutr.* 68:220–221, 1998.
21. American Institute for Cancer Research. The Diet and Cancer Link: Dietary Choices Play an Important Role in Reducing Cancer. Available online at www.aicr.org/diet.html/accessed June 28, 2004.
22. Voorrips, L. E., Brants, H. A., Kardinaal, A. F., et al. Intake of conjugated linoleic acid, fat and other fatty acids in relation to post menopausal breast cancer: the Netherlands Study on Diet and Cancer. *Am. J. Clin. Nutr.* 76:873–882, 2002.
23. Willett, W.C., and Leibel, R.L. Dietary fat is not a major determinant of body fat. *Am. J. Med.* 113:47S–59S, 2002.
24. Centers for Disease Control and Prevention. Trends in intake of energy and macronutrients—United States, 1971–2000. *MMWR* 53:80–82, 2004. Available online at www.cdc.gov/mmwr/preview/mmwrhtml/mm5304a3.htm/accessed June 22, 2004.
25. Revealing trans fats. *FDA Consumer* Sept/Oct, 37:20–26, 2003.
26. American Academy of Pediatrics Committee on Nutrition. Statement on cholesterol. *Pediatrics* 101:141–147, 1998.
27. American Dietetic Association. Position of the American Dietetic Association: Fat replacers. *J. Am. Diet. Assoc.* 98:463–468, 1998.

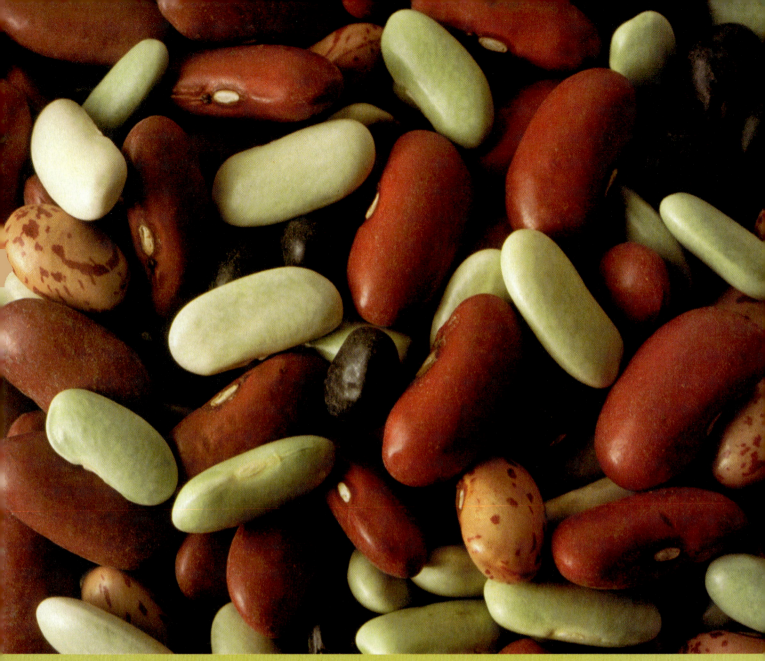

(Isabelle Rozenbaum/Age Fotostock America, Inc.)

CHAPTER 6 CONCEPTS

- Both plant and animal foods provide protein.
- Proteins are made up of chains of amino acids folded into three-dimensional shapes.
- Amino acids that cannot be made by the body in amounts sufficient to meet needs are essential in the diet.
- Amino acids can be used to synthesize body proteins, to make nonprotein molecules, and to provide energy.
- Protein is necessary to allow for growth as well as to maintain structure and regulate functions in the body.
- Animal sources of protein are generally of higher quality than plant sources.
- Plant sources of protein can meet needs if complementary proteins are chosen.
- Well-planned vegetarian diets can meet nutrient needs and promote health.

Just A Taste

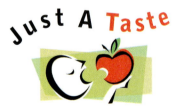

Are high-protein diets unhealthy?

Does eating extra protein make your muscles bigger?

Do you need protein supplements?

Can you stay healthy eating a vegetarian diet?

Proteins and Amino Acids

6

INTRODUCTION

Bicycling Magazine

Meatless Power
Carnivores May Be King of the Jungle,
but Veggie Lovers Can Rule the Road

By *Selene Yeager*

April 2003—Back in the day, bleu steak (so raw it's almost squirming) was a staple of the pro-cycling diet. But just as more Americans have embraced vegetarianism, so have more cyclists.

"Vegetarians tend to have lower body-mass indexes, lower cancer rates and lower cholesterol levels than meat-eaters," says Liz Applegate, Ph.D., consultant to the U.S. Olympic Cycling Team and author of the *Encyclopedia of Sports and Fitness Nutrition.* "They also tend to live longer. More athletes ask me questions about vegetarianism than any other diet topic. And they all want to know the same thing: Can I still ride as strong?"

Veggie-chowers such as six-time Ironman champ Dave Scott and Tour de France stage winner Sean Yates prove that you don't lose muscle when you go meatless. But you do have to eat smarter when you put the steak knife away.

For more information on this article, go to www.bicycling.com/article/0,5073,5921,00.html?category_id=363.

Do you need to eat muscle to build muscle? The power in the legs of these cyclists demonstrates that you don't. This is not to say protein isn't important. Evidence of its essentiality is seen in the sunken cheeks and swollen bellies of protein-deficient children around the world. But protein doesn't need to come from steaks and burgers. Peanut butter and tofu also provide protein. As this article tells us, athletes who avoid the flesh of animals can still cycle as fast and run as far as meat eaters.

Both Plant and Animal Foods Provide Protein

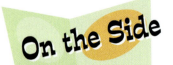

On the Side

Peanuts aren't nuts. They are legumes, which are members of the bean family and include all types of dried beans and peas as well as peanuts.

When we think of protein we usually think of a big steak, a plate of scrambled eggs, or a tall glass of milk. These animal foods provide the most concentrated sources of protein in our diet. One egg contains about 7 grams of protein, a cup of milk contains 8 grams, and a 3-ounce serving of meat provides over 20 grams (Figure 6.1). But plant foods such as grains and legumes are also important sources of dietary protein. Legumes, such as lentils, soybeans, peanuts, black-eyed peas, chickpeas, and dried beans, provide about 6 to 10 grams of protein per half-cup serving. Nuts and seeds provide about 5 to 10 grams per quarter cup. Even bread, rice, and pasta provide protein: about 2 to 3 grams per slice or half cup. Although most plant proteins are not used as efficiently as animal sources to build proteins in the human body, a diet including a variety of plant proteins can easily meet most people's needs.

Animal protein intake increases with prosperity

In the United States most people can afford to eat meat. About two-thirds of our dietary protein comes from meat, poultry, fish, eggs, dairy products, and other animal sources.[1] This is not the case in other parts of the world. Animal sources of protein are typically scarce in the diet of impoverished populations. These foods require more land and resources to produce and are more expensive to purchase. Instead, the developing world relies on plant foods such as grains and vegetables to meet protein needs. For example, in rural Mexico, most of the protein in the diet comes from beans, rice, and tortillas; in India, protein comes from lentils and rice; in China, rice with small amounts of meat and soy provides the protein. As the economic prosperity of a population grows, the proportion of animal foods in its diet typically increases. Since animal products are more concentrated sources of protein, as their intake increases so does the total amount of protein consumed in the diet. The typical American diet provides about 100 grams of protein a day, which is nearly twice what we actually need.

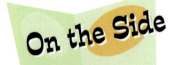

On the Side

For every 100 Calories of plant material a cow eats, only 10 Calories are stored in the cow and can be consumed by a person.

Different protein sources provide different combinations of nutrients

The source of the protein in your diet determines what other nutrients you consume along with it. Animal products provide B vitamins and minerals such as iron, zinc, and calcium. But animal products are low in fiber and are often high in saturated fat

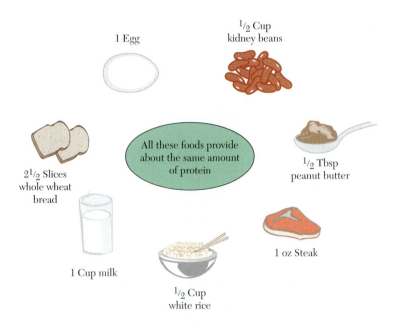

1 Egg

½ Cup kidney beans

2½ Slices whole wheat bread

All these foods provide about the same amount of protein

½ Tbsp peanut butter

1 Cup milk

½ Cup white rice

1 oz Steak

FIGURE 6.1

Each of these foods provides about the same amount of protein, although the animal proteins are used more efficiently by the body.

and cholesterol—a nutrient mix that increases the risk of heart disease. Plant sources of protein provide most but not all B vitamins, and also supply iron, zinc, and calcium but in less-absorbable forms. These foods also contain fiber, phytochemicals, and unsaturated fats—nutrients that should be increased in our diets to promote health. Recommendations for a healthy diet, such as the Dietary Guidelines and the Food Guide Pyramid, suggest that our diets be based on whole grain products, vegetables, and fruits and include smaller amounts of meats and dairy products. Following these guidelines will provide plenty of protein without an over-reliance on animal protein.

Proteins Are Made of Amino Acids

What do the proteins in a lamb chop, a kidney bean, and your thigh muscle have in common? They are all constructed of **amino acids** linked together in one or more folded, chainlike strands. There are approximately 20 amino acids commonly found in proteins. Each different protein contains a different number, combination and order of these amino acids. It is these differences that give specific proteins their unique functions in living organisms and unique characteristics in foods.

Amino acids The building blocks of proteins. Each contains a central carbon atom bound to a hydrogen atom, an amino group, an acid group, and a side chain.

Each amino acid has a unique structure

Each amino acid consists of a carbon atom bound to four chemical groups: a hydrogen atom; an amino group, which contains nitrogen; an acid group; and a fourth group called a side chain (Figure 6.2). The nitrogen in amino acids distinguishes protein from carbohydrate and fat; all three contain carbon, hydrogen, and oxygen, but only protein contains nitrogen. The side chains of amino acids vary in length and structure; they are what give different amino acids their different properties.

Some amino acids are essential in the diet

Nine of the amino acids needed by the adult human body must be consumed in the diet because they cannot be made in the body (Table 6.1). If the diet is deficient in one or more of these **essential** or **indispensable amino acids**, new proteins cannot be

Essential or **indispensable amino acids** Amino acids that cannot be synthesized by the human body in sufficient amounts to meet needs and therefore must be included in the diet.

TABLE 6.1
There are 20 Amino Acids in Proteins

Essential Amino Acids	Nonessential Amino Acids
Histidine	Alanine
Isoleucine	Arginine*
Leucine	Asparagine
Lysine	Aspartic acid (aspartate)
Methionine	Cysteine (cystine)*
Phenylalanine	Glutamic acid (glutamate)
Threonine	Glutamine*
Tryptophan	Glycine*
Valine	Proline*
	Serine
	Tyrosine*

*These amino acids are considered conditionally essential by the Institute of Medicine, Food and Nutrition Board (*Dietary Reference Intakes for Energy, Carbohydrates, Fiber, Fat, Protein and Amino Acids.* Washington, DC: National Academy Press, 2002).

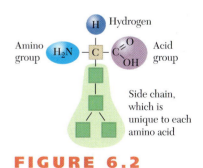

FIGURE 6.2

All amino acids have a similar structure, but each has a unique side chain.

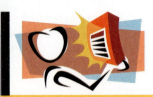

Off the Label: "Phenylketonurics: Contains Phenylalanine"

Did you ever read a can of diet soda? If you look closely you will see a warning that says "Phenylketonurics: Contains phenylalanine." Should you be worried? What's a phenylketonuric? A phenylketonuric is someone with a rare genetic disease called phenylketonuria (PKU), which prevents them from metabolizing the amino acid phenylalanine properly. If they eat foods high in this amino acid, compounds called phenylketones build up in their blood. High levels of these in infants and young children can interfere with brain development. High levels in pregnant women can cause mental retardation and other birth defects in their babies.[1]

PKU afflicts about 1 in 12,000 newborns.[2] Infants are tested for this disorder soon after birth because its symptoms can be prevented by a special low-phenylalanine diet. This diet must provide just enough of the essential amino acid phenylalanine to meet the body's needs but not so much that the buildup of phenylketones occurs. It must also provide sufficient tyrosine because people with PKU can't convert phenylalanine to tyrosine, so the conditionally essential amino acid tyrosine becomes an essential amino acid. There are special low-phenylalanine formulas for infants; children and adults must plan their diet carefully to limit protein, which is the source of most phenylalanine.

So why the warning on diet soda? It's not on milk cartons or packages of meat—foods that are high in proteins that contain phenylalanine. The reason is that someone with PKU would expect to find phenylalanine in any food containing protein, but they would not expect it in a can of diet soda. Diet sodas don't contain protein, but they do contain the artificial sweetener aspartame, which releases phenylalanine when it is broken down. The warning is included because soda is an unexpected source of phenylalanine, a compound that is harmless to most of us but can be hazardous to a phenylketonuric.

References
1. Brown, A. Barriers to control among pregnant women with phenylketonuria: United States 1998–2000. *MMWR Morb. Mortal Wkly. Rep.* February 15, 2002.
2. Seymour, C. A., Cockburn, F., Thomason, M. J., et al. Newborn screening for inborn errors of metabolism: A systematic review. *Health Technol. Assess.* I:1–95, 1997.

▲ **Conditionally essential amino acids** Amino acids that are essential in the diet only under certain conditions or at certain times of life.

▲ **Nonessential** or **dispensable amino acids** Amino acids that can be synthesized by the human body in sufficient amounts to meet needs.

made in the body without breaking down other body proteins to provide the needed amino acids. Some amino acids are **conditionally essential**, that is, they are essential only under certain conditions. For example, the amino acid tyrosine can be made in the body from the essential amino acid phenylalanine. As long as there is plenty of phenylalanine, tyrosine is nonessential. However, if there is not enough phenylalanine to make tyrosine, it becomes essential. Tyrosine is essential in the diets of individuals with the genetic disease phenylketonuria because their bodies are unable to convert phenylalanine to tyrosine.

The other amino acids commonly found in protein are **nonessential** or **dispensable amino acids** because they can be made in the human body. Most are made by a

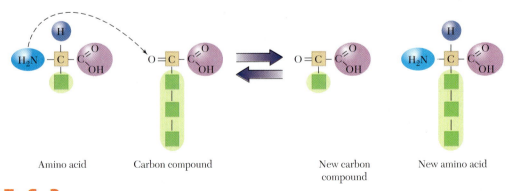

Amino acid   Carbon compound   New carbon compound   New amino acid

FIGURE 6.3

The process of transamination, transfers the amino group from a nonessential amino acid to a carbon compound to form a new amino acid and a new carbon compound.

process called **transamination**, which involves transferring the amino group from one amino acid to a carbon-containing molecule to form the needed amino acid (Figure 6.3).

★ **Transamination** The process by which an amino group from one amino acid is transferred to a carbon compound to form a new amino acid.

A protein's shape and function are determined by its amino acids

The amino acids in proteins are linked together by a chemical bond formed between the acid group of one amino acid and the nitrogen from the amino group of the next amino acid. This linkage is called a peptide bond. Two amino acids linked with a peptide bond are called a dipeptide; when three amino acids are linked, they form a tripeptide. Many amino acids bonded together constitute a polypeptide. A protein is made of one or more polypeptide chains folded into a three-dimensional shape (Figure 6.4).

The three-dimensional shape of a protein is determined by the amino acids it contains and the order in which they are linked together. Hair provides a simple example

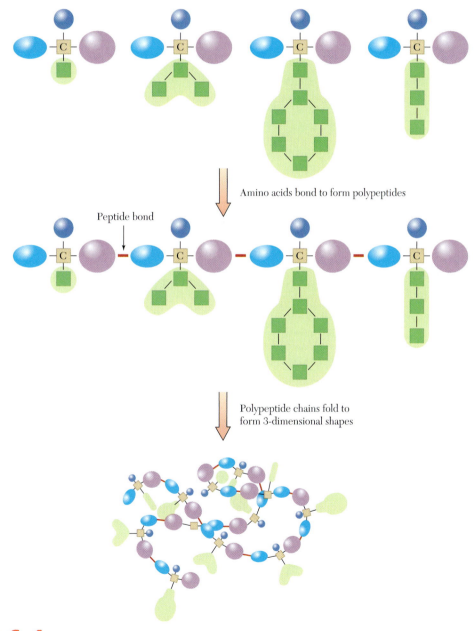

Amino acids bond to form polypeptides

Peptide bond

Polypeptide chains fold to form 3-dimensional shapes

FIGURE 6.4

When many amino acids are linked by peptide bonds, they form a polypeptide. When the polypeptide chains fold, the three-dimensional structure of a protein is created.

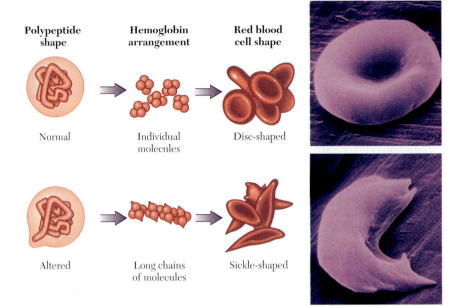

Polypeptide shape | Hemoglobin arrangement | Red blood cell shape

Normal — Individual molecules — Disc-shaped

Altered — Long chains of molecules — Sickle-shaped

FIGURE 6.5

In sickle-cell anemia, an abnormality in the sequence of amino acids in hemoglobin alters the shape and function of the protein molecule. Sickle-cell hemoglobin forms long chains that distort the shape of red blood cells. (Stan Fleger/Visuals Unlimited)

of how amino acids determine protein shape; interactions between the amino acids in the hair protein determine whether it is straight or curly. When the order of the amino acids in a protein changes, the protein's shape and function can be affected. For example, the disease sickle-cell anemia is caused by an abnormality in the amino acid sequence of the protein hemoglobin, which carries oxygen in the blood. The hemoglobin in a person with sickle-cell anemia has one amino acid that is different from normal hemoglobin. This one change causes the protein to fold differently, taking on a slightly different shape. These abnormally shaped hemoglobin molecules bind together, forming long chains and causing the red blood cells to take on a sickle shape (Figure 6.5). Sickle-shaped cells block capillaries, causing inflammation and pain. They also rupture easily, leading to a deficiency of red blood cells and a decreased ability to transport oxygen, which is called anemia.

The abnormality in sickle-cell hemoglobin is caused by an inherited error in the way hemoglobin is made, but the structure of a protein can also be altered after it is made, most often by environmental factors such as heat or acid. This change in structure is called **denaturation**, a change from the natural. When an egg is cooked, the heat denatures the protein. A raw egg white is clear and liquid, but once it has been denatured by cooking, it becomes white and firm and cannot be restored to its original form (Figure 6.6).

★ **Denaturation** The alteration of a protein's three-dimensional structure.

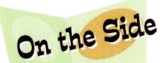

Mad cow disease is caused by a protein that is folded abnormally. This rogue protein is able to corrupt neighboring proteins by snuggling up against them and forcing them to change shape. The oddly folded proteins are not broken down normally, so they accumulate, forming clumps called plaques. These plaques damage nervous tissue, eventually killing the animal. For more information on mad cow disease, see Chapter 14.

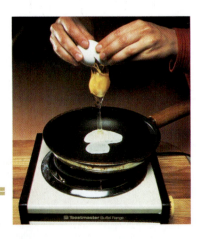

FIGURE 6.6

The protein in egg white is denatured by heat when the egg is cooked. (Charles D. Winters)

Proteins Must Be Digested to Be Absorbed

Like other nutrients, proteins must be digested before they can be absorbed into the body. Protein digestion begins in the acid environment of the stomach. Here, hydrochloric acid denatures proteins, opening up their folded structure to make the polypeptide chains more accessible to breakdown by enzymes. Stomach acid also activates the protein-digesting enzyme pepsin, which breaks some of the peptide bonds of the amino acid chains, leaving shorter polypeptides and amino acids. When the polypeptides enter the small intestine, they are broken into even smaller peptides and amino acids by protein-digesting enzymes produced by the pancreas and small intestine. Single amino acids, dipeptides, and tripeptides can be absorbed into the mucosal cells of the small intestine. Once inside these cells, dipeptides and tripeptides are broken into single amino acids (Figure 6.7).

Amino acids with similar structures compete for absorption

Amino acids enter your body by crossing from the lumen of the small intestine into the bloodstream. This is accomplished by one of several energy-requiring amino acid transport systems; amino acids with similar structures share the same transport system. Because of this, amino acids may compete with each other for absorption. If there is an excess of any one of the amino acids sharing a transport system, more of it will be absorbed, slowing the absorption of the other competing amino acids. This is generally not a concern when foods are eaten, because they contain a variety of amino acids and are not excessive in any one. However, if someone is taking an amino acid

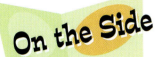

To observe protein denaturation first hand, add some lemon juice to a glass of milk. The acidic juice denatures the milk proteins, causing them to form white clumps that sink to the bottom of the glass. The same thing happens to the protein in your diet when it comes in contact with the acid in your stomach.

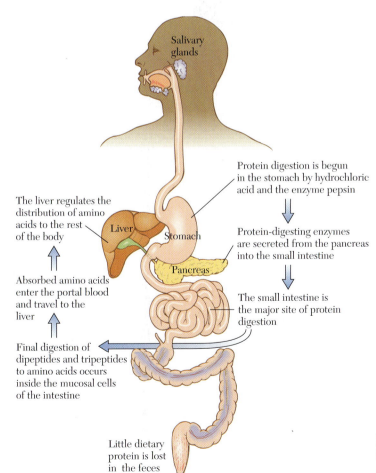

Salivary glands

The liver regulates the distribution of amino acids to the rest of the body

Liver

Stomach

Pancreas

Absorbed amino acids enter the portal blood and travel to the liver

Final digestion of dipeptides and tripeptides to amino acids occurs inside the mucosal cells of the intestine

Little dietary protein is lost in the feces

Protein digestion is begun in the stomach by hydrochloric acid and the enzyme pepsin

Protein-digesting enzymes are secreted from the pancreas into the small intestine

The small intestine is the major site of protein digestion

FIGURE 6.7

An overview of protein digestion and absorption.

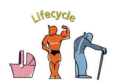

Amino acids that share the same transport system

Outside cell

Cell membrane

Inside cell

FIGURE 6.8

The amino acids in this figure share the same transport system, and since there are more of the purple ones than the green ones, more of the purple amino acids are able to cross the membrane into the cell.

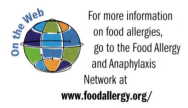

Severe allergic reactions to food are believed to cause about 30,000 trips to the hospital and between 150 and 200 deaths each year. There is no cure for a food allergy. The only way to avoid symptoms is to avoid the food.

For more information on food allergies, go to the Food Allergy and Anaphylaxis Network at **www.foodallergy.org/**

supplement, the supplemented amino acid hogs the transport system, and the absorption of other amino acids that share the same system may be impaired (Figure 6.8). For example, weight lifters often take supplements of the amino acid arginine. Because arginine shares a transport system with lysine, large doses of arginine can inhibit the absorption of lysine, upsetting the balance of amino acids in the body.

Absorption of protein fragments can cause allergies

Food allergies are triggered when a protein from the diet is absorbed without being completely digested. The proteins from milk, eggs, peanuts, tree nuts, wheat, soy, fish, and shellfish are common causes of food allergies. The first time the protein is consumed and a piece of it is absorbed intact, it stimulates the immune system. When the protein is consumed again, the immune system sees it as a foreign substance and mounts an attack, causing an allergic reaction. Allergic reactions to food can cause symptoms throughout the body. These can involve the digestive system, causing vomiting or diarrhea; the skin, causing a rash or hives; the respiratory tract, causing difficulty breathing; or the cardiovascular system, causing a drop in blood pressure. Reactions that are rapid and severe and involve more than one part of the body are called anaphylaxis and can be fatal. A severe anaphylactic reaction can cause breathing difficulty or a dangerous drop in blood pressure (see Chapter 3, Your Choice: When Food is the Foe).

Allergies commonly develop in infants because their gastrointestinal tracts and immune systems are immature. Once an infant's intestines mature, absorption of whole proteins is less likely and food allergies are sometimes outgrown. The absorption of whole proteins by very young infants, however, is also beneficial since antibody proteins absorbed from breast milk can provide temporary protection against certain diseases (see Chapter 12).

The Protein We Eat Provides Amino Acids to the Body

The protein in our diet provides us with amino acids. Once inside the body, amino acids provide the raw material needed to make all the various types of proteins we need. They are also used to make other nitrogen-containing molecules and, in some cases, to produce energy.

Amino acids are the building blocks of proteins

The amino acids available for protein synthesis come from those we consume in foods and those released by the breakdown of body proteins. All of the amino acids available to the body, including those present in tissues and body fluids, are referred to collec-

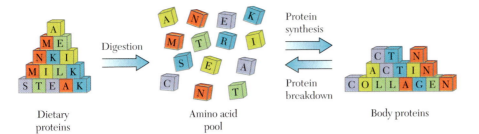

Dietary proteins   Amino acid pool   Body proteins

FIGURE 6.9

Amino acids can literally be thought of as building blocks. Protein consumed in the diet and body proteins that are broken down supply these building blocks to the amino acid pool. They are then used to construct new body proteins.

Amino acid pool All of the amino acids in body tissues and fluids that are available for protein synthesis.

tively as the body **amino acid pool**. Of the approximately 300 grams of protein synthesized by the body each day, only about 100 grams are made from amino acids consumed in the diet. The other 200 grams are made from amino acids recycled from protein broken down in the body (Figure 6.9).

DNA provides the instructions for making proteins The instructions that dictate which amino acids are needed and in what order they should be combined to produce a protein are contained in stretches of DNA called **genes**. When a protein is needed, the process of protein synthesis is turned on, and this information is used to make the necessary protein.

The first step in protein synthesis involves transferring, or transcribing, the blueprint or code for the protein from the gene into a molecule of messenger RNA (mRNA) (Figure 6.10). The mRNA then takes this information from the nucleus of the cell, where the gene is located, to ribosomes in the cytoplasm of the cell, where the protein is made. Here the information in mRNA is translated via another type of RNA, called transfer RNA (tRNA). Transfer RNA reads the code and delivers the needed amino acids to the ribosomes. Here the polypeptide chains that make up a protein are assembled.

Gene A length of DNA that codes for the synthesis of a protein.

Protein synthesis is carefully regulated Which body proteins are made is carefully regulated by the turning on and turning off of the genes that code for proteins. When a gene is turned on the protein is made, and the gene is said to be expressed. Not all genes are expressed in all cells or at all times, and therefore only

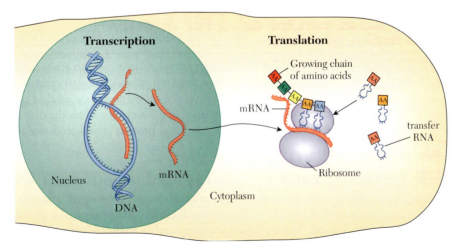

FIGURE 6.10

DNA in the nucleus of cells provides a blueprint for the sequence of amino acids in proteins. In the process of transcription, the information in DNA is copied into a strand of mRNA. The mRNA leaves the nucleus and travels to the cytoplasm, where it binds to a ribosome where translation occurs. Transfer RNA molecules in the cytoplasm collect amino acids and deliver them to the mRNA strand. The sequence in the mRNA dictates which transfer RNA will bind, and hence which amino acid, will be added to the growing amino acid strand. As each amino acid is added, its transfer RNA is released to collect another amino acid. As the strand grows, the ribosome moves along the mRNA to read the next part of the code.

The most abundant protein in the body is collagen; it holds cells together and forms the protein framework of bones and teeth. Protein also provides structure to individual cells; it is found in membranes, fluids, and organelles.

When the diet is deficient in protein, protein-based structures break down. The muscles become smaller, the skin loses its elasticity, and the hair becomes thin and can easily be pulled out by the roots. These outward signs of dietary protein deficiency have become marketing strategies for cosmetic companies. Shampoo and hand lotion manufacturers add protein to their products, suggesting that protein applied to the hair or skin will improve its structure. However, the proteins that make up hair and skin and other body structures can be made only inside the body, so a healthy diet will do more for hair and skin quality than expensive protein shampoos or lotions.

Enzyme proteins speed up metabolic reactions

The chemical reactions that break down molecules to produce energy and build molecules needed by the body require the help of enzymes. Enzymes are proteins that speed up metabolic reactions but are not used up or destroyed in the process. Without enzymes, metabolic reactions would occur too slowly to support life. Each of the reactions involved in the production of ATP and the synthesis and breakdown of carbohydrates, lipids, and proteins requires a specific enzyme with a specific structure. If the structure of the enzyme molecule is changed, it can no longer function in the reaction it is designed to accelerate.

Enzymes that function in the body are made by the body and therefore do not need to be consumed in the diet. The enzymes that we do consume in foods are broken down during digestion and are absorbed from the gastrointestinal tract as amino acids. Purified enzymes sold as dietary supplements are also broken down in the gut. These may provide some function before they are broken down. For example, people with lactose intolerance often take lactase, the enzyme that breaks down milk sugar. Lactase supplements break down lactose that is consumed while the lactase is in the gut. Eventually, these enzymes are also digested and absorbed as amino acids.

Proteins transport molecules throughout our body

Transport proteins act as shuttles. In the blood they carry substances from one organ to another. For example, hemoglobin, the protein that gives red blood cells their red color, picks up oxygen in the lungs and transports it to other organs of the body. The proteins in lipoproteins are needed to transport lipids from the intestines and liver to body cells. Some vitamins, such as vitamin A, require specific proteins to be transported in the blood. When protein is deficient, the vitamin A transport protein is not available and tissues become deficient in vitamin A even if it is consumed in the diet. For this reason, a protein deficiency can cause a vitamin A deficiency.

Some transport proteins shuttle substances across cell membranes to get them into and out of individual cells. For instance, proteins are needed to move glucose across the cell membrane. Transport proteins in the intestinal mucosa are needed to absorb amino acids from the intestinal lumen.

Proteins protect us from injury and infection

Proteins are an important part of the body's defense mechanisms. Skin, which is made up primarily of protein, is the first barrier against infection and injury. Foreign particles such as dirt or bacteria that are on the skin cannot enter the body and can be washed away. If the skin is broken and blood vessels are injured, blood-clotting proteins help prevent too much blood from being lost. If a foreign particle such as a virus or bacterium enters the body, the immune system fights it off by synthesizing proteins called **antibodies**. Each antibody has a unique structure that allows it to attach to a specific invader. When an antibody binds to an invading substance, the production of more of the same type of antibody is stimulated, and other parts of the immune sys-

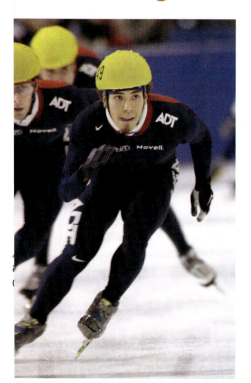

FIGURE 6.12

The extra muscle protein in Apollo Ohno's thigh muscles gives them extra size and strength and helped him to win gold in the 2002 Winter Olympics. (© AP/Wide World Photos)

✳ Remember

To be transported in the bloodstream, water-insoluble lipids must be packaged with protein as lipoproteins. The lipoprotein particles have a water-soluble envelope and can be transported in the blood. This is discussed in Chapter 5.

▲ Antibodies Proteins produced by cells of the immune system that destroy or inactivate foreign substances in the body.

tem are signaled to help destroy the invader. The next time the same type of invading bacterium or virus enters the body, the immune system is already primed to produce specific antibodies to fight off the infection. This is also how immunizations against diseases, such as measles, work. A small amount of dead or inactivated virus is injected into the body; the injected material does not cause disease, but it does stimulate the immune system to produce antibodies to the virus. When the body comes in contact with the live virus, a large-scale immune attack is mounted and the infection is prevented. When the immune system malfunctions as a result of protein deficiency or other causes, such as HIV infection, the ability to protect the body from infection is compromised.

Proteins help us move

Some proteins give cells and organisms the ability to move, contract, and change shape. When you climb a flight of stairs, walk across the room, or run around the block, you are relying on the muscle proteins actin and myosin. These two proteins slide past each other to shorten the muscle and cause contraction (Figure 6.13). A similar process causes contraction in the heart muscle and in the muscles of the digestive tract, blood vessels, and body glands. Actin and myosin can also cause contraction in non-muscle cells. This contraction helps individual cells, such as white blood cells of the immune system, change shape and move. The energy for contraction comes from ATP, which is derived primarily from the metabolism of carbohydrate and fat.

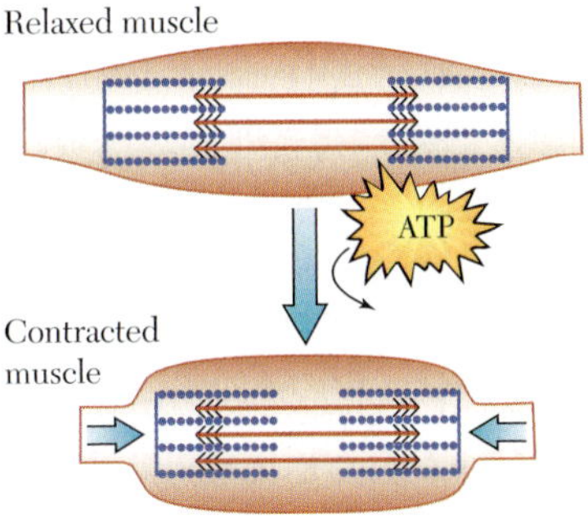

Some hormones are proteins

Hormones are chemical messengers that are secreted into the blood by one tissue or organ and act on target cells in other parts of the body. Hormones made from cholesterol are steroid hormones; those made of amino acids are classified as protein or peptide hormones. Insulin and glucagon are protein hormones involved in maintaining a steady level of blood glucose.

Proteins help regulate fluid balance

The distribution of fluids in body cells, in the bloodstream, and in the spaces between cells is important for homeostasis. Fluid moves back and forth across membranes to maintain appropriate concentrations of particles and fluids inside and outside cells and tissues (see Chapter 9). Proteins help regulate this fluid balance in two ways. First, protein transporters located in cell membranes pump particles from one side of a membrane to another. Fluid then follows to keep the concentration of particles equal. Second, large protein molecules present in the blood keep fluid in the blood, both by preventing it from being forced into tissues and by attracting fluid in tissues back into blood vessels.

Proteins help regulate acidity

The chemical reactions of metabolism require a specific level of acidity, or **pH**, to function properly. In the gastrointestinal tract, acid levels vary widely. The digestive enzyme pepsin works best in the acid environment of the stomach, whereas the pancreatic enzymes operate best in the more neutral environment of the small intestine. Inside the body, pH must be maintained at a relatively neutral level in order to allow metabolic reactions to proceed normally. If the pH changes, these reactions slow or stop. For instance, during strenuous exercise, lactic acid builds up in the muscles, making them more acidic. The increased acidity makes the metabolic reactions needed to fuel activity less efficient and contributes to fatigue (see Chapter 11). Proteins both within cells and in the blood help prevent large changes in acidity. For instance, the protein hemoglobin in red blood cells helps neutralize acid produced when carbon dioxide, a waste product of cellular respiration, reacts with water.

Relaxed muscle

ATP

Contracted muscle

FIGURE 6.13

The proteins actin and myosin cause muscles to contract. They use the energy in ATP to slide past each other and shorten the muscle.

On the Side

Genes code for the synthesis of specific proteins. By cutting the gene for the hormone insulin out of human cells and pasting it into bacterial cells, genetic engineers are able to make bacteria that produce human insulin. More than 80% of people with diabetes who inject insulin use a genetically engineered form. Before genetically engineered insulin was available, the major source of insulin was the pancreases of slaughtered pigs.

 pH A measure of acidity.

Adequate Protein Is Essential to Health

We need to eat protein to stay healthy. If we don't eat enough, body proteins that are broken down each day can't be replaced. The consequences of too little protein can be dramatic and devastating. But is there such a thing as too much protein? We plan our meals around meat, buy high-protein bars, and drink protein-rich shakes and smoothies. Do we need all this protein to stay healthy?

Protein deficiency is a world health problem

Although protein deficiency is uncommon in the United States and other developed nations, in developing countries it is a serious public health problem. Usually, protein deficiency occurs with a general lack of food and nutrients, but if the diet is extremely limited or protein needs are high as they are in young children, a pure protein deficiency can occur. The term **protein-energy malnutrition (PEM)** is used to refer to the continuum of conditions ranging from pure protein deficiency, called **kwashiorkor**, to energy deficiency, called **marasmus**.

Kwashiorkor is a deficiency of protein Kwashiorkor is typically a disease of children. The word "kwashiorkor" comes from the Ga tribe of the African Gold Coast. It means the disease that the first child gets when a second child is born.[2] When the new baby is born, the older child is no longer breast-fed. Rather than receiving protein-rich breast milk, the young child is fed a watered-down version of the diet eaten by the rest of the family. This diet is low in protein and is often high in fiber and difficult to digest. The child, even if able to get adequate energy, is not able to eat a large enough quantity to get adequate protein. Because children are growing, their protein needs per unit of body weight are higher than those of adults, and the effects of a deficiency become evident much more quickly.

The symptoms of kwashiorkor can be explained by examining the roles that proteins play in the body. Because protein is needed for the synthesis of new tissue, growth in both height and weight are hampered. Because proteins are important in immune function, there is an increased susceptibility to infection. There are changes in hair color because the pigment melanin is not made, and the skin flakes because structural proteins are not available to provide elasticity and support. Cells lining the digestive tract die and cannot be replaced, so nutrient absorption is impaired. The bloated belly typical of this condition is a result of both fat accumulating in the liver because there is not enough protein to transport it and fluid accumulating in the abdomen because there is not enough protein to keep fluid in the blood (Figure 6.14a).

★ Protein-energy malnutrition (PEM) A condition characterized by wasting and an increased susceptibility to infection that results from the long-term consumption of insufficient amounts of energy and protein to meet needs.

★ Kwashiorkor A form of protein-energy malnutrition in which only protein is deficient.

★ Marasmus A form of protein-energy malnutrition in which a deficiency of energy in the diet causes severe body wasting.

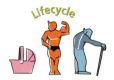
Lifecycle

On the Web
For more information on protein-energy malnutrition, and other world nutrition health issues, go to the World Health Organization at **www.who.int/nut/**

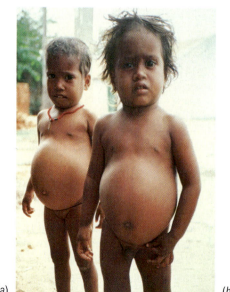
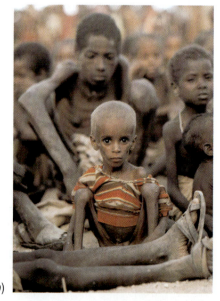

(a)   (b)

FIGURE 6.14

Kwashiorkor (a) is characterized by a bloated belly, whereas marasmus (b) presents as severe wasting. Most protein-energy malnutrition is a combination of the two (a: Courtesy Food and Agriculture Organization of the United Nations; b: Peter Turnley/Corbis Images)

Kwashiorkor occurs most commonly in Africa, South and Central America, the Near East, and the Far East. It has also been reported in poverty-stricken areas in the United States. Although kwashiorkor is typically a disease of children, it is seen in hospitalized adults who have high protein needs due to infection or trauma and a low protein intake because they are unable to eat.

Marasmus is a deficiency of calories and protein At the other end of the continuum of protein-energy malnutrition is marasmus, meaning to waste away. Marasmus is due to starvation; the diet doesn't supply enough calories or nutrients to meet needs. Marasmus may have some of the same symptoms as kwashiorkor, but there are also differences. In kwashiorkor, some fat stores are retained, since energy intake is adequate. In marasmus, individuals appear emaciated because their body fat stores have been depleted to provide energy (Figure 6.14b). Ketosis may occur in marasmus because fat is a major energy source and carbohydrate is limited. This is not so in kwashiorkor because carbohydrate intake is adequate; only protein is deficient.

Marasmus occurs in individuals of all ages. It has devastating effects in infants because most brain growth takes place in the first year of life; malnutrition in the first year of life causes decreases in intelligence and learning ability that persist throughout life. Marasmus often occurs in children who are fed diluted infant formula prepared by caregivers trying to stretch limited supplies. It occurs less often in breast-fed infants.

Too much protein may cause health problems

Adequate protein intake is absolutely essential to life. But consuming too much protein may also cause problems. Are all those high-protein dieters putting their health at risk? For a healthy person there are no short-term problems associated with consuming a diet very high in protein, but we are still investigating whether the same is true in the long term.

As protein intake increases above the amount needed, so does the production of protein-breakdown products, such as urea, which must be eliminated from the body by the kidneys. To do this, more water must be added to the urine. High-protein diets therefore increase water loss. Although not a concern for most people, this can be a problem if the kidneys are not able to concentrate urine. For example, the immature kidneys of newborn infants are not able to concentrate urine and therefore excrete more water than adults. Feeding a newborn infant formula that is too high in protein can increase fluid losses and lead to dehydration. High-protein diets are also a risk for people with kidney disease. The increased wastes produced by a high protein diet may speed the progression of renal failure in these individuals.[3] Despite this, there is little evidence that a high-protein diet will precipitate kidney disease in a healthy person.[5]

Increasing the amount of protein in the diet increases the excretion of calcium in the urine. This has led to speculation that high-protein diets may increase the risk of kidney stones and cause bone loss. High intakes of animal protein have been shown to increase the risk of kidney stones, but protein intake is not the only factor affecting risk, so further investigation is needed before conclusions can be drawn. High protein diets increase calcium loss in the urine, but this is probably not a concern because high-protein diets are also high in calcium, and bone loss does not occur as long as calcium intake is adequate.[5] Poor protein status rather than too much protein is probably more of a risk for bone loss.

Another concern with high-protein diets is related more to the rest of the diet than to the amount of protein. Typically, high-protein diets are also high in animal products; this dietary pattern is high in saturated fat and cholesterol and low in fiber and therefore increases the risk of heart disease. These diets are also typically low in grains, vegetables, and fruits, a pattern associated with a greater risk of cancer.[4] Such diets are also usually high in energy and total fat, which may promote excess weight gain.

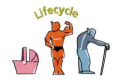

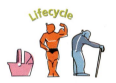

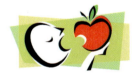

If followed for a short period of time, such as a few weeks, high-protein diets are not dangerous for healthy people. There is little information on the safety of these diets for longer periods of time. If you wish to consume a high-protein diet for longer, it should include sources of unrefined carbohydrates such as whole grains, vegetables, and fruits, and the animal sources of proteins should be from lean meats and low-fat dairy products.

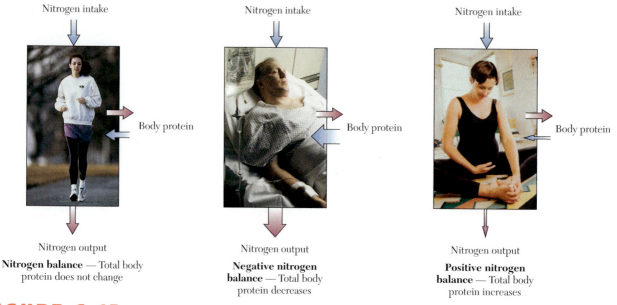

Nitrogen intake

Body protein

Nitrogen output

Nitrogen balance — Total body protein does not change

Nitrogen intake

Body protein

Nitrogen output

Negative nitrogen balance — Total body protein decreases

Nitrogen intake

Body protein

Nitrogen output

Positive nitrogen balance — Total body protein increases

FIGURE 6.15

In nitrogen balance, nitrogen intake is equal to the nitrogen output; in negative nitrogen balance, output exceeds intake because more body proteins are broken down than synthesized and the nitrogen is excreted; in positive nitrogen balance, intake exceeds output because more protein is used to synthesize body proteins than is lost from protein breakdown. (*Left*: Dennis Drenner; *center*: Brian Yarvin/Photo Researchers; *right*: Donna Day/Stone/Getty Images)

Protein Intake Must Balance Protein Losses

In order to stay healthy, you have to eat enough protein to replace the amount you use. Unlike other nutrients, the amount of protein you use can be estimated fairly accurately. This is because protein is the major source of nitrogen in the diet. And when body proteins are used and broken down, the nitrogen is excreted, primarily in urine. Therefore, comparing the amount of nitrogen you consume with the amount you excrete can be used to estimate how much protein your body is using. If your nitrogen intake equals your nitrogen excretion, it indicates that you are consuming enough protein to balance losses. Any excess dietary protein is simply broken down and used for energy; the nitrogen is removed and excreted. In this situation you are said to be in nitrogen balance. You are not gaining or losing body protein; you are just maintaining your body. If you are excreting more nitrogen than you consume, this extra nitrogen has come from body protein that has been broken down to meet needs. This situation is called negative nitrogen balance; protein is being lost from your body. It occurs due to injury or illness as well as when you are consuming a low-protein or low-calorie diet. Other conditions cause your body to excrete less nitrogen than you consume. This positive nitrogen balance occurs when your body is gaining protein. For example, when you grow, your body is adding protein as it builds new muscle, bone, and skin. Nitrogen balance is also positive during pregnancy and in individuals who are body-building to increase muscle mass (Figure 6.15).

Although these measures of nitrogen balance are accurate, it is impractical to assess each person's protein needs this way; therefore, the Dietary Reference Intakes (DRIs) include several types of recommendations for protein intake.[5]

The RDA is small compared to what we eat

Most of us eat more protein than we need: A typical American diet contains about 100 grams of protein. The RDA for protein for adults is 0.8 gram per kilogram of body weight.[6] For a person weighing 70 kilograms (154 pounds) the RDA is 56 grams of protein per day (Table 6.2). This recommendation is expressed per unit of body

TABLE 6.2
How Much Protein Do You Need?

First, find your body weight in kilograms:
   weight in kilograms = weight in pounds ÷ 2.2 pounds
Next, look up your RDA for protein:

Gender or condition	Age (years)	RDA (g/kg)
Male or female	0–0.5	1.52 (AI value)
	0.5–1	1.5
	1–3	1.1
	4–8	0.95
	9–13	0.95
	14–18	0.85
	≥19	0.8
Pregnancy		Nonpregnant RDA + 25 g/day
Lactation	first 6 months	Nonlactation RDA + 25 g/day

Now, do the math: Multiply your weight in kilograms by your RDA.
For example, a 23-year-old female weighing 68 kg would require 68 kg ×
0.8 g/kg = 54.4 grams of protein.

weight because protein is needed to maintain and repair the body. The more a person weighs, the more protein they need for these purposes.

RDAs have also been developed for each of the essential amino acids; these are not a concern in a typical diet but are important when developing solutions for intravenous feeding.

Protein needs are increased by growth To grow you must synthesize new body proteins. During the first year of life, growth is rapid, so a large amount of protein is required. Thus, an AI for the first 6 months of life has been set at 1.52 grams per kilogram of body weight per day; for the second 6 months, the RDA is 1.5 grams per kilogram. As the growth rate slows, requirements per unit of body weight decrease but continue to be greater than adult requirements until 19 years of age.

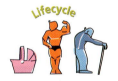

Lifecycle

During pregnancy both the mother and her unborn baby are growing. The mother's diet must supply enough protein to provide for the expansion of her blood volume, enlargement of her uterus and breasts, development of the placenta, and growth and development of the fetus. The RDA for pregnant women is 25 grams of protein per day higher than the nonpregnant recommendation. Most women in North America already consume this much protein in their typical diets.

Protein needs are also increased during lactation. The woman's body is not growing, but she is producing breast milk. The body needs protein to produce this high-protein fluid. The RDA during lactation is also 25 grams greater than that for a nonlactating woman per day.

Protein needs are increased by illness and injury Extreme stresses on the body such as infections, fevers, burns, or surgery increase protein breakdown. For the body to heal and rebuild, these losses must be replaced by dietary protein. The extra amount needed for healing depends on the injury. A severe infection may increase needs by about 30%, whereas a serious burn can increase requirements by 200 to 400%.

Protein needs are increased by some types of exercise Do athletes need more protein than the rest of us? If you base your answer on the number of high-protein beverages and amino acid supplements marketed to athletes, it might be yes. In fact, most athletes can meet their protein needs by consuming the RDA of 0.8 gram per kilogram of body weight. Only endurance athletes and strength athletes

SUMMARY

1. Dietary protein comes from both animal and plant sources. More prosperous populations usually consume more animal protein sources. These tend to be higher in iron, zinc, and calcium as well as saturated fat and cholesterol. Plant sources of protein are higher in unsaturated fat, fiber, and phytochemicals.

2. Amino acids are the building blocks from which proteins are made. The amino acids that the body is unable to make in sufficient amounts are called essential amino acids and must be consumed in the diet. Proteins are made of amino acid chains that fold over on themselves to create unique three-dimensional structures. The shape of a protein determines its function.

3. Amino acids, from the diet and the body, are used by cells to synthesize proteins according to instructions provided by DNA. Amino acids can also be used for energy and to synthesize glucose and non-protein molecules that contain nitrogen.

4. Digestion breaks dietary protein into small peptides and amino acids that can be absorbed. Amino acids that share the same transport system compete for absorption, so an excess of one can inhibit the absorption of another. If absorbed without being digested, proteins can cause food allergies.

5. In the body, protein molecules form structures, regulate body functions, transport molecules through the blood and in and out of cells, function in the immune system, and aid in muscle contraction, fluid balance, and acid balance.

6. Protein-energy malnutrition is a health concern, primarily in developing countries. Kwashiorkor occurs when the protein content of the diet is deficient but energy is adequate. It is most common in children. Marasmus occurs when total energy intake is deficient.

7. Protein requirements are determined by looking at the amount of nitrogen consumed as dietary protein and the amount excreted as protein waste products. For healthy adults, the RDA for protein is 0.8 gram per kilogram of body weight. Growth, pregnancy, lactation, illness, injury, and certain types of physical exercise can increase requirements. Recommendations for a healthy diet are to ingest 10 to 35% of calories from protein.

8. Animal proteins are considered high-quality complete proteins because their amino acid composition matches that needed to make body proteins. Plant proteins are limited in one or more of the amino acids needed to make body protein; therefore, they are considered incomplete proteins.

9. Vegetarian diets that include little or no animal protein can provide adequate protein if the sources of protein are complemented to supply enough of all the essential amino acids. Vegetarian diets are lower in saturated fat and cholesterol and higher in fiber, certain vitamins and minerals, antioxidants, and phytochemicals than meat-based diets. People consuming vegan diets must plan their diets carefully to meet their needs for vitamin B_{12}, calcium, vitamin D, iron, zinc, and omega-3 fatty acids.

REVIEW QUESTIONS

1. List some good dietary sources of animal protein and plant protein. Are these foods high in fat? How about fiber?
2. What are amino acids?
3. What is an essential amino acid?
4. What molecules contain the information needed to make a protein?
5. Describe the general structure of a protein.
6. List six functions provided by proteins in the body.
7. Why is protein deficiency most common in infants and children?
8. How does the typical protein intake in North America compare to recommendations?
9. What effect does moderate exercise have on protein needs?
10. What is protein quality?
11. What is protein complementation?
12. List three pairs of complementary protein sources.
13. Do vegans need to take vitamin supplements?

REFERENCES

1. Smit, E., Nieto, F. J., Crespo, C. J., and Mitchell, P. Estimates of animal and plant protein intake in U.S. adults: Results from the Third National Health and Nutrition Examination Survey, 1988–1991. *J. Am. Diet. Assoc.* 99:813–820, 1999.
2. Williams, C. D. Kwashiorkor: Nutritional disease of children associated with maize diet. *Lancet* 2:1151–1154, 1935.
3. Alebiosu, C. O. An update on 'progression promoters' in renal diseases. *J. Natl. Med. Assoc.* 95:30–42, 2003.
4. van't Veer, P., Jansen, M. C., Klerk, M., and Kok, F. J. Fruits and vegetables in the prevention of cancer and cardiovascular disease. *Public Health Nutr.* 3:103–107, 2000.
5. Institute of Medicine, Food and Nutrition Board. *Dietary Reference*

Intakes for Energy, Carbohydrates, Fiber, Fat, Protein and Amino Acids. Washington, DC: National Academy Press, 2002.

6. American Dietetic Association. Nutrition and athletic performance: Position of the American Dietetic Association, the Canadian Dietetic Association and the American College of Sports Medicine. *J. Am. Diet. Assoc.* 100:1543–1556, 2000.

7. Fuller, M.F. Protein and amino acid requirements. In *Biochemical and Physiological Aspects of Human Nutrition.* Stipanik, M.H., ed. Philadelphia: WB Saunders, 2000: 287–304.

8. American Dietetic Association. Position of the American Dietetic Association and Dietitians of Canada: Vegetarian diets. *J. Am. Diet. Assoc.* 103:748–765, 2003.

9. Messina, V., Melina, V., and Mangels, A.R. A new food guide for North American vegetarians *J. Am. Diet. Assoc.* 103: 771–775, 2003.

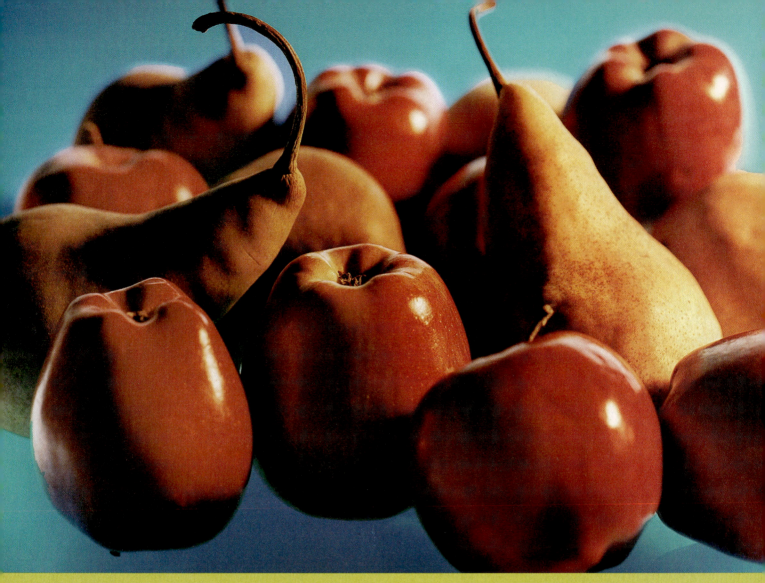

(©Johner/Phototonica)

CHAPTER 7 CONCEPTS

- More than half of the adults in the United States weigh more than is healthy.
- Keeping body weight healthy requires balancing calorie intake with calorie expenditure.
- The energy you obtain from food is used to keep you alive and moving and to process food.
- Energy consumed in excess of needs is stored as fat; this stored fat is used when you eat fewer calories than you burn.
- Genetics affect your propensity for storing excess body fat, but your food intake and activity level determine what you actually weigh.
- The goal of weight management is to reduce body fat to a healthy level and maintain that level throughout life.
- Weight loss requires reducing food intake and increasing activity; maintaining weight loss requires a permanent change in eating and exercise habits.
- Eating disorders are psychological disorders that involve abnormal eating behaviors in response to an excessive concern with body size and weight.

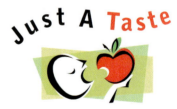

Just A Taste

Do overweight people eat more than thin people?

Is obesity inherited?

Can we stop the obesity epidemic?

Can an eating disorder be life-threatening?

Managing Your Weight

7

INTRODUCTION

The Washington Post

Is Obesity a Disease?
Insurance, Drug Access May Hinge on Answer

By *Rob Stein, Staff Writer*

Monday, Nov. 10, 2003—The rising number of Americans who are seriously overweight has triggered intense debate among scientists, advocacy groups, federal agencies, insurance companies and drug makers about whether obesity should be declared a "disease," a move that could open up insurance coverage to millions who need treatment for weight problems and could speed the approval of new diet drugs.

To read the entire article, go to www.washingtonpost.com.

ancer, diabetes, and atherosclerosis are diseases. How could weighing too much be a disease? Isn't it simply the result of eating too much and exercising too little? Some feel obesity fits the definition of a disease because it is a condition that affects health in a negative way, but many argue that it is really a risk factor, like smoking or high blood cholesterol, that predisposes to illness but is not itself a disease. Whether or not it is a disease, the health consequences of being obese are serious. Carrying excess body fat increases the risk of other health problems, shortens life expectancy, and increases health care costs. About 400,000 people die each year in the United States from obesity-related diseases.[1] Weight-related health problems are now second only to tobacco use as the leading cause of preventable death in the United States.[2] Estimates suggest that obesity costs about $99.2 billion—more than the health-care costs incurred by daily smokers and heavy drinkers.[3] The more people who are obese, the higher the nation's health care expenses and the cost to society as a whole in terms of lost wages and productivity. To solve the obesity problem, we need to understand why so many of us are overweight and what we can do to change this trend.

We Are in the Midst of an Obesity Epidemic

⚹ Overweight A condition in which body mass index is 25 to 29.9 kg/m².

⚹ Obesity A condition characterized by excess body fat. It is defined as a Body Mass Index of 30 kg/m² or greater.

In 1960, 13.4% of adults were obese; in 1991, 23% were obese; and now, a decade later, 31% are obese (Figure 7.1). The dramatic rise in the incidence of **overweight** and **obesity** that has occurred in the United States over the last few decades has led medical and public health officials to call the situation epidemic. Obesity-related health complications directly affect a greater proportion of the population than either the Black Death, a plague that killed about half the population of Europe in the 14th century, or the influenza epidemic of 1918, which infected a fifth of the world's population. Sixty-four percent of American adults are overweight, and about half of these people carry enough extra fat to be considered obese.[4] The obesity epidemic affects both men and women and spans every culture in the nation. Among African Americans, over 60% of men and 78% of women are overweight; among Mexican Americans, over 74% of men and 71% of women are overweight. The problem is not limited to adults. Ten percent of children between 2 and 5 years of age are overweight, and 15% of children and teens 6 to 19 years of age are overweight.[4]

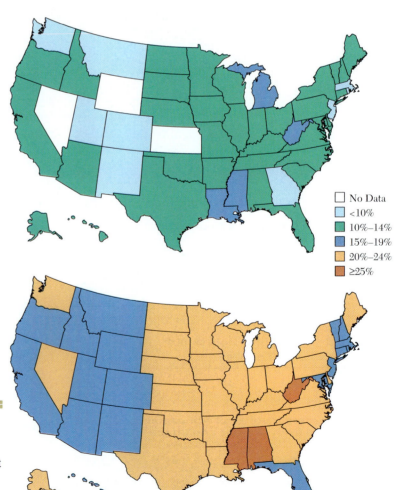

☐ No Data
☐ <10%
☐ 10%–14%
☐ 15%–19%
☐ 20%–24%
☐ ≥25%

FIGURE 7.1

These maps, which show the percentage of the adult population that was obese in each state in 1991 (top map) and 2002 (bottom map), illustrate the dramatic rise in the incidence of obesity. In 1991 there were no states that had rates of obesity that exceeded 19%. By 2002 over half the states had rates of 20% or greater. (*Obesity Trends Among US Adults, BRFSS, 1991-2002,* Centers for Disease Control)

Although the numbers are most striking for the United States, obesity is a growing concern worldwide. In Canada between 1978 and 1992, obesity increased from 8 to 12% among women and from 9 to 14% among men. In Europe, the incidence of obesity has increased by 10 to 40% in the last 10 years.[5] Obesity is even becoming a problem in developing nations, where we typically think of undernutrition as the main concern. In Brazil between 1974 and 1997, obesity increased from 4.1 to 13.9%.[6] In Western Samoa, where a strong genetic predisposition toward obesity had already made obesity rates high, it increased still further between 1978 and 1991, from 39 to 58% among men and from 60 to 77% among women.[7]

Excess body fat increases disease risk

Your body weight is the sum of the weight of your fat and your lean tissue or **lean body mass**, which includes muscles, organs, and bones. A high body weight may be due to large muscles or to excess body fat. If the extra weight is due to excess fat, then it increases your risk of a host of chronic health problems, including high blood pressure, heart disease, high blood cholesterol, diabetes, stroke, gallbladder disease, arthritis, sleep disorders, respiratory problems, and cancers of the breast, uterus, prostate, and colon (Table 7.1). Obesity also increases the incidence and severity of infectious disease and has been linked to poor wound healing and surgical complications. It increases pregnancy risks for both the mother and child. The more overweight you are, the greater your health risks. The longer you are overweight, the greater the risks;

TABLE 7.1
Excess Weight Increases Health Risks

Cardiovascular disease is more likely when body weight is elevated
- Blood pressure increases as body weight increases
- Triglyceride levels increase as body weight increases
- LDL cholesterol increases as body weight increases
- HDL cholesterol falls as body weight increases

Type 2 diabetes risk increases with body weight
- Fasting blood sugar increases with increasing body weight
- Eighty percent of people with type 2 diabetes are obese
- Incidence increases as much as 30-fold with a BMI >35

Respiratory problems are more common in overweight people
- Sleep apnea is more common in overweight people
- The workload of muscles used for breathing increases
- Asthma is worse

Gallbladder disease is more common in overweight people

Osteoarthritis and degenerative joint disease increase with increasing weight

Menstrual irregularities are increased in overweight women

Cancer risk is higher in overweight people
- Obese women are at increased risk for cancers of the endometrium, breast, cervix, and ovaries
- Obese men are at increased risk for colorectal and prostate cancer

A sedentary lifestyle further increases risk
- Obese individuals who are inactive have higher risks of illness and death
- Inactivity increases the likelihood of developing diabetes and heart disease

On the Side

For the first time in human history, the number of overweight people in the world rivals the number of underweight people. According to the Worldwatch Institute, a Washington, D.C.–based research organization, the number of underfed people has declined slightly since 1980 to about 1.1 billion, while the number of overweight people has surged to 1.1 billion.

Lean body mass Body mass attributed to nonfat body components such as bone, muscle, and internal organs. It is also called fat-free mass.

those who gain excess weight at a young age and remain overweight throughout life have the greatest health risks.

Carrying excess body fat also has psychological and social consequences. Our society puts a high value on physical appearance. Being thin is considered attractive and being fat is not. Those who do not conform to standards may pay a high psychological and social price. For example, overweight children are often teased and ostracized. This teasing about body weight is associated with low body satisfaction, low self-esteem, depression, social isolation, and thinking about and attempting suicide.[8,9] If obese children grow into obese adolescents and adults, and most of them do, they may experience discrimination in college admissions and in the job market, in the workplace, and even on public transportation. Obese individuals of every age are more likely to experience depression, a negative self-image, and feelings of inadequacy.[10] The physical health consequences of obesity may not manifest themselves as disease for years, but the psychological and social problems experienced by the obese are felt every day.

A change in lifestyle can help stem the obesity epidemic

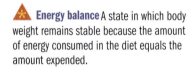 **Energy balance** A state in which body weight remains stable because the amount of energy consumed in the diet equals the amount expended.

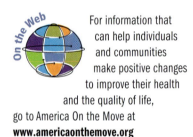 For information that can help individuals and communities make positive changes to improve their health and the quality of life, go to America On the Move at **www.americaonthemove.org**

Reversing the obesity epidemic is a monumental but not insurmountable task. Obesity is caused by consuming more calories than you burn in activity over a long period of time. Preventing obesity requires maintaining **energy balance** by matching intake with output in the short term and in the long term. On a personal level, this means paying attention to which foods you choose, how much you eat, and what you do. It involves choosing more nutrient-dense foods, consuming smaller portions than we are accustomed to, and learning to incorporate exercise into our recreation and everyday life. As a society we need to make this doable by transforming cities and communities into places where it is easy to walk or bike to the store, school, or office; by manufacturing healthier foods and packaging and serving them in more reasonable portion sizes; and by incorporating exercise into the school day and the work day. The only way to stop the obesity epidemic is to change the way we eat and the way we live, the factors that caused average American body weight to increase in the first place. The causes of obesity and solutions to the problem for individuals and the population are discussed more throughout the chapter.

Body Fat: How Much and Where Determines the Risk

Some body fat is essential for health; it cushions our organs, insulates us from changes in temperature and provides stored energy for times of need, but how much is too much? The answer depends on who you are. In general, women store more body fat than men, so the level that is healthy for women is somewhat higher. A healthy level of body fat for a young adult female is between 21 and 33% of total weight; for young adult males, it is between 8 and 20%.[11] With aging, lean body mass decreases and body fat increases, even if body weight remains the same (Appendix B). Some of this change may be prevented by physical activity.

There are many techniques for measuring body composition

 Bioelectric impedance analysis A technique for estimating body composition that measures current flow through the body and calculates resistance to flow.

The proportion of body weight that is fat compared to lean, or body composition, can be measured by a variety of different techniques (Table 7.2). Some of these measurements can be made in a doctor's office or at a health club; others require expensive, sophisticated equipment and are most often used in research settings. Currently the easiest and therefore most popular way to measure body composition is with a technique that measures current flow through the body, called **bioelectric impedance analysis**. This involves holding a meter or standing on a scale that passes a painless, low-energy electrical current through the body; the rate of current flow can be used to calculate the ratio of lean tissue to fat. Although this measurement is quick and easy

TABLE 7.2
Measuring Body Composition

Method	How Does It Work?	Pros and Cons
Bioelectric impedance	Measures current flow through the body; since fat resists current flow, more fat means more resistance to flow	Fast, easy, and inexpensive; inaccurate if body water is not normal, such as after heavy exercise
Skinfold thickness	Measures subcutaneous fat at several locations, based on the assumption that subcutaneous fat is representative of total body fat	Fast, easy, inexpensive; can be inaccurate if not performed by a trained observer
Underwater weighing	Uses the difference between weight on land and weight under water to calculate body density; if you are more dense, you have less fat	Accurate; can't be used for children or ill or frail adults
Air displacement (Bod Pod)	Measures air displacement in a closed chamber and uses this to calculate body density; if you are more dense, you have less fat	Accurate and easy for the subject; expensive, not readily available
Dilution	Measures the concentration of a detectable water-soluble substance that has been ingested or injected into the bloodstream and allowed to mix with the water throughout the body; the more it has been diluted by body water, the greater the amount of lean tissue	Accurate; expensive, invasive, and may involve the use of radioactive substances
Dual-energy X-ray absorptiometry (DEXA)	Uses low-energy X-rays for assessing body composition	A single investigation can accurately determine total body mass, bone mineral mass, and percent body fat; expensive and it does not distinguish between visceral and subcutaneous fat
Computerized tomography (CT)	Uses X-rays to visualize fat and lean tissue	Useful for measuring the amount of visceral fat; expensive
Magnetic resonance imaging (MRI)	Uses magnetic fields to create an internal body image	Accurately measures visceral fat; expensive

and available at many gyms and health clubs, it is not always accurate. To be accurate, measurements need to be made when your stomach and bladder are empty and you are normally hydrated. Measurements are less accurate after a meal or exercise session. Another inexpensive and non-invasive technique for estimating body composition is measuring **skinfold thickness**. The thickness of the skin and fat layer that lies over the muscles is measured at several locations on the arms, legs, and/or abdomen using a caliper (Figure 7.2). These measurements are accurate if they are done by someone trained in the technique. A more precise method is underwater weighing. This involves weighing someone on land and under water to calculate body density and, subsequently, the amount of body fat. Although this method is accurate, it cannot be

⭐ **Skinfold thickness** A technique that measures the thickness of the subcutaneous fat layer, which is used to estimate total body fat.

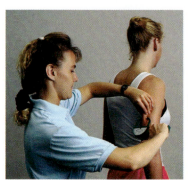

FIGURE 7.2

Measurements of skinfold thickness at several locations can be used to estimate total body fat. The triceps skinfold shown here is measured at the midpoint of the back of the arm. (David Young-Wolff/PhotoEdit)

used for small children or frail adults, and it is less portable than skinfold or impedance measures. Other methods for measuring the amount of fat are listed in Table 7.2; most of these are more expensive and invasive.

Body Mass Index can determine if your weight is in the healthy range

Body Mass Index (BMI) An index of weight in relation to height that is used to compare body size with a standard.

Body Mass Index (BMI) is an index of body weight in relation to height. Although BMI is not actually a measure of body fat, it is recommended as a better way to assess body fatness than measuring weight alone.[12] BMI is calculated according to the following equation:

$$BMI = \text{weight in kg}/(\text{height in m})^2$$

or

$$BMI = \text{weight in pounds}/(\text{height in inches})^2 \times 703$$

For example, someone who is 6 feet (72 inches) tall and weighs 180 pounds has a Body Mass Index of 24.5 kg/m² (180/72² × 703 = 24.5 kg/m²).

Figure 7.3 can be used to determine BMI and see if it is in the healthy range for adults. A healthy BMI for adults is between 18.5 and 24.9 kg/m². In general, people

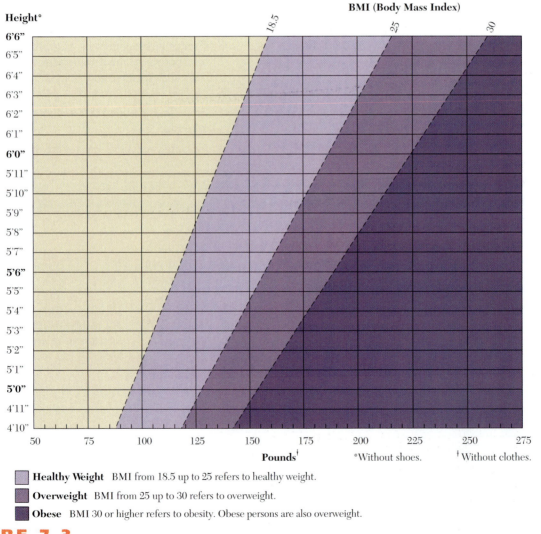

Healthy Weight BMI from 18.5 up to 25 refers to healthy weight.

Overweight BMI from 25 up to 30 refers to overweight.

Obese BMI 30 or higher refers to obesity. Obese persons are also overweight.

FIGURE 7.3

To determine your BMI range, locate your weight (in pounds) on the bottom scale and draw a vertical line up from this point. Locate your height (in feet and inches) on the left scale and draw a horizontal line that extends into the graph. The point where these two lines meet indicates your BMI status. (*Report of the Dietary Advisory Committee on the Dietary Guidelines for Americans, 2000.*)

with a BMI in this range have the lowest health risks. Those with a BMI of less than 18.5 kg/m² are considered **underweight**. Those whose BMI is between 25 and 29.9 kg/m² are overweight, and those with a BMI of 30 kg/m² or greater are obese.[12] A BMI of 40 or over is classified as **extreme** or **morbid obesity**.

Being underweight leaves no body reserves Some people are naturally lean, and this reduces their health risks. Research has suggested that being on the low side of the body weight standard may reduce the risk of diabetes and other chronic diseases and may even increase longevity (see chapter 13).[13] But body fat is needed for cushioning, as an insulator, and as a reserve for periods of illness. People with little energy reserves are at a disadvantage during a famine or when battling a disease such as cancer that causes wasting and malnutrition.

When leanness is due to intentional or forced food restriction rather than a lifetime of being lean, the health consequences could be severe. Substantial reductions in body weight due to starvation or eating disorders decrease the ability of the immune system to fight disease, and very low body weight is associated with an increased risk of early death.[14] Too little body fat can cause problems at all stages of life. During adolescence it can delay sexual development. During pregnancy, too little weight gain increases the risk that the baby will have health complications, and in the elderly too little body fat increases the risk of malnutrition. Therefore, statistically a low body weight is associated with an increased risk of early death.

A high BMI doesn't always mean you have too much fat
Even though BMI correlates well with body fat, it is not a perfect tool for evaluating the health risks associated with obesity. This is particularly true in athletes who have highly developed muscles; their BMI may be high because they have an unusually large amount of lean body mass. In these individuals BMI is high, but body fat and hence disease risk are low (Figure 7.4). BMI is also not suitable to evaluate weight in pregnant and lactating women, because a higher body weight is normal. It is also not accurate in individuals who have lost muscle, such as many older adults. Although BMI can be a useful tool, because of these limitations, other information is also needed to determine nutritional health and fitness. Someone who is in the overweight category on the basis of BMI but consumes a healthy diet and exercises regularly may be more fit and have a lower risk of chronic disease than someone with a BMI in the healthy range who is sedentary and eats a poor diet.

Where your body fat is located affects your health risks

Where you store your body fat affects the health risks associated with having too much. Fat that is located under the skin, called **subcutaneous fat**, carries less risk than fat that is deposited around the organs in the abdomen, called **visceral fat**. An increase in visceral fat is associated with a higher incidence of heart disease, high blood pressure, stroke, diabetes, and breast cancer. Generally, fat in the hips and lower body is subcutaneous, whereas fat deposited around the waist in the abdominal region is primarily visceral fat. Therefore, people who carry their excess fat around and above the waist have more visceral fat. Those who carry their extra fat below the waist in the hips and thighs have more subcutaneous fat. In the popular literature, these body types have been dubbed apples and pears, respectively (Figure 7.5).

Where your extra fat is deposited is determined primarily by your genes.[15] Visceral fat storage is more common in men than women. African American women store less visceral fat than Caucasian women, even though they have a higher overall incidence of obesity.[16] Age and environment also influence where fat is stored.[17] After menopause, visceral fat increases in women. Stress, tobacco use, and alcohol consumption predispose people to visceral fat deposition, whereas physical activity reduces it.

To determine if your body fat is a concern, you can measure your BMI and waist circumference. For males, a BMI of 25 to 34.9 kg/m² and a waist circumference greater than 40 inches indicates abdominal fat storage and is associated with increased risk. For

⚠ **Underweight** A BMI of less than 18.5 kg/m².

⚠ **Extreme** or **morbid obesity** A condition in which BMI is greater than 40 kg/m².

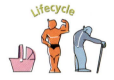
Lifecycle

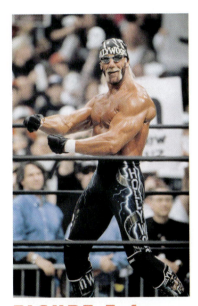

FIGURE 7.4

Wrestler/actor Hulk Hogan, at 6 feet 8 inches tall and 275 pounds, has a BMI of 30.3, which falls into the category of obese. However, it is unlikely that his high BMI is due to excess body fat or that it indicates an increased risk of disease. (Duomo/Corbis)

⚠ **Subcutaneous fat** Body fat that lies under the skin.

⚠ **Visceral fat** Body fat that lies around internal organs.

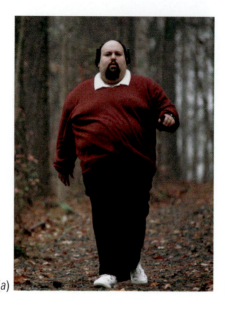
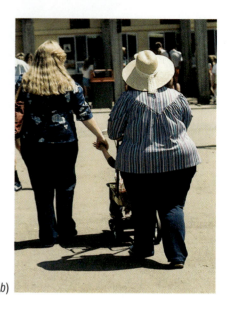

FIGURE 7.5

(*a*): Overweight individuals with apple-shaped body types deposit more fat in the abdominal region and are at greater risk of developing heart disease and diabetes. (*b*): Overweight individuals with pear-shaped body types deposit more fat in the hips and thighs, where it is primarily subcutaneous. (*a*, Corbis; *b*, © Tom McHugh/Photo Researchers)

(*a*)   (*b*)

females in this BMI range, waist circumference of greater than 35 inches increases risks (Table 7.3). In order to monitor body weight and risk, the Dietary Guidelines for Americans, 2000, recommends that all Americans keep track of their weight and their waists and avoid increases in both.

Your Genes Affect Your Body Size and Composition

Genes A length of DNA that contains the information needed to synthesize a protein.

Are you shaped like your mother or your father? The information that determines body size and shape is contained in the **genes** you inherit from your parents. Some of us inherit tall, slender bodies with long, thin bones. Others inherit stocky bodies with short bones. Some people have broad hips and others broad shoulders (Figure 7.6). These characteristics don't change much over time. Even body weight tends to remain at a particular level or set point for long periods despite changes in the amounts we eat or exercise. When energy intake or activity level changes, the body compensates to

TABLE 7.3
Does Your Body Mass Index Increase Your Disease Risk?

Weight Class	BMI[a]	Disease Risk[b]	
		Men: waist ≤40 in Women: waist ≤35 in	Men: waist >40 in Women: waist >35 in
Underweight	<18.5		
Normal weight	18.5–24.9		
Overweight	25.0–29.9	Increased	High
Obesity (class I)	30.0–34.9	High	Very high
Obesity (class II)	35.0–39.9	Very high	Very high
Extreme or morbid obesity (class III)	≥40	Extremely high	Extremely high

[a]BMI = Body Mass Index: body weight (kg)/height squared (m²)
[b]Disease risk for type 2 diabetes, hypertension, and cardiovascular disease relative to individuals with a normal weight and normal waist circumference.

Data are from National Institutes of Health, National Heart, Lung, and Blood Institute. *Clinical Guidelines on the Identification, Evaluation, and Treatment of Overweight and Obesity in Adults. Executive Summary.* Available online at: www.nhlbi.nih.gov/guidelines/obesity/ob_home.htm.

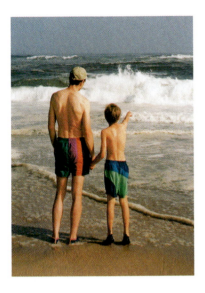
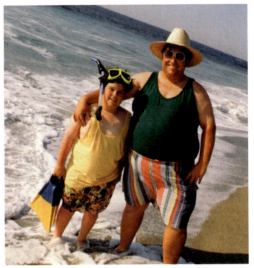

FIGURE 7.6

The genes we inherit from our parents are important determinants of our body size and shape. Some of us inherit long, lean bodies and others a huskier build and a tendency to put on pounds. (*left*: Courtesy Lori Smolin; *right*: Bruce Ayres/Stone/Getty Images)

prevent significant changes in weight or fat. This is why your weight remains fairly constant even when you increase your exercise level—perhaps on a weekend hiking trip. It is also why most people gain back weight that they lose when they follow a weight-loss diet.

Obesity genes regulate body weight and fatness

Genes involved in regulating body fatness have been called **obesity genes** because an abnormality in one or more of these could result in obesity. More than 300 genes and regions of human chromosomes have been linked to obesity.[18] These genes are responsible for the production of proteins that affect how much food you eat and how much energy you expend and regulate the way fat is stored in your body. The combined effects of all these genes help to determine and regulate what you weigh and how much fat you carry.

To regulate weight and fatness at a constant level, the body must be able to respond both to changes in food intake that occur over a short time frame as well as to more long-term changes in the amount of stored body fat. Signals related to food intake affect **hunger** or **satiety** over a short period of time—from meal to meal—whereas signals from the **adipose tissue** trigger the brain to adjust both food intake and energy expenditure for long-term regulation.

How much you eat at each meal is affected by internal signals How do you know how much to eat for breakfast or when it is time to eat lunch? The physical sensations of hunger or satiety that determine how much you eat at each meal are triggered by signals from the gastrointestinal tract, levels of circulating nutrients, and messages from the brain.[19] Some signals are sent before we eat to tell us we are hungry, some are sent while food is in the GI tract, and some occur once nutrients are circulating in the bloodstream.

The simplest type of signal about how much food you have eaten comes from local nerves in the walls of the stomach and small intestine that sense the volume or pressure of food and send a message to your brain to either start or stop eating. Once you have eaten, nutrients in the GI tract send information directly to the brain and trigger the release of hormones that tell us to stop eating. Once nutrients have been absorbed, circulating levels of nutrients, including glucose, amino acids, ketones, and fatty acids, are monitored by the brain and may trigger signals to eat or not to eat. There are many different signals that regulate different aspects of food intake. For instance, the hormone insulin is released by the pancreas in response to the intake of carbohydrate. Insulin allows glucose to be taken up by cells, thereby reducing circulating levels of

Obesity genes Genes that code for proteins involved in the regulation of food intake, energy expenditure, or the deposition of body fat. When they are abnormal, the result is abnormal amounts of body fat.

Hunger The desire to acquire and consume food that occurs in response to physiological signals.

Satiety The feeling of fullness and satisfaction, caused by food consumption, that eliminates the desire to eat.

Adipose tissue Tissue composed primarily of fat-storing cells.

For more information on healthy weight management, go to the Weight Control Information Network at **www.niddk.nih.gov/health/nutrit/htm/**

Ghrelin A hormone produced by the stomach that stimulates food intake.

glucose and increasing hunger. The hormone **ghrelin** may be the reason you typically feel hungry around lunchtime, regardless of when and how much you had for breakfast. It is produced by the stomach and is believed to stimulate your desire to eat at usual meal times. Levels rise an hour or two before a meal and drop very low after a meal. Overproduction of ghrelin could contribute to obesity because levels have been found to increase in people who have lost weight, increasing their desire to eat more.[20] Another hormone (peptide PYY) causes a reduction in appetite. It is released from the gastrointestinal tract after a meal and the amount released is proportional to the calories in the meal.[21] Some food intake signals even trigger the consumption of specific nutrients. For example, when levels of the neurotransmitter serotonin are low, we have been found to crave carbohydrate, but when it is high, we prefer protein.

Long-term regulation monitors the amount of body fat

Sometimes we don't pay attention to whether or not we are full and make room for dessert anyway. If this happens often enough, it can cause an increase in body weight and fatness. To return fatness to a set level, the body must be able to monitor how much fat is present. Some of this information comes from hormones, such as insulin and **leptin** that are secreted in proportion to the amount of body fat.[22] Levels of insulin in the blood increase with the amount of body fat. Insulin affects food intake and body weight by sending appetite-suppressing signals to the brain and by affecting the amount of leptin produced and secreted. Leptin is a hormone produced by the **adipocytes**. The amount of leptin produced is proportional to the size of adipocytes, so more leptin is released as fat stores grow. Leptin travels in the blood to the **hypothalamus**, where it binds to proteins called leptin receptors. When leptin levels are high, mechanisms that cause an increase in energy expenditure and a decrease in food intake are stimulated, and pathways that promote food intake and, hence, weight gain are inhibited. When fat stores shrink, less leptin is released. Low leptin levels in the brain allow pathways that decrease energy expenditure and increase food intake to become active. Thus, leptin acts like a thermostat or lipostat to keep body fatness from changing (Figure 7.7).

 Leptin A protein hormone produced by adipocytes that signals information about the amount of body fat.

 Adipocytes Fat-storing cells.

 Hypothalamus The region of the brain that monitors and regulates conditions and activities in the body, including food intake and energy expenditure.

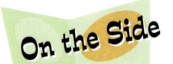

Throughout human history, starvation has threatened survival. Thus, over time the human body has developed ways to conserve body fat stores and prevent weight loss. Today more of us are concerned about eating too much than not enough. Unfortunately, preventing weight gain is not in our evolutionary repertoire. We complain about how hard it is to lose weight, but it is after all our ability to store and preserve body fat that has allowed us to survive the famines that have plagued us in the past.

FIGURE 7.7

Leptin helps maintain body fat at a preset level. When adipocytes gain fat, more leptin is released, triggering events that decrease food intake and increase energy expenditure. When fat is lost, less leptin is released, causing an increase in food intake and a decrease in energy expenditure.

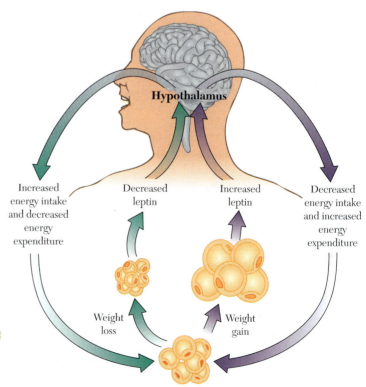

Your set point for body weight may change over time

If body weight is regulated at a particular set point, then why are so many of us getting fatter? It appears that the mechanisms that defend body weight are not absolute. Changes in physiological, psychological, and environmental circumstances do cause the level at which body weight is regulated to change, usually increasing it over time. For example, body weight increases in most adults between the ages of 30 and 60 years, and after having a baby, most women return to a weight that is 1 to 2 pounds higher than their pre-pregnancy weight. This suggests that the mechanisms that defend against weight loss are stronger than those that prevent weight gain.[23]

Defective obesity genes may promote excess fat storage

When a gene is defective, the protein it codes for is not made or is made incorrectly. When an obesity gene, such as the gene for leptin, is defective, the signals to decrease food intake and/or increase energy expenditure are not received, and weight gain results (Figure 7.8). A few cases of human obesity have been linked directly to defects in the genes for leptin and leptin receptors.[24] But mutations in single genes such as these are not responsible for most human obesity. Rather, variations in many genes interact with one another and affect metabolic rate, food intake, fat storage, and activity level. These in turn affect overall body shape and size.

Most overweight people do not have a slower metabolism
Many overweight people contend that they eat almost nothing and yet continue to gain weight. This would imply that they expend less energy than normal-weight individuals. One possible explanation for this is that overweight people use their calories very efficiently, so they don't need to eat as much to maintain their body weight. The results of studies comparing food intake and body weight have been mixed. Part of the problem is that overweight individuals are more likely to underreport their food intake than their lean counterparts. Studies measuring energy expenditure and body weight show that calorie use increases with increasing body weight; this suggests that overweight individuals need to eat more than their lean counterparts to maintain their higher body weight.[25] Although some individuals may need fewer calories than others to maintain weight, there is little evidence that an efficient metabolism is a factor in the majority of cases of human obesity.

Overweight people may be less efficient at burning off extra calories
Your body has mechanisms that are designed to keep your weight at a specific set point. When you overeat occasionally, your metabolism speeds up to burn the extra calories and prevent weight gain.[26] Conversely, when you decrease your food intake, the rate at which your body uses calories slows. These changes in the amount of energy you expend in response to changes in circumstance, such as overeating or undereating, changes in temperature, or trauma, are referred to as **adaptive thermogenesis**.

Several biochemical mechanisms have been proposed to explain adaptive thermogenesis. One mechanism simply wastes energy by allowing opposing biochemical reactions to occur simultaneously. For example, a molecule is formed and then broken down. The result is that calories are burned, but there is no net change in the number of molecules in the body and, therefore, no storage of energy as fat. Another mechanism that may explain adaptive thermogenesis is that excess energy is dissipated by separating or uncoupling the breakdown of energy-yielding nutrients from the production of ATP. When this occurs, energy is lost as heat. Animals have a specialized type of adipose tissue called **brown adipose tissue** that is particularly good at wasting energy as heat. It contains many more mitochondria (where aerobic metabolism occurs) than the more common white adipose tissue, and these mitochondria can be uncoupled to release the energy in food as heat. In rats, brown adipose tissue generates heat to prevent weight gain during overfeeding and to provide warmth when the environmental temperature is low. Brown adipose tissue is unlikely to play a major role in

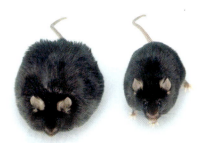

FIGURE 7.8

A mouse with a defect in the leptin gene may weigh three times as much as a normal mouse. Both of these mice have defective leptin genes, but the one on the right was treated with leptin injections. (Courtesy John Sholtis, Rockefeller University, New York/ © 1995 Amgen, Inc.)

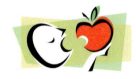

Overweight people must eat more than lean individuals of the same age and height because they have more tissue to fuel and maintain. This is frustrating to dieters because, as they lose weight, the amount they can eat without weight gain decreases.

Adaptive thermogenesis The change in energy expenditure induced by factors such as changes in ambient temperature and food intake.

Brown adipose tissue A type of fat tissue that has a greater number of mitochondria than the more common white adipose tissue. It can waste energy by producing heat and is believed to be responsible for some of the change in energy expenditure in adaptive thermogenesis in rodents.

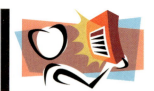

Off the Label: How Many Calories in that Bowl, Box, or Bar?

Are you looking for foods that will help you maintain a healthy weight? Fresh fruits and vegetables are always a good choice. But for packaged foods, you need to check the label. Be sure you know what the terms mean.

The Nutrition Facts portion of a food label lists the Calories per serving, but it is also important to check the serving size. For instance, the standard serving of cookies is usually one ounce, or about three cookies. If you eat 12 cookies, you are consuming four times the Calories listed on the label for a standard serving.

People tend to eat in units—one can of juice, one bottle of iced tea, one bag of potato chips—but food labels don't always reflect the calorie count for that unit. For example, on a hot day a bottle of iced tea or fruit juice may be just what you need to cool off. The label says that a serving has only 100 Calories. Take a closer look. The serving size is 8 ounces and the bottle is 20 ounces. So your cool gulp of iced tea may be giving you 250 Calories, mostly as added sugars. One of the recommendations of the FDA's Working Group on Obesity is to label as single servings those foods for which the entire contents of the package typically are consumed at one time. For example, a 20-ounce bottle of soda would be labeled as containing 275 Calories per bottle rather than 110 Calories per 8 ounces.[1] It has also been suggested that the label design be changed so that the number of Calories is more prominent on the food label.

In evaluating the calorie content of a food, you may also see descriptors such as "low-calorie," "calorie-free," "reduced-calorie," and "light." These terms are defined so they can be helpful in selecting foods. A food labeled "low-calorie" must have no more than 40 Calories per serving. A product labeled "calorie-free," must contain fewer than 5 Calories in a serving. "Reduced-calorie" or "fewer calories" on the label means the product contains at least 25% fewer calories per serving than a reference food. "Light" or "lite" may be used to describe foods that contain one-third fewer calories or half the fat of a comparable product. For example, the label on "lite" microwave popcorn or "light" corn chips must state both the number

Nutrition Facts		
Serving Size 3 cookies (32g)		
Servings Per Container About 11		
Amount Per Serving		
Calories 160	Calories from Fat 70	
		% Daily Value*
Total Fat 8g		12%
Saturated Fat 2.5g		12%
Cholesterol 0mg		0%
Sodium 105mg		4%
Total Carbohydrate 21g		7%
Dietary Fiber 1g		3%
Sugars 5g		

of Calories per serving and the fact that this is 30% fewer than the regular product. The terms "light" and "lite" are also used to describe food properties such as texture and color. For example, a label that says "light in texture" means just that; it does not mean that the calories are reduced. The term "light" may also appear without explanation on foods like brown sugar, cream, or molasses, which have traditionally included the term as part of their name.

Watch out for low-fat and low-carbohydrate products. These are often popular choices among dieters, but they should be chosen with care. Low-fat foods may contain fewer calories than the full-fat version, but the difference may be minimal. The FDA has not yet defined "low-carb" or "low-carbohydrate," so these terms are at the discretion of the manufacturer. The bottom line on using food labels is to read and understand the entire label before assuming that you are making the best choice.

Reference
1. U.S. Food and Drug Administration. *FDA Proposes Action Plan to Confront Nation's Obesity Problem.* Available online at www.fda.gov/oc/inititives/obesity/ Accessed July 13, 2004.

or Bar?). The energy content of foods in a diet can also be estimated from the Exchange Lists shown in Table 7.4. For example, one starch exchange, whether a slice of bread, one-half cup of cereal, or six saltines, provides about 80 Calories.

▲ **Total energy expenditure (TEE)** The sum of basal energy expenditure, thermic effect of food (TEF), and the energy used in physical activity, regulation of body temperature, deposition of new tissue, and production of milk.

We use energy to keep us alive and moving and to process our food

The total amount of energy used by the body each day is called **total energy expenditure (TEE)**. It includes the energy needed to maintain basic bodily functions such as the beating of your heart, as well as that needed to process food and to fuel physical

TABLE 7.4
Exchange Lists Estimate the Calories in Your Diet

Exchange Groups/Lists	Foods	Serving Size	Energy (Cal)
Carbohydrate Group			
Starch	Rice, cereal, potatoes	1/2 cup	80
	Bread	1 slice	
Fruit	Apple, peach, pear	1 small	60
	Banana	1/2 medium	
	Canned fruit	1/2 cup	
Milk	Milk or yogurt	1 cup	
Fat-free or low-fat			90–110
Reduced-fat			120
Whole			150
Vegetables	Cooked vegetables	1/2 cup	Varies
	Raw vegetables	1 cup	
Meat Group	Meat	1 ounce	
Very lean			35
Lean			55
Medium fat			75
High fat			100
Fat Group	Butter, oil, margarine	1 tsp	45

activity. In individuals who are growing or pregnant, total energy expenditure also includes the energy used to deposit new tissues. In women who are lactating, it includes the energy used to produce milk. There is also a small amount of energy used to maintain body temperature in a cold environment.

Most of our energy is used to maintain basic body functions About 60 to 75% of the body's total energy expenditure is for **basal metabolism**. Basal metabolism includes all of the involuntary things your body does to keep you alive such as breathing, circulating blood, regulating body temperature, synthesizing tissues, removing waste products, and sending nerve signals. The rate at which energy is used for these basic functions is called **basal metabolic rate (BMR)** and is often expressed in Calories per hour. Basal needs include the energy necessary for essential metabolic reactions and life-sustaining functions but do not include the energy needed for physical activity or for the digestion and absorption of food. BMR is measured in the morning in a warm room before the subject rises and at least 12 hours after food intake or activity in order to minimize residual energy being used for activity or processing food. Because of the difficulty of achieving these conditions, measures are often made after about 5 to 6 hours without food or exercise. When determined under these conditions, the rate of energy expenditure is referred to as **resting metabolic rate (RMR)**. RMR values are about 10 to 20% higher than BMR values.[33]

Basal needs are affected by how much you weigh and how much of your weight is lean tissue. It increases with increasing body weight and thus is higher in heavier individuals. It also rises with the amount of lean body mass; BMR is generally higher in men than in women because men have greater lean body mass. BMR decreases with age, partly because of the decrease in lean body mass that usually occurs in older adults.

Basal needs can be altered by certain conditions. For instance, BMR is decreased when calorie intake is consistently below needs.[34] This drop in BMR decreases the amount of energy needed to maintain weight. It is a beneficial adaptation in someone who is starving, but in someone who is trying to lose weight it is frustrating because it

Basal metabolism The energy expended to maintain an awake resting body.

Basal metabolic rate (BMR) The rate of energy expenditure under resting conditions. It is measured after 12 hours without food or exercise.

Resting metabolic rate (RMR) The rate of energy expenditure at rest. It is measured after 5 to 6 hours without food or exercise.

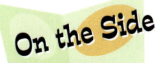
On the Side

Someone whose total energy expenditure is 2500 Cal/day may use 1500 to 1800 of this for basic body functions.

makes weight loss more difficult. Abnormal levels of thyroid hormones can also affect basal needs. Individuals who overproduce these hormones require more energy, and those who underproduce them require less energy. The fact that thyroid hormones, produced by the thyroid gland, affect energy expenditure is the reason obesity was once explained as a glandular problem. It is now known that obesity due to a lack of thyroid hormones is rare. An elevation in body temperature, such as that which occurs with a fever, increases energy needs. It is estimated that for every 1 degree Fahrenheit above normal body temperature, there is a 7% increase in BMR. This extra energy use explains why people often lose weight when they have a fever.

Energy expended in physical activity varies greatly

Physical activity is the second major component of energy expenditure. In most people it accounts for a smaller proportion of total energy expenditure than basal metabolism: about 15 to 30% of energy requirements in most cases. In some athletes and laborers it may account for a higher percentage of total energy expenditure. The energy expended for activity is the one component of our total energy needs over which we have control. It includes the energy we use for planned exercise as well as for performing the activities of daily life, such as cooking, gardening, and walking the dog. Often a person's occupation has a great effect on their energy needs. For example, a construction worker who spends 8 hours a day doing physical labor uses a great deal more energy in his daily activities than does an office worker who spends most of his day sitting at a desk (Figure 7.11).

The amount of energy expended for various activities depends on how strenuous the activity is and the length of time it is performed. Jogging for 30 minutes uses more energy than walking for 30 minutes, but if you walk for an hour you will probably burn as many calories as you would jogging for 30 minutes. Energy expenditure is also affected by body size. Because it takes more energy to move a heavier object, the amount of energy expended for many activities increases as body weight increases. For example, a 120-pound person uses about 190 Calories walking for an hour, but a 180-pound person will expend 290 Calories for the same walk. The energy costs of specific activities are listed in Appendix J.

A small amount of energy is needed to digest, absorb, and use the nutrients in food

Our energy comes from food, but we also need energy to digest food and to absorb, metabolize, and store the nutrients from this food. The energy used for these processes is called the **thermic effect of food (TEF)** or **diet-induced thermogenesis**. This increase in energy expenditure causes body temperature to rise slightly for several hours after eating. The energy required for TEF is estimated to be about 10% of energy intake but can vary, depending on the amounts and types of nutrients consumed. Because it takes energy to store nutrients, TEF increases with the size of the meal. The composition of meals also affects TEF. A meal that is high in fat has a lower TEF than a meal high in carbohydrate or protein because dietary fat can be efficiently stored as body fat. This difference in the energy cost of storing energy means a diet high in fat may produce more body fat than a diet high in carbohydrate.[35]

Thermic effect of food (TEF) or **diet-induced thermogenesis** The energy required for the digestion, absorption, metabolism, and storage of food and the nutrients it provides. It is equal to approximately 10% of daily energy intake.

FIGURE 7.11

The type of job you have has a huge impact on your daily energy expenditure. A carpenter may burn about 2800 Calories in an 8-hour work day, whereas a computer technician burns less than half of this. (a: Ryan McVay/ PhotoDisc, Inc./Getty Images; b: Rubberball Productions/Getty Images)

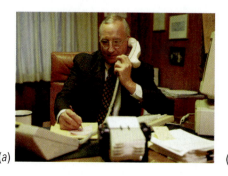
(a)

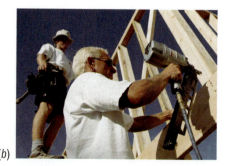
(b)

Energy can be added to or removed from body stores

When you eat a meal, the energy contained in that meal is used to fuel your body. When you consume more than you need the extra is stored. Your body stores a small amount of energy as glycogen and a large amount as fat. Between meals or when you reduce your intake for a longer time, you still need energy, and some of it must come from glucose. To get this energy, our bodies rely on energy stores.

When your energy intake exceeds your needs, body stores get bigger People typically eat three to six times during the day. The sum of the intake for all of these meals and snacks must meet energy needs for weight to remain stable, but each time we eat we are likely to consume more energy than is needed at that moment in time. The body must therefore decide which nutrients it will use immediately and which it will store for later. This is determined on the basis of what the body needs, which nutrients can be stored, and how efficiently they can be stored. When alcohol is consumed, it is quickly broken down and used for energy. This is because it is toxic and the body cannot store it. When protein is consumed, its constituent amino acids are used to synthesize body proteins and other nitrogen-containing molecules. Then, any excess amino acids are broken down and used for energy. When carbohydrate is consumed, it is used to supply blood glucose and to build glycogen stores in the liver and in muscles. Once glycogen stores are full, the remaining carbohydrate is used for energy. When fat is consumed, it is used to meet immediate energy needs and any remaining dietary fat is stored as triglycerides, primarily in adipose tissue. These cells grow as they accumulate more fat (Figure 7.12). The greater the number of adipocytes an individual has, the greater the ability to store fat. Most adipocytes are formed between infancy and adolescence. In adulthood, only excessive weight gain can cause the production of new fat cells.

Most of the fat that is stored in the body comes from fat consumed in the diet (Figure 7.13). This is because excess dietary fat is easy to store as body fat. Dietary fat can be transported directly to the adipose tissue, where the enzyme lipoprotein lipase breaks the triglycerides into fatty acids and glycerol, which can then enter the adipocytes, where they are reassembled into triglycerides for storage. The body is capable of converting excess carbohydrate and amino acids into fat for storage. However, under normal dietary circumstances, this doesn't occur because it involves numerous metabolic reactions and the body must expend energy in the conversion process.[36]

When your energy intake does not meet your needs, body stores are used When your diet doesn't provide enough energy, you must use your body stores. Between meals, you break down liver glycogen in order to maintain a steady supply of blood glucose. But liver glycogen is limited. When you

✳ Remember

As discussed in Chapter 5, the ability of the body to store excess triglycerides is theoretically limitless. Adipocytes can increase in weight by about 50 times, and new fat cells can be made when existing cells reach their maximum size.

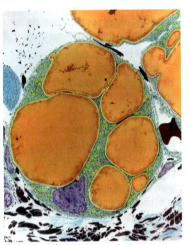

FIGURE 7.12

Adipocytes contain droplets of fat surrounded by other cell components. As body fat is gained, the size of the fat droplets increases. (Ed Reschke/Peter Arnold, Inc.)

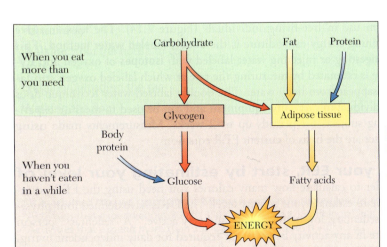

FIGURE 7.13

When you eat more than you need at that time, some energy is put into body stores. Dietary fat is easily stored as body fat. Carbohydrate can be stored as glycogen or converted into fat and excess energy as protein can also be converted into body fat. When you haven't eaten in a while, you retrieve energy from these stores. A small amount of body protein is also broken down to make glucose. If you don't eat for a long time, there are other metabolic changes that occur to ensure your energy needs are met.

The physical symptoms of anorexia are those of starvation The first obvious physical symptom of anorexia is weight loss. As weight loss becomes severe, symptoms of starvation begin to appear. Starvation affects mental function, causing anorexics to become apathetic, dull, exhausted, and depressed. Physical symptoms include depletion of fat stores; wasting of muscles; inflammation and swelling of the lips; flaking and peeling of skin; growth of fine hair on the body, and dry, thin, brittle hair on the head that may fall out. In females, estrogen levels drop, and menstruation becomes irregular or stops.[6] This can delay sexual maturation and can have long-term effects on bone density. In males, testosterone levels decrease. In the final stages of starvation, symptoms include abnormalities in electrolyte balance, dehydration, edema, cardiac abnormalities, absence of ketones due to fat-store depletion, and infection, which further increases nutritional needs.

Treatment of anorexia nervosa must restore nutritional health The goal of treatment for anorexia nervosa is to help resolve the psychological and behavioral problems while providing for physical and nutritional rehabilitation. Early treatment of anorexia is important because starvation may cause irreversible damage. The goal of nutrition intervention is to promote weight gain by increasing energy intake and expanding dietary choices.[57] Nutritional rehabilitation in mild cases involves learning about nutrition and meal planning in order to develop healthy eating patterns. In more severe cases, anorexics are hospitalized, and their food intake and exercise behaviors are carefully controlled. Intravenous nutrition may be necessary to keep the individual alive. Some anorexics make full recoveries but about half have poor long-term outcomes—remaining irrationally concerned about weight gain and never achieving normal body weight.

Bulimia nervosa is characterized by cycles of bingeing and purging

"Bulimia" is from the Greek *bous* (ox) and *limos* (hunger), denoting hunger of such intensity that a person could eat an entire ox. The modern concept of bulimia nervosa as an eating disorder arose in the early 1970's, when a set of symptoms was identified and distinguished from anorexia and obesity. Many different names were used for this disorder, including dysorexia, bulimarexia, thin-fat syndrome, binge/purge syndrome, and dietary chaos syndrome. The term bulimia nervosa was coined in 1979 by a British psychiatrist who suggested that bulimia consisted of powerful urges to overeat in combination with a morbid fear of becoming fat and the avoidance of the fattening effects of food by inducing vomiting or abusing purgatives or both.[58] It currently occurs in 2 to 5% of the population.[59] Bulimia nervosa is a disorder that involves frequent episodes of **binge eating** or **bingeing** that are almost always followed by purging and other inappropriate compensatory behaviors. A diagnosis of bulimia is based on the frequency with which episodes of binge eating and inappropriate compensatory behaviors occur. Bulimia is subdivided into nonpurging and purging types. Nonpurging bulimics use behaviors such as fasting or excessive exercise to prevent weight gain. Purging bulimics regularly engage in behaviors that may include self-induced vomiting and misuse of enemas, laxatives, diuretics, or other medications.

Preoccupation with body weight dominates bulimia nervosa As with anorexia, people with bulimia have an intense fear of becoming fat. They have a negative body image accompanied by a distorted perception of their body size. Their self-esteem is highly tied to their impressions of their body shape and weight. They are preoccupied with the fear that once they start eating they will not be able to stop. They may engage in continuous dieting, which leads to a preoccupation with food.

People with bulimia blame all of their problems on their appearance; this allows them to avoid things that are real problems. A bulimic also thinks he or she is the only person in the world with this problem. As a result they are often socially isolated. They may avoid situations that will expose them to food, such as going to parties or out to dinner, further isolating them socially.

Binge eating or **bingeing** The rapid consumption of a large amount of food in a discrete period of time associated with a feeling that eating is out of control.

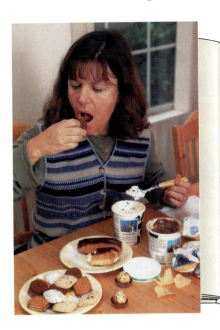

Dear Diary,

Today started well. I stuck to my diet through breakfast, lunch, and dinner, but by 8 PM I was feeling depressed and bored. I thought food would make me feel better. Before I knew it I was at the convenience store buying two pints of ice cream, a large bag of chips, a one pound package of cookies, half dozen candy bars, and a quart of milk. I told the clerk I was having a party. But it was a party of one. Alone in my dorm room I started by eating the chips, then polished off the cookies and the candy bars, washing them down with milk and finishing with the ice cream. Luckily no one was around so I was able to vomit without anyone hearing. I feel weak and guilty but also relieved that I got rid of all those calories. Tomorrow, I will start a new diet.

FIGURE 7.24

Bulimia is characterized by binge eating followed by purging. (David Young Wolff/ PhotoEdit)

The binge/purge behavior distinguishes bulimia Bulimia typically begins with dieting that is motivated by the desire to be thin. Overwhelming hunger may finally cause the dieting to be interrupted by a period of overeating. Eventually a pattern develops involving semi-starvation interrupted by periods of gorging. During a food binge, a bulimic experiences a sense of lack of control. The amount of food consumed during a binge varies but is typically on the order of 3400 Calories—as much as many teenagers eat in an entire day. One study found that bulimics consumed an average of about 7000 Calories in a 24-hour period.[60] Binges usually last less than 2 hours and occur in secrecy. They stop when the food runs out or when pain, fatigue, or an interruption intervenes (Figure 7.24).

After these binge episodes, most bulimics use purging techniques such as vomiting or abuse of laxatives or diuretics to eliminate the excess calories from their bodies. The most common behavior is self-induced vomiting. It is used at the end of a binge but also after normal eating to eliminate food before it is absorbed and the energy it provides can cause weight gain. Laxatives are taken to induce diarrhea. Although the patients believe the diarrhea prevents calories from being absorbed, in fact, nutrient absorption is almost complete before food enters the colon where laxatives work. The weight loss associated with laxative abuse is due to dehydration. Diuretics also cause water loss, but via the kidney. They do not cause fat loss. A smaller number of bulimia sufferers resort to other methods of eliminating these excess calories, such as extreme exercise or fasting. A few bulimics use a combination of purging and non-purging methods.

Purging can damage the gastrointestinal tract It is the purging of the binge-purge cycle that is most hazardous to health in bulimia nervosa. Purging by vomiting brings stomach acid into the mouth. Frequent vomiting affects the gastrointestinal tract by causing tooth decay, sores in the mouth and on the lips, swollen jaws and salivary glands, irritation of the throat, esophageal inflammation, and changes in stomach capacity and stomach emptying.[61] It also causes broken blood vessels in the face from the force of vomiting, electrolyte imbalance, dehydration, muscle weakness, and menstrual irregularities. Laxative and diuretic abuse can also cause dehydration and electrolyte imbalance. Rectal bleeding may occur from laxative overuse.

Treatment of bulimia nervosa must separate eating from emotions The overall goal of therapy for people with bulimia nervosa is to separate eating from their emotions and from their perceptions of success and to promote eating in response to hunger and satiety. Psychological issues related to body

On the Side

In a study that measured the food from a binge that remained in the stomach after vomiting, it was found that on average 1209 Calories were retained after a binge containing 3530 Calories.

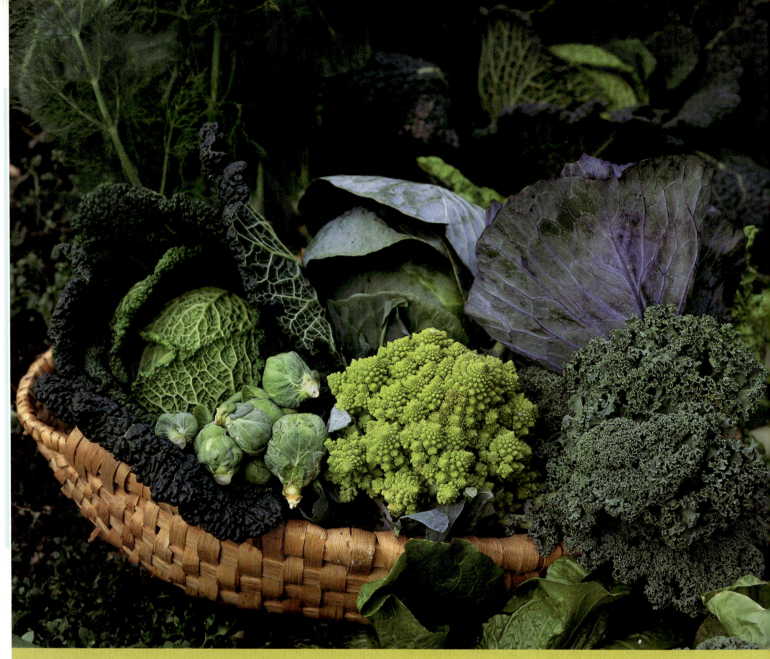

(©Reinhard/Age Fotostock America, Inc.)

- Thiamin, riboflavin, niacin, biotin, and pantothenic acid are B vitamins needed to produce ATP from carbohydrate, fat, and protein.
- Vitamin B_6 is important for amino acid metabolism as well as energy production.
- Folate is a coenzyme that is needed for cell division.
- Vitamin B_{12}, only found in animal foods, is needed for nerve function and to activate folate.
- Vitamin C is needed to form connective tissue and acts as a water-soluble antioxidant.
- Vitamin A is essential for vision, and it regulates cell differentiation and growth.
- Vitamin D is necessary for bone health.
- Vitamin E is a fat-soluble antioxidant.
- Vitamin K is essential for blood clotting.

Just A Taste

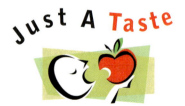

Do vitamins give you extra energy?

Should everyone take folate supplements?

Does eating carrots improve your vision?

Can vitamin E protect you from heart disease?

The Vitamins

8

INTRODUCTION

Vitamin D Concerns on the Rise

By *Karen Collins, R.D.*

Dec. 5, 2003—A lack of vitamin D—thought to be a problem of a bygone era—is showing up in growing numbers of women, children, and the elderly, increasing the risk of bone disease and possibly other health problems.

Exposing only the face, hands, and forearms to sunlight for 10 to 30 minutes, just two or three days a week, can usually produce all the vitamin D we need. Longer exposure doesn't produce more of this vitamin. Yet today, many people's lifestyles and locations do not allow them to produce enough, making dietary sources vital.

For more information on vitamin D concerns go to www.msnbc.msn.com/id/3660416.

Aren't vitamin deficiency diseases a thing of the past? After all, the vitamins have been identified, characterized, and purified. We get them from foods that are natural sources and they are added to our breakfast cereal and sold in pill form. For over 100 years scientists have been experimenting with how much of which ones we need to stay healthy and public health officials have been providing us with guidelines as to how best to get enough from our diets. How can anyone have a deficiency?

Despite advances in vitamin research over the last century, millions of people around the globe still suffer from vitamin deficiency diseases. In the United States, the plentiful and

235

varied food supply make severe vitamin deficiencies unlikely but this doesn't mean everyone gets enough of everything all the time. Marginal deficiencies often go unnoticed and can be mistaken for other conditions.

Vitamins Are Vital to Your Health

⚠️ **Vitamins** Organic compounds needed in the diet in small amounts to promote and regulate the chemical reactions and processes needed for growth, reproduction, and the maintenance of health.

Vitamins are essential to your health. You only need very small quantities but if you don't get enough your body cannot function optimally. Severe deficiencies cause debilitating diseases but even marginal intakes can cause subtle changes that affect your health today and your risk of chronic disease tomorrow. An organic substance is classified as a vitamin if lack of it in the diet causes symptoms that are relieved by adding it back to the diet.

The fact that the vitamins we eat in food are essential to health seems simple and obvious, but it was not always so. For centuries, people knew that some diseases could be cured by certain foods. But it was a long time before we understood why particular foods relieved specific ailments. Cures attributed to foods seemed like nothing short of a miracle. People too weak to rise from their beds, those with bleeding wounds that would not heal, those too mentally disturbed to function in society, and those with other serious ailments were cured with changes in diet. Even before the chemistry of these substances was unraveled, the civilized world was enchanted with the magic of vitamins. They brought hope that incurable diseases could be remedied by simple dietary additions.

Today we understand what vitamins do and why they cure deficiency diseases, but we still hold out hope for more miracles from these small molecules. And we might get a few. Scientists continue to discover important links between vitamins and the risk of developing illnesses such as heart disease, cancer, osteoporosis, and high blood pressure. What is being uncovered is far subtler than the miracle cures of the 19th-century deficiency diseases, but people cling to the belief that taking more vitamins will cure what ails them. As a result of this "more is always better" attitude vitamin toxicities have become a concern. A toxic reaction can be as devastating as a deficiency. Trying to get the right amount of each of the vitamins may sound analogous to walking a tightrope between not enough and too much. In reality it is not that hard to get enough of most vitamins from a well-planned diet and most toxicities are not caused by foods but rather by excessive use of supplements.

Vitamins provide many different functions in the body

To date, 13 substances have been identified as vitamins essential in the diet (Table 8.1). They were named alphabetically in approximately the order in which they were identified: A, B, C, D, and E. The B vitamins were first thought to be one chemical substance but were later found to be many different substances, so the alphabetical name was broken down by numbers. Vitamins B_6 and B_{12} are the only ones that are still commonly referred to by their numbers. Thiamin, riboflavin, and niacin were originally referred to as vitamin B_1, B_2, and B_3, respectively, but today they are not typically called by these names.

Vitamins each have a unique role in the body. For instance, vitamin A is needed for vision, vitamin K is needed for blood clotting, and vitamin C is needed to synthesize connective tissue. Many body processes require the presence of more than one vitamin. For example the B vitamins thiamin, riboflavin, niacin, biotin, and pantothenic acid are all needed to produce ATP from carbohydrate, fat, and protein. In some cases adequate amounts of one vitamin depend on the presence of another. For example, vitamin B_{12} is needed to provide the form of folate needed for cell division and vitamin C helps restore vitamin E to its active form.

TABLE 8.1
Where Does Each Vitamin Fit?

Water-Soluble Vitamins	Fat-Soluble Vitamins
B Vitamins	Vitamin A
• Thiamin (B$_1$)	Vitamin D
• Riboflavin (B$_2$)	Vitamin E
• Niacin (B$_3$)	Vitamin K
• Biotin	
• Pantothenic acid	
• Vitamin B$_6$	
• Folate	
• Vitamin B$_{12}$	
Vitamin C	

Vitamins are found in almost everything you eat

Almost all foods contain some vitamins (Figure 8.1). Grain products are good sources of the B vitamins thiamin, niacin, riboflavin, pantothenic acid, and vitamin B$_6$. Meats, such as beef, pork, and chicken, and fish are good sources of all of the B vitamins. Milk provides riboflavin and vitamins A and D; leafy greens, such as spinach and kale, provide folate, vitamin A, vitamin E, and vitamin K; citrus fruits like oranges and grapefruit provide vitamin C; and vegetable oils, such as corn and safflower oil, are high in vitamin E.

Processing affects vitamin content The amount of a vitamin in a food depends on the amount naturally found in that food as well as how the food is cooked, stored, and processed. The vitamins naturally found in foods can be washed away during preparation, destroyed by cooking, or damaged by exposure to light or oxygen. Thus, processing steps such as canning vegetables, refining grains, and drying fruits can cause nutrient losses. However, other processing steps such as **fortification** and **enrichment** add nutrients to foods. Some nutrients are added to foods to prevent vitamin or mineral deficiencies and promote health in the population (see Chapter 10). For example, milk is fortified with vitamin D to promote bone health, and grains are fortified with folic acid to reduce the incidence of birth defects. Some foods are also fortified with nutrients to help increase product sales.

Dietary supplements can boost vitamin intake We also get vitamins in **dietary supplements**. Currently about half of adult Americans take some form of dietary supplement on a daily basis and 80% take them occasionally.[1] While supplements provide specific nutrients, they do not provide all the benefits of foods. A pill that meets vitamin needs does not provide the energy, protein, minerals, fiber, or phytochemicals that would have been supplied by food sources of these vitamins (see Chapter 10).

Not all of what you eat can be used by the body The vitamins that we consume in our diets are needed in the cells and fluids of our body. In order to provide their essential functions, vitamins must get to the target tissues. The amount of a nutrient consumed that can be used by the body is referred to as its **bioavailability**. Bioavailability is affected by the composition of individual foods, the diet as a whole, and conditions in the body. For example, the thiamin in certain individual foods such as blueberries and red cabbage cannot be used by the body because these foods contain antithiamin factors that destroy the thiamin. An example of how

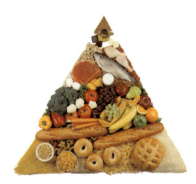

FIGURE 8.1

All the food groups contain choices that are good sources of vitamins. (© Topic Photo Agency) (PhotoDisc, Inc./Getty Images)

Fortification A term used generally to describe the addition of nutrients to foods, such as the addition of vitamin D to milk.

Enrichment The addition of specific nutrients to a food to restore those lost in processing to a level equal to or higher than originally present.

Dietary supplement A product intended for ingestion in the diet that contains one or more of the following: vitamins, minerals, plant-derived substances, amino acids, or concentrates or extracts.

Bioavailability A general term that refers to how well a nutrient can be absorbed and used by the body.

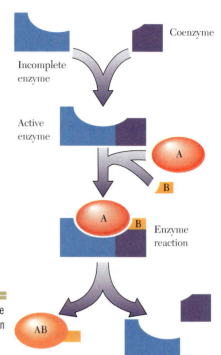

FIGURE 8.4

The B vitamins serve as coenzymes. This figure shows that the coenzyme must bind to form an active enzyme. The enzyme in this example can then join A and B to form a new molecule, shown here as AB.

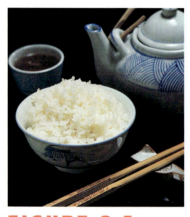

FIGURE 8.5

Unenriched white rice is a poor source of thiamin. (Charles D. Winters)

⚠ **Wernicke-Korsakoff syndrome** A form of thiamin deficiency associated with alcohol abuse that is characterized by mental confusion, disorientation, loss of memory, and a staggering gait.

to find the cause of beriberi. His success came as a twist of fate. He ran out of food for his experimental chickens and instead of the usual brown rice, he fed them white rice. Shortly thereafter, the chickens came down with beriberi-like symptoms. When he fed them brown rice again, they got well. What did this mean? To Eijkman it provided evidence that the cause of beriberi was not a poison or a microorganism, but rather something missing from the chicken feed.

The incidence of beriberi in East Asia increased dramatically the 1800s due to the rising popularity of polished rice. Polished or white rice is produced by polishing off the bran layer of brown rice creating a more uniform product. However, polishing off the bran also removes the vitamin-rich portion of the grain (Figure 8.5). Therefore, in populations where white rice was the staple of the diet, beriberi, became a common health problem.

Thiamin is needed to produce energy from glucose The reason thiamin is needed for nerve cells to obtain energy is because it is a coenzyme for some of the important energy-yielding reactions in the body. One of these is essential for the production of energy from glucose, the energy source for nerve cells. In addition to its role in energy production it is needed for neurotransmitter synthesis and is also essential for the metabolism of other sugars and certain amino acids, and for the synthesis of ribose, a sugar that is part of the structure of RNA (ribonucleic acid).

Thiamin deficiency affects the nervous and cardiovascular systems. Without thiamin, glucose, which is the primary fuel for the brain and nerve cells, cannot be used normally and nerve impulses cannot be transmitted normally. This leads to weakness and depression, which are the first symptoms of beriberi; other neurological symptoms include poor coordination, tingling sensations, and paralysis. The reason deficiency affects the cardiovascular system is not well understood, but symptoms include rapid heartbeat and enlargement of the heart.

Overt beriberi is rare in North America today, but a form of thiamin deficiency called **Wernicke-Korsakoff syndrome** does occur in alcoholics. People with this condition experience mental confusion, psychosis, memory disturbances, and eventually coma. They are particularly vulnerable because thiamin absorption is decreased due to the effect of alcohol on the gastrointestinal tract. In addition, thiamin intake is low because alcohol contributes calories to the alcoholic's diet but brings with it almost no nutrients.

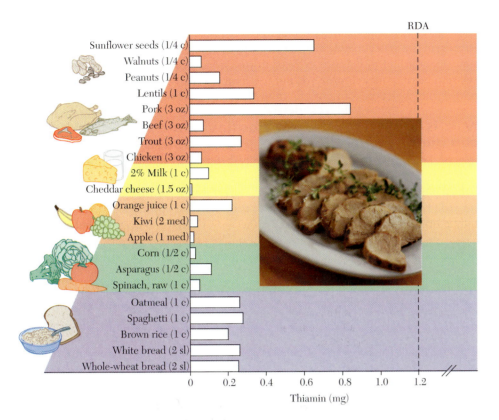

RDA

Sunflower seeds (1/4 c)
Walnuts (1/4 c)
Peanuts (1/4 c)
Lentils (1 c)
Pork (3 oz)
Beef (3 oz)
Trout (3 oz)
Chicken (3 oz)
2% Milk (1 c)
Cheddar cheese (1.5 oz)
Orange juice (1 c)
Kiwi (2 med)
Apple (1 med)
Corn (1/2 c)
Asparagus (1/2 c)
Spinach, raw (1 c)
Oatmeal (1 c)
Spaghetti (1 c)
Brown rice (1 c)
White bread (2 sl)
Whole-wheat bread (2 sl)

0   0.2   0.4   0.6   0.8   1.0   1.2

Thiamin (mg)

FIGURE 8.6

Thiamin content of selections from each group of the Food Guide Pyramid. The dashed line represents the RDA for adult men. Pork is a better source of thiamin than other meats. (Randy Mayor/Foodpix/PictureArts Corp.)

The recommended intake for thiamin can be met by eating a varied diet You can meet your needs for thiamin by snacking on sunflower seeds and having a serving of roast pork for dinner. These foods are exceptionally good sources of thiamin. Together 3 ounces of pork and a quarter cup of sunflower seeds provide 1.5 mg of thiamin, well above the RDA, which is 1.2 mg per day for adult men age 19 and older and 1.1 mg per day for adult women 19 and older.[2] But even a diet that doesn't include these foods can meet your thiamin needs as long as you make nutritious choices such as those recommended by the Food Guide Pyramid (Figure 8.6). Legumes, nuts, and seeds are good sources. Grains are also good sources; thiamin is found in the bran of whole grains and it is added to enriched refined grains. A large proportion of the thiamin consumed in the United States comes from enriched grains used in foods such as baked goods. Some breakfast cereals are fortified with so much additional thiamin that a single bowlful contains more than the RDA.

Although it is easy to meet thiamin needs some of the thiamin in foods may be destroyed during cooking or storage because it is sensitive to heat, oxygen, and low-acid conditions. Thiamin availability is also affected by the presence of antithiamin factors that destroy the vitamin. There are enzymes in raw shellfish and freshwater fish that degrade thiamin during food storage and preparation and during passage through the gastrointestinal tract. These enzymes are destroyed by cooking so they are only a concern in foods consumed raw. Other antithiamin factors that are not inactivated by cooking are found in tea, coffee, betel nuts, blueberries, and red cabbage. Habitual consumption of foods containing antithiamin factors increases the risk of thiamin deficiency.[2]

Despite the fact that intakes of thiamin above the RDA have not been shown to be beneficial, many supplements contain up to 50 mg of thiamin and promise that they will provide "more energy." Although thiamin is needed to produce energy, unless it is deficient, increasing thiamin intake does not increase the ability to produce energy. There is no UL for thiamin since no toxicity has been reported when excess is consumed from either food or supplements.[2]

✱ Remember

Enriched grains have thiamin as well as riboflavin, niacin, and iron added to them (see Chapter 4).

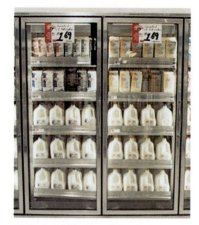

Riboflavin: a bright yellow vitamin

Riboflavin is a water-soluble vitamin that provides a visible indicator when you consume too much of it. Excess is excreted in your urine—turning it a bright fluorescent yellow. The color may surprise you but it is harmless. No adverse effects have been reported from high doses of riboflavin from foods or supplements.

Milk is the best source of riboflavin in the North American diet

Ever wonder why milk comes in opaque cardboard or cloudy plastic containers? The reason is that it is one of the best sources of riboflavin in our diet and riboflavin is destroyed by light. If your milk was in a clear glass bottle and sat in a lighted grocery store display case for several days much of the riboflavin would be destroyed. The most riboflavin-friendly milk containers are opaque so the riboflavin is fully protected from light (Figure 8.7). Other major dietary sources of riboflavin include other dairy products, liver, red meat, poultry, fish, whole grains, and enriched breads and cereals. Vegetable sources include asparagus, broccoli, mushrooms, and leafy green vegetables such as spinach.

The RDA for riboflavin for adult men age 19 and older is 1.3 mg per day and for adult women 19 and older, 1.1 mg per day.[3] Two cups of milk provide about half the amount of riboflavin recommended for a typical adult. If you do not include milk in your diet you can meet your riboflavin needs by including two to three servings of meat and four to five servings of enriched grain products and high-riboflavin vegetables such as spinach (Figure 8.8).

Riboflavin is needed to produce energy from carbohydrate, fat, and protein

Riboflavin has two active coenzyme forms that function in producing energy from carbohydrate, fat, and protein. Riboflavin is also involved directly or indirectly in converting a number of other vitamins, including folate, niacin, vitamin B$_6$, and vitamin K, into their active forms.

When riboflavin is deficient, injuries heal poorly because new cells cannot grow to replace the damaged ones. Tissues that grow most rapidly, such as the skin and the lin-

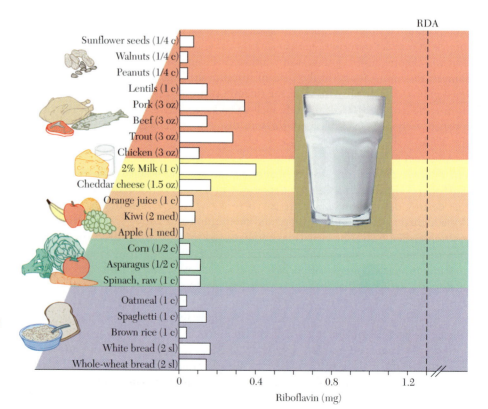

ings of the eyes, mouth, and tongue, are the first to be affected. This causes symptoms such as cracking of the lips and at the corners of the mouth; increased sensitivity to light; burning, tearing, and itching of the eyes; and flaking of the skin around the nose, eyebrows, and earlobes.

A deficiency of riboflavin rarely occurs alone; it usually occurs in conjunction with deficiencies of other B vitamins. This is because the same foods provide many of the B vitamins. Because riboflavin is needed to convert other vitamins into their active forms, some of the symptoms seen with riboflavin deficiency reflect deficiencies of these other nutrients.

Niacin: deficiency caused an epidemic of mental illness

In the early 1900's psychiatric hospitals in the southeastern United States were filled with patients with the niacin-deficiency disease **pellagra**. At the time, no one knew what caused it but the prime suspects were toxins or microorganisms. The mystery of pellagra was finally unraveled by Dr. Joseph Goldberger, who was sent by the U.S. Public Health Service to investigate the pellagra epidemic. He observed that individuals in institutions such as hospitals, orphanages, and prisons suffered from pellagra, but the staff did not. If pellagra were an infectious disease, both populations would be equally affected. Dr. Goldberger proposed that pellagra was due to a deficiency in the diet. To test his hypothesis, he added nutritious foods such as fresh meats, milk, and eggs to the diet of children in orphanages. The symptoms of pellagra disappeared, supporting his hypothesis that pellagra is due to a deficiency of something in the diet. In another experiment he was able to induce pellagra in healthy prison inmates by feeding them an unhealthy diet. The missing dietary component was later identified as the water-soluble B vitamin niacin.

A niacin deficiency causes dermatitis, diarrhea, and dementia
The need for niacin is so widespread in metabolism that a deficiency causes major changes throughout the body. The early symptoms of pellagra include fatigue, decreased appetite, and indigestion. These are followed by symptoms that can be remembered as the three D's: dermatitis, diarrhea, dementia. If left untreated, niacin deficiency results in a fourth D—death.

Niacin coenzymes function in glucose metabolism and in reactions that synthesize fatty acids and cholesterol (see Figure 8.3). There are two forms of niacin: nicotinic acid and nicotinamide. Either form can be used by the body to make the active coenzyme forms.

Niacin is found in meats, legumes, and grains
Meat and fish are good sources of niacin (Figure 8.9). Other sources include legumes, wheat bran, and peanuts. Niacin added to enriched grains provides much of the usable niacin in the North American diet. Niacin can also be synthesized in the body from the essential amino acid tryptophan. Tryptophan, however, is only used to make niacin if enough is available to first meet the needs of protein synthesis. When the diet is low in tryptophan, it is not used to synthesize niacin.

The reason pellagra was prevalent in the South in the early 1900's is because the local diet among the poor consisted of corn meal, molasses, and fatback or salt pork—all poor sources of both niacin and protein. Corn is low in tryptophan and the niacin found naturally in corn is bound to other molecules and therefore not well absorbed. Molasses contains essentially no protein or niacin and salt pork is almost pure fat, so it does not contain enough protein to both meet protein needs and synthesize niacin. Although corn-based diets such as this one are historically associated with the appearance of niacin deficiency it has not been a problem in Mexico and Central American countries. One reason may be because the treatment of corn with lime water, as is done during the making of tortillas, enhances the availability of niacin (Figure 8.10). The diet in these regions also includes legumes, which provide both niacin and a source of tryptophan for the synthesis of niacin.

Pellagra The disease resulting from a deficiency of niacin.

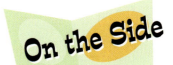

On the Side

In searching for the cause of pellagra, Dr. Goldberger and his coworkers ingested blood, nasal secretions, feces, and urine from patients with the disease—none of them developed pellagra. This helped to disprove the hypothesis that pellagra was an infectious disease.

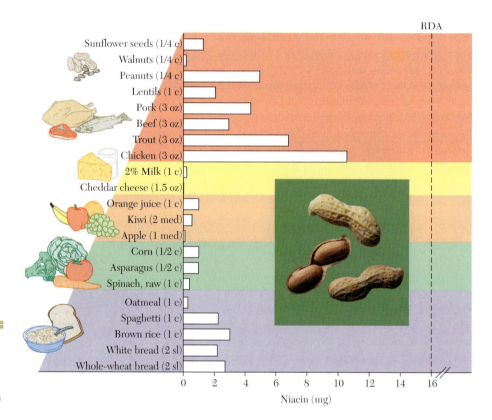

FIGURE 8.9

Niacin content of selections from each group of the Food Guide Pyramid. The dashed line represents the RDA for adult men. Meat, legumes, and grains are good sources of the vitamin. (PhotoDisc, Inc./Getty Images)

Today, as a result of the enrichment of grains, including corn meal, with niacin, thiamin, riboflavin, and iron, pellagra is rare in the United States but it remains common in India and parts of China and Africa. Efforts to eradicate this deficiency include the development of new varieties of corn that provide more available niacin and more tryptophan than traditional varieties.

Because some of the requirement for niacin can be met by the synthesis of niacin from tryptophan, the RDA is expressed as **niacin equivalents (NEs)**. One NE is equal to 1 mg of niacin or 60 mg of tryptophan, the amount needed to make 1 mg of niacin.[3] To estimate the niacin contributed by high-protein foods, protein is considered to be about 1% tryptophan. The RDA for adult men and women of all ages is 16 and 14 mg NE per day, respectively. A medium chicken breast and a cup of steamed asparagus provide this amount.

⚠ **Niacin equivalents (NEs)** The measure used to express the amount of niacin present in food, including that which can be made from its precursor, tryptophan. One NE is equal to 1 mg of niacin or 60 mg of tryptophan.

FIGURE 8.10

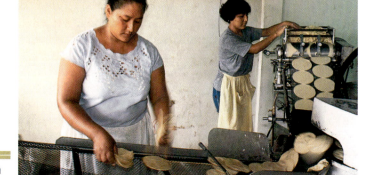

Tortillas, eaten in Mexico and other Latin American countries, provide niacin because the corn is treated with lime water, making the niacin available for absorption. (Jeff Greenberg/Photo Researchers)

High-dose niacin supplements can be toxic There is no evidence of any adverse effects from consumption of niacin naturally occurring in foods, but supplements can be toxic. The adverse effects of high intakes of niacin include flushing of the skin, a tingling sensation in the hands and feet, a red skin rash, nausea, vomiting, diarrhea, high blood sugar levels, abnormalities in liver function, and blurred vision. The UL for adults is 35 mg, but high-dose supplements of one form of niacin (50 mg or greater) are used under medical supervision to treat elevated blood cholesterol (see Chapter 5). Another form is under investigation for its benefits in the prevention and treatment of diabetes. When vitamins are taken in large doses to treat diseases that are not due to vitamin deficiencies, they are really being used as drugs rather than vitamins.

Biotin: eggs contain it but can block its use

You probably know that you shouldn't eat raw eggs because they can contain harmful bacteria, but did you know that eating raw eggs could cause a biotin deficiency? Raw egg whites contain a protein called avidin that tightly binds biotin and prevents its absorption. Biotin was discovered when rats fed protein derived from raw egg whites developed a syndrome of hair loss, dermatitis, and neuromuscular dysfunction. Thoroughly cooking eggs kills bacteria and denatures avidin so that it cannot bind biotin (Figure 8.11).

Biotin is important in energy production and glucose synthesis Biotin is a coenzyme for a group of enzymes that add an acid group to molecules. It functions in energy production and in glucose synthesis. It is also important in the metabolism of fatty acids and amino acids (see Figure 8.3). Although biotin deficiency is uncommon, it has been observed in those frequently consuming raw egg whites as well as people with malabsorption or protein-energy malnutrition, those receiving intravenous feedings lacking biotin, and those taking certain anticonvulsant drugs for long periods.[3] Biotin deficiency in humans causes nausea, thinning hair, loss of hair color, a red skin rash, depression, lethargy, hallucinations, and tingling of the extremities.

Biotin is consumed in the diet and made by bacteria in the gut Good sources of biotin in the diet include cooked eggs, liver, yogurt, and nuts. Fruit and meat are poor sources. Biotin is also synthesized by bacteria in the gastrointestinal tract. Some of this is absorbed into the body and contributes to our biotin needs. An AI of 30 mg per day has been established for adults based on the amount of biotin found in a typical North American diet. High doses of biotin have not resulted in toxicity symptoms; there is no UL for biotin.

Pantothenic acid: widely distributed in food and widely used in the body

Pantothenic acid, which gets its name from the Greek word *pantos* (meaning "from everywhere"), is widely distributed in foods. It is particularly abundant in meat, eggs, whole grains, and legumes. It is found in lesser amounts in milk, vegetables, and fruits.

In addition to being "from everywhere" in the diet, pantothenic acid seems to be needed everywhere in the body. It is part of a key coenzyme needed for the breakdown of carbohydrates, fatty acids, and amino acids as well as the modification of proteins and the synthesis of neurotransmitters, steroid hormones, and hemoglobin. Pantothenic acid is also part of a coenzyme essential for the synthesis of cholesterol and fatty acids (see Figure 8.3).

The wide distribution of pantothenic acid in foods makes deficiency rare in humans. It may occur as part of a multiple B vitamin deficiency resulting from malnutrition or chronic alcoholism. The AI is 5 mg per day for adults. Pantothenic acid is relatively nontoxic and there are not sufficient data to establish a UL.[3]

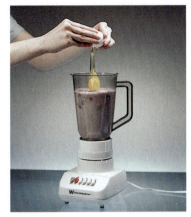

FIGURE 8.11

Raw eggs are often used to make high-protein health drinks. This is not recommended because raw eggs may contain bacteria that can make you sick, and egg whites contain a protein that makes biotin unavailable. (Charles D. Winters)

Vitamin B₆ Is Important in Protein Metabolism

Vitamin B₆ is one of only two B vitamins that we still know by its number. The chemical name for vitamin B₆ is pyridoxine but we rarely hear it called this. The important role of vitamin B₆ in amino acid metabolism distinguishes it from the other B vitamins.

Vitamin B₆ is needed to synthesize and break down amino acids

Vitamin B₆ has three forms—pyridoxal, pyridoxine, and pyridoxamine. These can be converted into the active coenzyme form, pyridoxal phosphate, which is needed for the activity of more than 100 enzymes involved in the metabolism of carbohydrate, fat, and protein. It is particularly important in amino acid synthesis and breakdown; without vitamin B₆ the non-essential amino acids cannot be made in the body (Figure 8.12). Pyridoxal phosphate is needed to synthesize hemoglobin, the oxygen-carrying protein in red blood cells, and is important for the immune system because it is needed to form white blood cells. It is also needed for the conversion of tryptophan to niacin, the release of glucose from the carbohydrate storage molecule glycogen, the synthesis of certain neurotransmitters, and the synthesis of the lipids that are part of the myelin coating on nerves, which is essential for normal transmission of nerve signals.

Vitamin B₆ deficiency causes numbness and tingling
Vitamin B₆ deficiency causes neurological symptoms including numbness and tingling in the hands and feet as well as depression, headaches, confusion, and seizures. These symptoms may be related to the role of vitamin B₆ in neurotransmitter synthesis and myelin formation. Anemia also occurs in vitamin B₆ deficiency, because without B₆ hemoglobin cannot be synthesized normally. Other deficiency symptoms such as poor growth, skin lesions, and decreased antibody formation may occur because of the central role vitamin B₆ plays in protein and energy metabolism. Since vitamin B₆ is needed for amino acid metabolism, the onset of a deficiency can be hastened by a diet that is low in vitamin B₆ but high in protein.

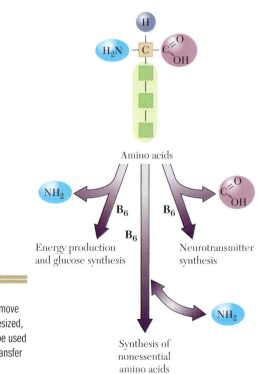

FIGURE 8.12

Vitamin B₆ is essential for many different types of reactions involving amino acids. It is needed to remove the acid group so neurotransmitters can be synthesized, to remove the amino group so what remains can be used to produce energy or synthesize glucose, and to transfer an amino group to make a new amino acid.

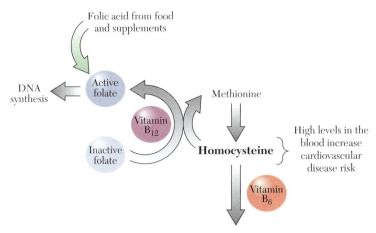

FIGURE 8.13

The accumulation of homocysteine in the blood is associated with an increased risk of heart disease. Vitamins B₆, B₁₂, and folate, are needed to keep homocysteine levels in the normal range. Vitamin B₆ is needed to break down homocysteine. Vitamin B₁₂ and folate are needed to convert homocysteine to methionine.

Vitamin B₆ status is related to heart disease risk Vitamin B₆ is needed to break down the amino acid homocysteine. If B₆ levels are low, homocysteine can't be broken down and levels rise. Even a mild elevation in blood homocysteine levels has been shown to be a risk factor for heart disease (Figure 8.13).[4] Two other B vitamins, folate and vitamin B₁₂ are also involved in homocysteine metabolism. These are needed to convert homocysteine to the amino acid methionine. If they are unavailable, homocysteine levels will increase. A study that examined the effect of folate and vitamin B₆ intake in women found that those with the highest levels in their diets had about half the risk of coronary heart disease as women with the lowest levels.[5]

Both animal and plant foods are good sources of vitamin B₆

Animal sources of vitamin B₆ include chicken, fish, pork, and organ meats. Good plant sources include whole wheat products, brown rice, soybeans, sunflower seeds, and some fruits and vegetables such as bananas, broccoli, and spinach (Figure 8.14). Refined grains, like white rice and white bread, are not good sources of vitamin B₆, because the vitamin is lost in refining whole grains but is not added back in enrichment. It is added to many fortified breakfast cereals; these make an important contribution to vitamin B₆ intake.[6] It is destroyed by heat and light, so it can easily be lost in processing.

The RDA for vitamin B₆ is 1.3 mg per day for both adult men and women 19 to 50 years of age.[3] A 3-ounce (85-g) serving of chicken, fish, or pork, or half a baked potato, provides about one-fourth of the RDA for an average adult; a banana provides about one-third.

Too much vitamin B₆ is toxic

For years people assumed that because water-soluble vitamins were excreted in the urine they could not cause toxic reactions. However, reports in the 1980's of severe nerve impairment in individuals taking 2 to 6 g of pyridoxine per day showed these assumptions to be false.[7] The reactions of some supplement users were so severe that they were unable to walk; symptoms improved when the pyridoxine supplements were stopped. The UL for adults is set at 100 mg per day from food and supplements.[3] Despite the potential for toxicity, high-dose supplements of vitamin B₆ containing 100 mg per dose (5000% of the Daily Value) are available over the counter, making it easy to obtain a dose that exceeds the UL. These supplements are taken to reduce the symptoms of premenstrual syndrome (PMS), treat carpal tunnel syndrome, and strengthen immune function. Although studies have not found a relationship between carpal tunnel syndrome and vitamin B₆ status, some studies report that low-dose supplements of vitamin B₆ may reduce symptoms of PMS and improve immune function.[8]

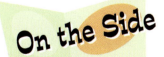

Individuals with an inherited disease called homocysteinuria have extremely high levels of homocysteine in their blood and may have heart attacks and strokes by the age of 2.

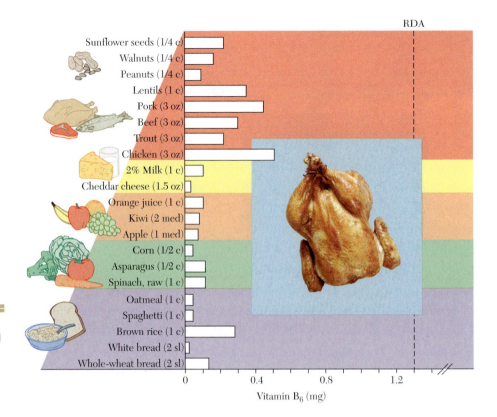

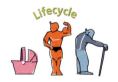

FIGURE 8.14

Vitamin B$_6$ content of selections from each group of the Food Guide Pyramid. The dashed line represents the RDA for men and women up to 50 years of age. The best sources are meats, legumes, and whole grains. (David Bishop/Foodpix/PictureArts Corp.)

PMS causes mood swings, food cravings, bloating, tension, depression, headaches, acne, breast tenderness, anxiety, temper outbursts, and over 100 other symptoms. Because vitamin B$_6$ is needed for the synthesis of the neurotransmitters serotonin and dopamine, insufficient vitamin B$_6$ has been suggested to cause the anxiety, irritability, and depression associated with PMS by reducing levels of these neurotransmitters. Trials on the effect of vitamin B$_6$ supplements on PMS have had conflicting results—in some cases low-dose supplements appear to be effective in reducing symptoms.[9]

Vitamin B$_6$ supplements have been found to improve immune function in older adults, but the reason for the improvement is unclear.[10] Immune function can be impaired by a deficiency of any nutrient that hinders cell growth and division. Therefore, one of the most common claims for vitamin supplements in general is that they improve immune function. Vitamin B$_6$ is no exception. Since the elderly frequently have low intakes of vitamin B$_6$, it is unclear whether the beneficial effects of supplements are due to an improvement in vitamin B$_6$ status or immune system stimulation.

Folate and Vitamin B$_{12}$ Are Needed for Cell Division

Inside the nucleus of every cell is the DNA that holds the genetic code. Before a cell can divide it must make a copy of its DNA. The B vitamin folate is needed for the synthesis of DNA and vitamin B$_{12}$ is needed to keep folate active. Therefore if either B$_{12}$ or folate is missing, DNA cannot be copied and new cells cannot be made correctly. As a result of this interdependency, many of the same symptoms are seen when either vitamin B$_{12}$ or folate are deficient.

Folate: important for rapidly dividing cells

A number of different forms of folate are needed for the synthesis of DNA and the metabolism of some amino acids. Because folate is needed for cells to replicate, it is particularly important in tissues where cells are dividing rapidly such the bone marrow, where red blood cells are made, and the developing tissues of an unborn baby.

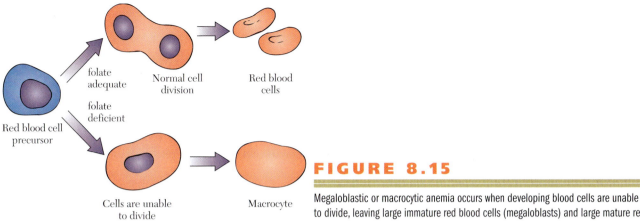

FIGURE 8.15

Megaloblastic or macrocytic anemia occurs when developing blood cells are unable to divide, leaving large immature red blood cells (megaloblasts) and large mature red blood cells (macrocytes).

Folate deficiency results in anemia One of the most notable symptoms of folate deficiency is anemia. Without folate, developing red blood cells cannot divide. Instead, they just grow bigger (Figure 8.15). Fewer mature red cells are produced so the oxygen-carrying capacity of the blood is reduced. This condition is called **megaloblastic** or **macrocytic anemia**. Other symptoms of folate deficiency include poor growth, problems in nerve development and function, diarrhea, and inflammation of the tongue. Groups most at risk of a folate deficiency include pregnant women and premature infants because of their rapid rate of cell division and growth; the elderly because of their limited intake of foods high in folate; alcoholics because alcohol inhibits folate absorption; and tobacco smokers because smoke inactivates folate in the cells lining the lungs.[2]

Megaloblastic or **macrocytic anemia** A condition in which there are abnormally large immature and mature red blood cells and a reduction in the total number of red blood cells and the oxygen-carrying capacity of the blood.

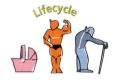

Folate intake is related to neural tube defects A low folate intake increases the risk of birth defects that affect the brain and spinal cord called **neural tube defects** (Figure 8.16). The exact role of folate in neural tube development is not known, but it is necessary for a critical step called neural tube closure. Neural tube closure occurs very early in pregnancy—only 28 days after conception—when most women may not yet even know they are pregnant. Therefore to reduce the risk of these defects, folate status must be adequate before a pregnancy begins and during the early critical days of pregnancy (see Chapter 12). However, folate is not the only factor contributing to neural tube defects. Not every pregnant woman with low folate levels gives birth to a child with a neural tube defect. Instead, these birth defects are probably due to a combination of factors that are aggravated by low folate levels.

Neural tube defects Irregularities in the formation of the portion of the embryo that develops into the brain and spinal cord. These occur early in development and result in brain and spinal cord abnormalities.

Folate status may affect heart disease and cancer risk Low folate intake may increase the risk of heart disease because of its relation to homocysteine levels (see Figure 8.13). Low folate status may also increase the risk of developing cancer

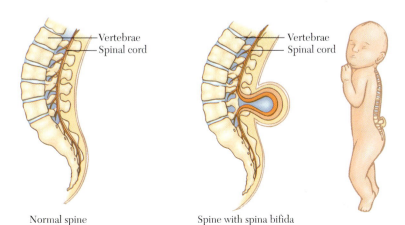

FIGURE 8.16

Early in pregnancy, the neural tube develops into the brain and spinal cord. If folate is inadequate during neural tube closure, neural tube defects such as spina bifida, shown here, occur more frequently. In spina bifida the bones that make up the back do not completely surround the spinal cord, allowing membranes, fluid, and, in severe cases, the nerves of the spinal cord to bulge out where they are unprotected.

On the Web

For more information on folic acid and birth defects, go to the Spina Bifida Association of America at **www.sbaa.org**

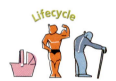

Lifecycle

⚠ **Dietary folate equivalent (DFE)** A unit used to express the amount of folate available to the body that accounts for the higher bioavailability of folic acid in supplements and enriched foods compared to folate found naturally in foods. One DFE is equivalent to 1 μg of folate naturally occurring in food, 0.6 μg of synthetic folic acid from fortified food or supplements consumed with food, or 0.5 μg of synthetic folic acid consumed on an empty stomach.

of the uterus, cervix, lungs, stomach, esophagus, and colon. Although folate deficiency does not cause cancer, it has been hypothesized that low folate intake enhances an underlying predisposition to cancer. The relation between folate and cancer is strongest for colon cancer. Alcohol consumption greatly increases the cancer risk associated with a low folate diet.[11]

Vegetables, legumes, oranges, and grains are good sources of folate
Asparagus, oranges, legumes, liver, and yeast are excellent food sources of folate. Fair sources include grains, corn, snap beans, mustard greens, and broccoli, as well as some nuts. Small amounts are found in meats, cheese, milk, fruits, and other vegetables (Figure 8.17).

Folic acid is added to enriched grain products, including enriched breads, flours, corn meal, pasta, grits, and rice. If you look at the label on a bag of enriched flour you will see that it is fortified with folic acid. Folic acid is a stable form of folate that rarely occurs naturally in food but is used in supplements and fortified foods; it is more easily absorbed than natural folate. In the 3-year period after the fortification of grain products with folic acid, the incidence of neural tube defects decreased by 25%.[12]

Women of childbearing age need extra folate
The RDA for folate is set at 400 μg **dietary folate equivalents (DFEs)** per day for adult men and women. Expressing needs in DFEs allows one unit to be used for all the forms of folate; one DFE is equal to 1 μg of food folate, 0.6 μg of synthetic folic acid from fortified food or supplements consumed with food, or 0.5 μg of synthetic folic acid consumed on an empty stomach. Because supplementing folic acid early in pregnancy has been shown to reduce neural tube defects, a special recommendation is made for women capable of becoming pregnant; 400 μg of synthetic folic acid from fortified foods and/or supplements is recommended in addition to the food folate consumed in

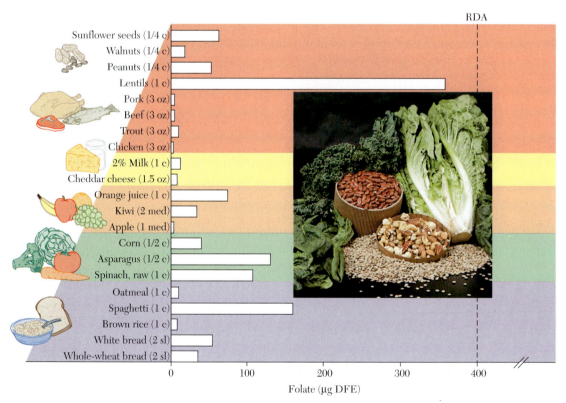

FIGURE 8.17

Folate content of selections from each group of the Food Guide Pyramid. The dashed line represents the RDA for adults. Legumes, fortified foods, and some fruits and vegetables are good sources. (George Semple)

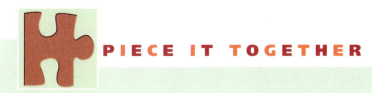

PIECE IT TOGETHER

Is It Hard to Meet Folate Recommendations?

Marcia would like to have a baby but before she tries to conceive, she wants to be sure she is in the best condition possible. She consults her physician who gives her a clean bill of health but suggests she make sure she is getting enough folate.

WHY IS FOLATE A CONCERN FOR WOMEN CAPABLE OF BECOMING PREGNANT?

Research shows that consuming extra folic acid can reduce the risk of a type of birth defect called a neural tube defect that affects an unborn child's brain or spinal cord. For the extra folic acid to be beneficial, it must be consumed for at least a month before conception and continued for a month after. Since many pregnancies are not planned, it is recommended that all women of childbearing age consume 400 µg of folic acid from fortified foods or supplements.

Marcia records her food intake for 1 day to determine her folate intake:

Food	Servings	Total Folate (µg)
Breakfast		
Oatmeal, regular	1 cup	2
Milk	1 cup	12
Banana	1 medium	22
Orange juice	8 ounces	75
Coffee	1 cup	0
Lunch		
Hamburger	1	11
Hamburger bun	1	32
French fries	20 pieces	24
Coke	12 ounces	0
Apple	1 medium	4
Dinner		
Chicken	3 ounces	4
Refried beans	1/2 cup	106
White rice	1 cup	80
Tortilla	1	60
Salad	1 cup	64
Salad dressing	1 Tbsp	1
Milk	1 cup	12
Cake	1 piece	32
Total		**541 µg**

DOES MARCIA'S FOLATE INTAKE MEET THE RDA?

Yes. Marica consumes 541 µg of folate, which is greater than the RDA of 400 µg DFE, but her doctor told her that

women who are capable of becoming pregnant should consume 400 µg of folic acid from fortified foods or supplements each day in addition to the folate found in a varied diet. Folic acid is added to enriched grains, so it can be found in any food that contains enriched grains; you can check the ingredient list to see if the food you have chosen contains added folic acid. The percent Daily Value includes both the natural folate and added folic acid.

WHICH FOODS IN MARCIA'S DIET ARE HIGHEST IN FOLATE? OF THESE, WHICH DO YOU THINK HAVE BEEN FORTIFIED WITH FOLIC ACID?

Food	Amount	Natural	Fortified
Rice	80 µg		√
Orange juice	75 µg	√	
Your answers:			

WHY IS THE OATMEAL LOW IN FOLATE BUT THE OTHER GRAIN PRODUCTS ARE GOOD FOLATE SOURCES?

Oatmeal is a whole grain, so it has not been fortified with folic acid. The other grain products in her diet, such as the white rice, tortilla, and hamburger bun, are refined so they contain added folic acid. Even though Marcia is trying to increase her intake of the folic acid form of this vitamin she should not pass up whole grains—they are good sources of most B vitamins, minerals, and fiber.

LIST SOME MODIFICATIONS MARCIA COULD MAKE IN HER DIET TO PROVIDE THE RECOMMENDED AMOUNTS AND FORMS OF FOLATE?

Your answer:

WOULD YOU RECOMMEND MARCIA TAKE A FOLATE SUPPLEMENT?

Your answer:

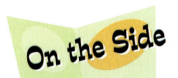

Not everyone needs a folate supplement. If you are male or a female who is too young or too old to have a baby, the amount of folate you get from a healthy diet will meet your needs. Even women of childbearing age can get enough folic acid without a supplement if they eat enough folic acid fortified foods.

⚠ **Pernicious anemia** An anemia resulting from vitamin B_{12} deficiency that occurs due to a lack of a protein called intrinsic factor needed to absorb dietary vitamin B_{12}.

⚠ **Intrinsic factor** A protein produced in the stomach that is needed for the absorption of adequate amounts of vitamin B_{12}.

⚠ **Cobalamin** The chemical term for vitamin B_{12}.

On the Side

The presence of a factor in stomach secretions that could cure pernicious anemia was demonstrated by William Castle in a rather disgusting experiment. He ate red meat, made himself vomit, and fed the stomach secretions to his patients. The intrinsic factor in his vomit allowed the patients to absorb vitamin B_{12} and their symptoms improved.

a varied diet. The folic acid form is recommended because it is the form that has been shown to reduce birth defects. This recommendation is made for all women of child-bearing age because folate is needed very early in a pregnancy—before most women are aware that they are pregnant. To get 400 μg of folic acid, you would need to eat 4 to 6 servings of fortified grain products each day or take a supplement containing folic acid.

Excess folate can mask anemia caused by vitamin B_{12} deficiency

Although extra folate is recommended for pregnant women, too much is a concern for some groups. There is no known folate toxicity, but a high intake may mask the early symptoms of vitamin B_{12} deficiency, allowing it to go untreated so irreversible nerve damage can occur. The UL for adults is set at 1000 μg per day of folate from supplements and/or fortified foods. This value was determined based on the progression of neurological symptoms seen in patients who are deficient in vitamin B_{12} and taking folate supplements.

Vitamin B_{12}: absorption requires intrinsic factor

If you lived in the early 1900's and developed a condition called **pernicious anemia**, it was a death sentence. There was no cure. In the 1920's researchers George Minot and William Murphy pursued their belief that pernicious anemia could be cured by something in the diet. Their experiments were able to restore good health to patients by feeding them about 4 to 8 ounces of slightly cooked liver at every meal.

Today we know that liver contains high levels of vitamin B_{12}. We also know that pernicious anemia is not actually caused by a lack of the vitamin in the diet, but rather an inability to absorb the vitamin. Vitamin B_{12} absorption requires a protein called **intrinsic factor** that is produced by cells in the stomach lining. With the help of stomach acid, intrinsic factor binds to vitamin B_{12} and this vitamin B_{12}-intrinsic factor complex is then absorbed in the small intestine. When very large amounts of the vitamin are consumed, some can be absorbed without intrinsic factor. This is why Minot and Murphy were able to cure pernicious anemia with extremely high dietary doses of the vitamin. Today, pernicious anemia is treated with injections of vitamin B_{12} rather than plates full of liver.

Vitamin B_{12} is needed for nerve function

Vitamin B_{12}, also known as **cobalamin**, is necessary for the maintenance of myelin, which is the coating that insulates nerves and is essential for nerve transmission. Vitamin B_{12} is also needed for the production of energy from certain fatty acids and to convert homocysteine to methionine (see Figure 8.13). This reaction also converts folate from an inactive form to a form that functions in DNA synthesis. Because of the need for vitamin B_{12} in folate metabolism, a deficiency can cause a secondary folate deficiency and, consequently, macrocytic anemia.

Symptoms of vitamin B_{12} deficiency include an increase in blood homocysteine levels and anemia that is indistinguishable from that seen in folate deficiency. Other symptoms include numbness and tingling, abnormalities in gait, memory loss, and disorientation due to degeneration of the myelin that coats the nerves, spinal cord, and brain. If not treated, this eventually causes paralysis and death.

Consuming extra folate can mask a vitamin B_{12} deficiency

When the diet is deficient in vitamin B_{12}, consuming extra folate can mask the vitamin B_{12} deficiency by preventing the appearance of anemia. If the deficiency is not treated, the other symptoms of B_{12} deficiency, such as nerve damage, progress and can be irreversible. This connection between folate and vitamin B_{12} has raised concerns that our folate-fortified food supply may allow B_{12} deficiencies to go unnoticed. So far, this has not been a problem in the population. The amounts of folate consumed from a typical diet are unlikely to be high enough for this to occur. However, the amounts of folate in supplements may be high enough to mask a vitamin B_{12} deficiency.[13]

Vitamin B$_{12}$ is not found in plants

Vitamin B$_{12}$ is found only in animal products—beef, pork, chicken, and fish are excellent sources. Plant foods do not provide this vitamin unless they have been fortified with the vitamin or contaminated by bacteria, soil, insects, or other sources of B$_{12}$ (Figure 8.18).

The RDA for adults of all ages for vitamin B$_{12}$ is 2.4 µg per day; the average intake for both adult men and women exceeds this.[3] No toxic effects have been reported with excess vitamin B$_{12}$ intakes of up to 100 µg per day from food or supplements. Sufficient data are not yet available to establish a UL for vitamin B$_{12}$.

Vegetarians and older adults are at risk for vitamin B$_{12}$ deficiency

Despite the fact that average intakes exceed the RDA for vitamin B$_{12}$ and blatant deficiencies of this vitamin are rare, marginal deficiencies are a concern in vegan vegetarians and older adults.

Vitamin B$_{12}$ deficiency is a concern among vegans—those who consume no animal products—because vitamin B$_{12}$ is only found in foods of animal origin. Diets that do not include animal products must include supplements or foods fortified with vitamin B$_{12}$ in order to meet needs.[14] Severe deficiency has been observed in breast-fed infants of vegan women, but marginal deficiency is a concern for all vegans if supplements or fortified foods are not included in the diet.

Vitamin B$_{12}$ deficiency is a concern in older adults because of a condition called **atrophic gastritis** that reduces vitamin B$_{12}$ absorption. Atrophic gastritis affects 10 to 30% of adults over age 50. It is an inflammation of the lining of the stomach that reduces stomach acid secretion and allows microbial overgrowth. Without sufficient stomach acid, the enzymes that release protein-bound vitamin B$_{12}$ cannot function properly so the bound vitamin B$_{12}$ cannot be released to bind to intrinsic factor for absorption. In addition, the large numbers of microbes in the gut compete for available vitamin B$_{12}$, reducing absorption. To ensure adequate B$_{12}$ absorption, individuals over the age of 50 should consume vitamin B$_{12}$ that is not bound to proteins; it is found in fortified foods such as breakfast cereals and vitamin B$_{12}$-containing supplements.

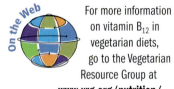

On the Web For more information on vitamin B$_{12}$ in vegetarian diets, go to the Vegetarian Resource Group at **www.vrg.org/nutrition/**

Atrophic gastritis An inflammation of the stomach lining. It causes a reduction in stomach acid and allows bacterial overgrowth.

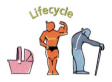

Lifecycle

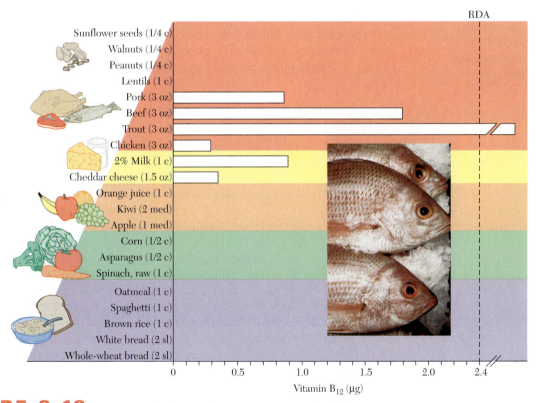

FIGURE 8.18

Vitamin B$_{12}$ content of selections from each food group of the Food Guide Pyramid. The dashed line represents the RDA for adult men and women. Vitamin B$_{12}$ is only found in foods of animal origin or foods that have been fortified with the vitamin. (Corbis Images)

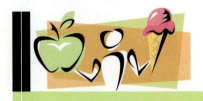

So, What Should I Eat?

B (vitamin) sure
- Choose meat, chicken, or fish—they are all good sources of B vitamins
- Choose whole grain bread to get vitamin B_6
- Enrich your diet with some enriched grains
- Have a bowl of fortified breakfast cereal for B_{12} insurance

Focus on folate
- Use leaf lettuce or spinach in your salad
- Add some beans—pinto beans, kidneys beans, baked beans are all are high in folate and fiber
- Snack on an orange—you'll get your folate as well as vitamin C

Vitamin C Saved Sailors from Scurvy

Scurvy The disease resulting from a deficiency of vitamin C.

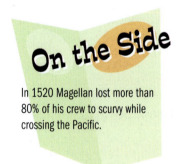

On the Side

In 1520 Magellan lost more than 80% of his crew to scurvy while crossing the Pacific.

Ascorbic acid The chemical term for vitamin C.

Collagen The major protein in connective tissue.

Throughout human history the disease **scurvy** has been the downfall of armies, navies, and explorers. Scurvy is caused by a deficiency of vitamin C. The reason this vitamin was a particular problem is that fresh fruits and vegetables are its main sources; these foods spoil quickly and don't transport well on long voyages. Sailors in the 17th and 18th centuries were far more likely to die of scurvy than be killed in shipwrecks or battles. In 1593 Sir Richard Hawkins observed that consuming citrus fruit could cure scurvy. Unfortunately, it took another 200 years before the observations of Hawkins and others after him were acted on, and meanwhile, thousands continued to suffer and die from scurvy. Finally, it became common practice to include a source of vitamin C in the shipboard diet. The mandatory inclusion of lime or lemon juice in the rations of British sailors protected them from scurvy and earned them the name "limeys."

Vitamin C is needed to maintain connective tissue

Vitamin C, also known as **ascorbic acid**, is a water-soluble vitamin needed in reactions that synthesize a number of compounds including neurotransmitters, hormones such as the thyroid and steroid hormones, bile acids, and carnitine, needed for fatty acid breakdown. But its best known role is in the synthesis and maintenance of **collagen**. Collagen is the most abundant protein in the body and forms the base of all connective tissue. Collagen can be thought of as the glue that holds the body together. It is in bones and teeth, ligaments and tendons; it forms the scars that bind a wound together, and gives structure to blood vessel walls. A vitamin C-requiring reaction is essential for the formation of bonds that hold adjacent collagen molecules together and give it strength (Figure 8.19). Like all body proteins collagen is continuously being broken down and reformed. Without vitamin C, the bonds holding adjacent collagen molecules together cannot be formed and maintained so the collagen that is broken down cannot be replaced. It is the inability to form healthy collagen that causes the symptoms of scurvy.

When vitamin C intake is below 10 mg per day, the symptoms of scurvy begin to appear. The capillary walls weaken and rupture causing bleeding under the skin and into the joints. This causes raised red spots on the skin, joint pain and weakness, and easy bruising. The gums bleed and break down and the teeth loosen and eventually

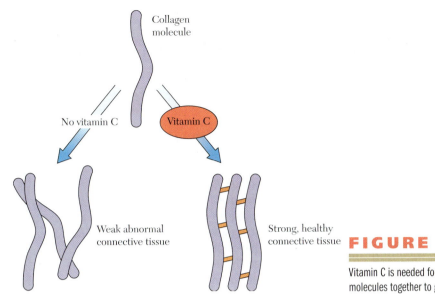

FIGURE 8.19

Vitamin C is needed for the formation of chemical bonds that link collagen molecules together to give connective tissue strength and stability.

fall out. Wounds do not heal and old wounds may reopen and bones fracture. Sufferers become tired, depressed, and suffer from hysteria.

Vitamin C is a water-soluble antioxidant

Vitamin C is also an **antioxidant**. Antioxidants are substances that protect against **oxidative damage** caused by reactive oxygen molecules. Reactive oxygen molecules such as **free radicals** can be generated by normal oxygen-requiring reactions inside the body or can come from environmental sources such as air pollution or cigarette smoke. Free radicals cause damage by snatching electrons from DNA, proteins, carbohydrates, or unsaturated fatty acids. This results in changes in the structure and function of these molecules. Antioxidants act by destroying reactive oxygen molecules before they can do damage. Some antioxidants are produced in the body; others, such as vitamin C, vitamin E, and the mineral selenium, are consumed in the diet.[15]

Vitamin C acts as an antioxidant in the blood and other body fluids. Its antioxidant properties help maintain the immune system so the ability to fight infection is decreased when this vitamin is deficient. Its antioxidant action also regenerates the active antioxidant form of vitamin E and enhances iron absorption by keeping iron in its more readily absorbed form. When about 50 mg of vitamin C—the amount contained in 5 ounces of orange juice—is consumed in a meal containing iron, iron absorption is enhanced (see Chapter 9).

Citrus fruit is one of the best sources of vitamin C

Citrus fruit, such as oranges, lemons, and limes, is an excellent source of vitamin C. A large orange has enough to meet the RDA of 90 mg per day for men and 75 mg per day for women. Other fruits that are high in vitamin C include strawberries, kiwis, and cantaloupe. Vegetables in the cabbage family, such as broccoli, cauliflower, bok choy, and Brussels sprouts, as well as green leafy vegetables, green and red peppers, okra, tomatoes, and potatoes, are also good sources (Figure 8.20). Meat, fish, poultry, eggs, dairy products, and grains are poor sources. Vitamin C is destroyed by oxygen, light, and heat, so it is readily lost in cooking. This loss is accelerated in low-acid foods and by the use of copper or iron cooking utensils.

Cigarette smoking increases the requirement for vitamin C because the vitamin is used to break down compounds in cigarette smoke.[15] It is recommended that cigarette

Antioxidant A substance that is able to neutralize reactive oxygen molecules and thereby reduce oxidative damage.

Oxidative damage Damage caused by highly reactive oxygen molecules that steal electrons from other compounds, causing changes in structure and function.

Free radical One type of highly reactive molecule that causes oxidative damage.

✳ Remember

The oxidation of LDL particles by free radicals discussed in Chapter 5 is an early step leading to the buildup of atherosclerotic plaque. Vitamin C helps prevent this oxidation.

On the Side

Most animals make vitamin C in their bodies. Humans and other primates, guinea pigs, the Indian fruit-eating bat, an Asian bird called the red-vented bulbul, rainbow trout, and Coho salmon are the only animal species that are unable to make their own vitamin C.

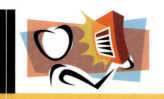

Off the Label: How Much Vitamin C Is in Your Orange Juice?

How much vitamin C is in your orange juice? How much folate is in your breakfast cereal? How much iron is in a box of raisins? Vitamins and minerals are important in your diet, but it can be difficult to tell from food labels exactly how much is in a food. It's easy to tell how much fat, carbohydrate, and even sodium are in a food because these are all listed by weight in the Nutrition Facts section of the food label. But the amounts of other micronutrients are listed only as a percent of the Daily Value.

Food labels are required to provide the % Daily Values for vitamin A, vitamin C, iron, and calcium. Amounts of other vitamins are often provided voluntarily. In order to determine the amount of one of these nutrients in a food, you need to know the Daily Value for that nutrient. The Daily Values for vitamins are given below (see Table 2.3 for values for other nutrients). Once you know the Daily Value, you can multiply it by the % Daily Value on the label to determine the amount in a serving of the food. So, to find out how much vitamin C is in your orange juice follow these steps:

1. Look up the Daily Value:

Nutrient	Daily Value	Nutrient	Daily Value
Vitamin A	5000 IU*	Thiamin	1.5 mg
Vitamin D	400 IU*	Riboflavin	1.7 mg
Vitamin E	30 IU*	Niacin	20 mg
Vitamin K	80 μg	Vitamin B$_6$	2.0 mg
Biotin	300 μg	Folic acid	400 μg
Pantothenic acid	10 mg	Vitamin B$_{12}$	6 μg
Vitamin C	60 mg		

*The Daily Values for some fat-soluble vitamins are expressed in International Units (IU). The DRIs use a newer system of measurement.

2. Find the % Daily Value on your food label
3. Multiply the % Daily Value by the Daily Value to find out how much is in a serving

60 mg × 120% of Daily Value = 60 × 1.2
= 72 mg vitamin C

Even if you don't look up the Daily Value and calculate the exact amount of vitamin C or some other vitamin in a food, the % Daily Value on the food label tells you if that food is a good source. As a general guideline, if the % Daily Value is 5% or less it is a poor source, if it is 10 to 19%, the food is a good source of that nutrient. If the % Daily Value is 20% or more, the food is an excellent source of that nutrient. Whether you are converting Daily Values into amounts of vitamins or just looking at the Daily Value, be sure to consider how many servings you plan to eat. Doubling the serving doubles the nutrients and calories.

Orange Juice

Nutrition Facts

Serving Size 8 fl oz (250 mL)
Servings Per Container 8

Amount Per Serving

Calories 110	Calories from Fat 0

	%Daily Value**
Total Fat 0g	**2%**
Sodium 0mg	**0%**
Potassium 450mg	**13%**
Total Carbohydrate 26g	**9%**
Sugars 7g	
Protein 2g	

Vitamin C 120%	•	Calcium	2%
Thiamin 10%	•	Riboflavin	4%
Niacin 4%	•	Vitamin B$_6$	6%
Folate 15%	•	Magnesium	6%

Not a significant source or saturated fat, cholesterol, dietary fiber, vitamin A and iron.

*Percent Daily Values are based on a 2,000 calorie diet.

Vitamin C is the most common vitamin supplement

One-third of the population of the United States takes supplements of vitamin C—usually in the hope that it will prevent the common cold. Although vitamin C does not prevent colds, it may help to reduce their duration and the severity of cold symptoms. Vitamin C supplements have also been suggested to reduce the risk of cardiovascular disease and cancer but there is not sufficient evidence to support this effect.[15]

Vitamin C, even in supplements, is considered nontoxic for most people. As the amount consumed increases, the amount absorbed decreases and the vitamin C absorbed in excess of need is excreted in the urine. However, excessive doses can cause unpleasant side effects in healthy individuals. The most common symptoms include diarrhea, nausea, and abdominal cramps. These are caused when unabsorbed vitamin C draws water into the intestine. Large doses of vitamin C in chewable supplements can also damage teeth. Vitamin C is an acid; it can actually dissolve tooth enamel when vitamin C tablets are chewed. High intakes of vitamin C can be a more serious concern for some individuals. In those prone to kidney stones, it can increase stone formation. In individuals who are unable to regulate iron absorption, it can increase absorption allowing amounts in the body to reach toxic levels. For those with sickle cell anemia, it can worsen symptoms. Other potential problems associated with vitamin C intakes greater than 3 grams per day include interference with drugs prescribed to slow blood clotting and, because the structure of vitamin C is similar to that of glucose, interference with urine tests used to monitor glucose levels in diabetes. The UL for vitamin C has been set at 2000 mg per day from food and supplements. At intakes above this level the likelihood of diarrhea and gastrointestinal disturbances increases.

Choline: Is It a Vitamin?

Choline is a dietary component that is needed to synthesize a number of important molecules in the body. However, it is not considered a dietary essential because it can be synthesized in the body. Nonetheless, the DRIs have set a recommended intake for this compound; 550 mg per day is recommended for men and 425 mg per day for women.[3]

Choline is found in many foods. Particularly good sources include egg yolks, organ meats, spinach, nuts, and wheat germ. The average daily choline intake in the United States is estimated to be 600 to 1000 mg per day; an amount well in excess of the recommended intake. Choline deficiency is unlikely in healthy humans.[3]

Experiments that fed people large doses of choline found that excesses can cause a fishy body odor. In addition, experiments have demonstrated that too much choline can cause excess sweating, reduced growth rate, low blood pressure, and liver damage. The amounts needed to cause these symptoms are much higher than can be obtained from foods. The UL for choline for adults is 3.5 grams per day.

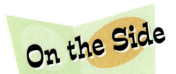

On the Side

Hippocrates, who lived 460–325 BC, recognized night blindness and recommended eating raw liver as a cure.

Vitamin A Is Needed for Healthy Eyes

Did anyone ever tell you that eating carrots would help you see in the dark? It turns out they were right. Carrots are a good source of **beta-carotene (β-carotene)**, a precursor that can be converted into vitamin A in your body. Vitamin A is a fat-soluble vitamin needed for night vision and healthy eyes; one of the first signs of a deficiency is difficulty seeing in dim light, a condition called **night blindness** (Table 8.3). Severe vitamin A deficiency is a world health problem that causes blindness in thousands of children each year.

Vitamin A comes preformed and in precursor forms

Vitamin A is found preformed and in precursor or provitamin forms in our diet. Preformed vitamin A compounds are known as **retinoids**. There are three retinoids that are active in the body: retinal, retinol, and retinoic acid. Retinoids are found in animal foods such as liver, fish, egg yolks, and dairy products. **Carotenoids**, including β-carotene, are yellow-orange pigments found in plants, some of which are vitamin A

Beta-carotene (β-carotene) A carotenoid that has more provitamin A activity than other carotenoids. It is also an antioxidant.

Night blindness Inability to see clearly in dim light.

Retinoids The chemical forms of preformed vitamin A: retinol, retinal, and retinoic acid.

Carotenoids Natural pigments synthesized by plants and many microorganisms. They give yellow-orange fruits and vegetables their color.

TABLE 8.3
A Quick Guide to the Fat-Soluble Vitamins

Vitamin	Food Sources	Recommended Intake for Adults	Major Functions	Deficiency Symptoms	Groups at Risk of Deficiency	Toxicity and UL
Vitamin A (retinol, retinal, retinoic acid, vitamin A acetate, vitamin A palmitate, retinyl palmitate, provitamin A, carotene, β-carotene, carotenoids)	Retinol: liver, fish, fortified milk and margarine, butter, eggs. Carotenoids: carrots, leafy greens, sweet potatoes, broccoli, apricots, cantaloupe	700–900 μg/day	Vision, health of cornea and other epithelial tissue, cell differentiation, reproduction, immunity	Night blindness, xeropthalmia, poor growth, dry skin, impaired immunity	Those who live in poverty (particularly children and pregnant women), those consuming very low-fat or low-protein diets	Headache, vomiting, hair loss, liver damage, skin changes, bone pain, birth defects. UL is 3000 μg of preformed vitamin A
Vitamin D (calciferol, cholecalciferol, ergocalciferol, dihydroxy vitamin D)	Egg yolk, liver, fish oils, tuna, salmon, fortified milk and margarine, synthesis from sunlight	5–15 μg/day	Absorption of calcium and phosphorous, maintenance of bone	Rickets in children: abnormal growth, misshaped bones, bowed legs, soft bones. Osteomalacia in adults: weak bones and bone pain	Some breast-fed infants, children, and elderly (especially those with dark skin and little sun exposure), people with kidney disease	Calcium deposits in soft tissues, growth retardation, kidney damage. UL is 50 μg
Vitamin E (tocopherol, alpha-tocopherol)	Vegetable oils, leafy greens, seeds, nuts, peanuts	15 mg/day	Antioxidant, protects cell membranes	Broken red blood cells, nerve damage	Those with poor fat absorption, premature infants	Inhibition of vitamin K activity. UL is 1000 mg from supplemental sources
Vitamin K (phylloquinones, menaquinone)	Vegetable oils, leafy greens, synthesis by intestinal bacteria	90–120 μg/day	Synthesis of blood clotting proteins	Hemorrhage	Newborns (especially premature), people on long-term antibiotics	Anemia, brain damage. No UL

UL, Tolerable Upper Intake Level

precursors; they can be converted into retinoids once inside the body. β-carotene, the most potent vitamin A precursor, is plentiful in carrots, squash, apricots, and other orange and yellow vegetables and fruits. It is also found in leafy green vegetables such as spinach and broccoli where the yellow-orange pigment is masked by green chlorophyll (Figure 8.21). Other carotenoids that provide some provitamin A activity include α-carotene found in leafy green vegetables, carrots, and squash, and β-cryptoxanthin found in corn, green peppers, and lemons. Generally the term vitamin A refers to both the retinoids and provitamin A carotenoids. All forms of vitamin A in the diet are fairly stable when heated but may be destroyed by exposure to light and oxygen.

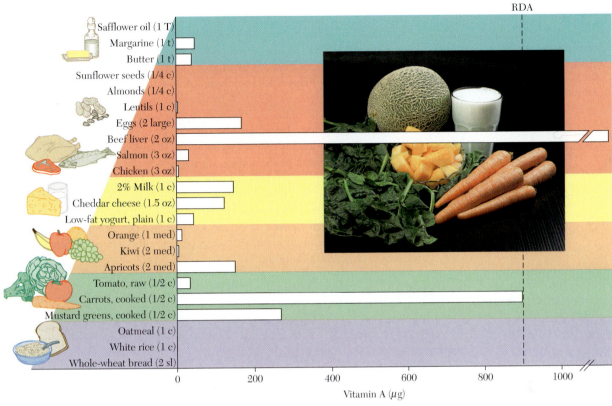

FIGURE 8.21

Vitamin A content of selections from each food group of the Food Guide Pyramid. The dashed line represents the RDA for adult men. Both plant and animal foods are good sources of vitamin A. (George Semple)

Vitamin A requires fat for absorption and protein for transport

Both retinoids and carotenoids are bound to proteins in foods. To be absorbed, they must be released from the protein by protein-digesting enzymes. Then the released carotenoids and retinoids must combine with bile acids and other dietary fats in order to be absorbed. Absorption of preformed vitamin A is efficient but carotenoids are less well absorbed, and absorption decreases as intake increases.[16]

When dietary fat intake is very low (less than 10 g/day), vitamin A absorption is impaired. This is rarely a problem in the United States and other industrialized countries, where typical fat intake is greater than 50 grams per day. However, in developing countries, vitamin A deficiency may occur not only because the diet is low in the vitamin but also because the diet is too low in fat for the vitamin to be absorbed efficiently. Diseases that cause fat malabsorption can also interfere with vitamin A absorption and cause a deficiency.

Like other dietary fats, retinoids and carotenoids are transported from the intestine in chylomicrons. These lipoproteins deliver the retinoids and carotenoids to body tissues such as bone marrow, blood cells, spleen, muscles, kidney, and liver. To move from liver stores to other body tissues, preformed vitamin A must be bound to a protein called **retinol-binding protein**. For this reason, vitamin A deficiency can also be caused by a protein deficiency. Without sufficient retinol-binding protein, vitamin A cannot be transported to the tissues where it is needed. Likewise, when zinc is deficient, a vitamin A deficiency may occur because zinc is needed to make proteins involved in vitamin A transport and metabolism.

There is no specific blood transport protein for carotenoids, but since they are fat-soluble, they are incorporated into lipoproteins to travel in the bloodstream.

✳ Retinol-binding protein A protein that is necessary to transport vitamin A from the liver to other tissues.

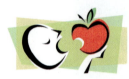

⚠️ **Rhodopsin** A light-sensitive compound found in the retina of the eye that is composed of the protein opsin loosely bound to retinal.

Eating carrots can improve your vision in low light if you are deficient in vitamin A. Carrots provide β-carotene, which can be converted into active vitamin A. If your vitamin A status is normal, eating more carrots will not cause further improvements in vision.

✳️ **Gene expression** Refers to the events of protein synthesis in which the information coded in a gene is used to synthesize a protein.

Vitamin A is necessary for vision

Vitamin A is involved in the perception of light. In the eye, the retinal form of the vitamin combines with the protein opsin to form the visual pigment **rhodopsin**. When light strikes rhodopsin, it changes from a curved molecule to a straight one (Figure 8.22). This change in shape initiates a series of events that cause a nerve signal to be sent to the brain allowing us to see. When it changes shape, retinal is released from opsin. After the light stimulus has passed, rhodopsin is regenerated. Because some retinal is lost in these reactions, it must be replaced by retinol from the blood. If blood levels of vitamin A are low, as they are in someone who is vitamin A deficient, there is a delay in the regeneration of rhodopsin, during which time no light can be seen. All of us are blinded for a few seconds after looking into the bright headlights of an approaching car at night, but someone with night blindness from vitamin A deficiency would take a lot longer to recover. Night blindness is one of the first and more easily reversible symptoms of vitamin A deficiency. If deficiency progresses, more serious and less reversible symptoms occur that are related to other essential roles that this vitamin plays throughout the body.

Vitamin A regulates gene expression

Vitamin A helps to regulate **gene expression**. This means that it can turn on or turn off certain genes. When a specific gene is turned on it instructs the cell to make a particular protein. Proteins regulate functions within cells and throughout the body. This turning on (or turning off) of genes increases (or decreases) the production of proteins and thereby affects various cellular functions. For example, vitamin A turns on a gene in liver cells that makes a protein that enables the liver to make glucose.

Vitamin A is needed to maintain epithelial tissue Vitamin A is necessary for the maintenance of epithelial tissue, which makes up the skin and the tissues that line the eyes, intestines, lungs, vagina, and bladder. Vitamin A maintains

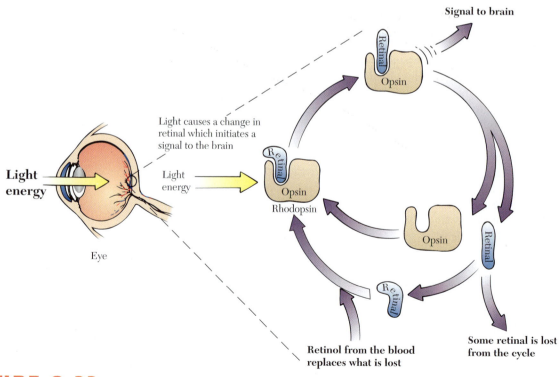

FIGURE 8.22

In the visual cycle of the eye, retinal binds to the protein opsin to form rhodopsin. When light strikes rhodopsin, it causes a change in retinal that sends a nerve signal to the brain that allows us to see. When the retinal is released from opsin, some retinal is lost and must be replaced by retinol from the blood.

this tissue through its role in **cell differentiation**, the process whereby immature cells change in structure and function to become mature cells that can perform specialized functions. When vitamin A is deficient, epithelial cells do not differentiate normally because vitamin A is not there to turn on or turn off the production of particular proteins. For example, the lining of the eye normally contains cells that secrete mucus to lubricate the eye. When these cells die, immature cells differentiate to become new mucus-secreting cells to replace the dead ones. Without vitamin A, the immature cells can't differentiate normally and instead of mucus-secreting cells they become cells that produce a protein called keratin. Keratin is a hard protein that makes up hair and fingernails. When mucus-secreting cells are replaced by keratin-producing cells, the surface of the eye becomes hard and dry, leaving the eye open to infection. This keratinization of the eye is an early stage of **xerophthalmia**, a spectrum of eye disorders that are associated with vitamin A deficiency. In the early stages, xeropthalmia can be treated by increasing vitamin A intake but if left untreated, it can result in a softening of the cornea, called keratomalacia, and permanent blindness.

Vitamin A is needed for reproduction, growth, and immunity

The ability of vitamin A to regulate the growth and differentiation of cells makes it essential throughout life for normal reproduction, growth, and immune function. In reproduction, vitamin A is needed to direct cells to differentiate and to form the shapes and patterns needed for a complete organism. In growing children, vitamin A affects the activity of cells that form and break down bone; a deficiency early in life can cause abnormal jawbone growth, resulting in crooked teeth and poor dental health. In the immune system, vitamin A is needed for the differentiation that produces the different types of immune cells. When vitamin A is deficient, the activity of specific immune cells cannot be stimulated leading to an increased susceptibility to all sorts of infections.

β-Carotene is a vitamin A precursor and an antioxidant

Some of the β-carotene and other carotenoids in our diet are converted to vitamin A, whereas others remain as carotenoids. Carotenoids are fat-soluble antioxidants, but their antioxidant role in the human body is still unclear. Populations that consume diets high in foods containing carotenoids have been shown to have a lower incidence of diseases in which oxidative processes play a role such as cancer, heart disease, and the eye disorders macular degeneration and cataracts. Although carotenoids might be a key reason for this reduction in certain diseases, there is not enough evidence to prove that the effect is due to the carotenoids and not some other component of the foods. Therefore it has not been possible to make a specific recommendation for the intake of carotenoids.[15]

Vitamin A needs can be met with plant and animal sources

You can meet your body's needs for vitamin A by eating animal products such as eggs and dairy products and by eating fruits and vegetables that are sources of carotenoids. Because carotenoids are not absorbed as well as preformed vitamin A and are not completely converted to vitamin A inside the body, you get less functional vitamin A from 1 μg of carotenoids than you do from 1 μg of retinoids. To account for this difference a correction factor, referred to as **retinol activity equivalents (RAE)**, is used to express the amount of usable vitamin A in foods; 1 RAE provides the same amount of usable vitamin A as 1 μg of retinol. It takes 12 μg of β-carotene to provide 1 RAE and 24 μg of α-carotene or β-cryptoxanthin to provide 1 RAE.[16] The RDA is set at 900 μg of vitamin A per day for men and 700 μg of vitamin A per day for women. No specific recommendations have been made for intakes of carotenoids; their intake is considered only with regard to the amount of retinol they provide.

Cell differentiation Structural and functional changes that cause cells to mature into specialized cells.

Xerophthalmia A spectrum of eye conditions resulting from vitamin A deficiency that may lead to blindness. An early symptom is night blindness, and as deficiency worsens, lack of mucus leaves the eye dry and vulnerable to cracking and infection.

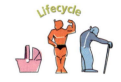

Lifecycle

Retinol activity equivalent (RAE) The amount of retinol, β-carotene, α-carotene, or β-cryptoxanthin that provides vitamin A activity equal to 1 μg of retinol.

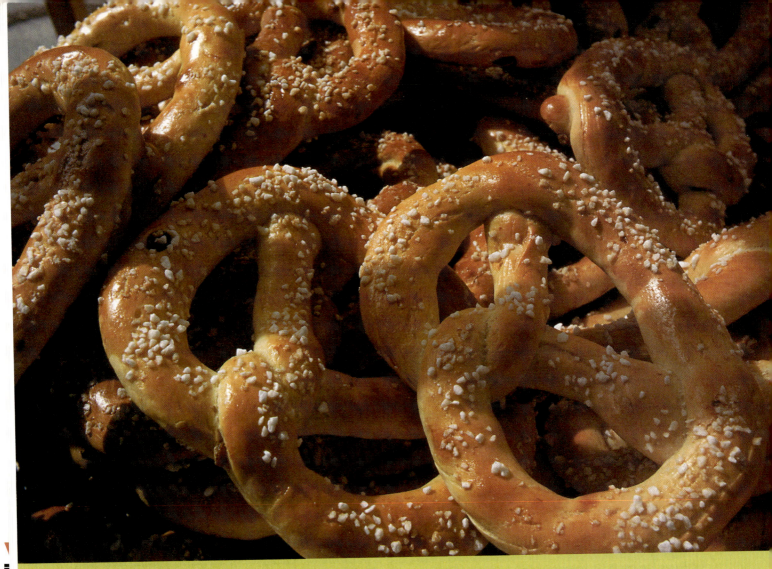

(© Corrine J. Humphrey/Index Stock)

CHAPTER 9 CONCEPTS

- Water is an essential macronutrient; to maintain fluid balance, intake must equal losses.
- Sodium, chloride, and potassium are electrolytes. These and other minerals are important in regulating blood pressure.
- Calcium, phosphorus, and magnesium are minerals needed for bone health.
- Iron is a component of the oxygen transport protein hemoglobin. Iron-deficiency anemia is the most common nutritional deficiency worldwide.
- Copper functions in iron transport, connective tissue synthesis, lipid metabolism, and antioxidant protection.
- Zinc is needed for many enzymes and for the activity of a number of vitamins and hormones.
- Selenium is an essential part of the antioxidant enzyme glutathione peroxidase.
- Iodine is essential for the synthesis of the thyroid hormones.
- Chromium helps insulin function.
- Fluoride is important for healthy teeth and bones.

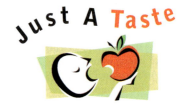

Just A Taste

Can taking a supplement of one mineral cause a deficiency of another?

How long can a person survive without water?

Does eating too much salt raise blood pressure?

Are iron supplements dangerous?

Water and Minerals

INTRODUCTION

Reuters Health

Study: Overweight Children Risk Iron Deficiency

Tuesday, July 6, 2004—Overweight children are at double the risk of being iron deficient, perhaps because of bad diet or lack of exercise, a study said on Tuesday. . . .

Iron deficiency is a global problem most commonly found in poorer people lacking proper nutrition, but the study concluded that the rising number of obese people in the developed world should be checked and treated for it.

Too little iron in the blood can cause anemia and lead to learning and behavioral problems as well as pose limits on work and exercise.

One out of seven U.S. children is overweight, a three-fold increase in the past 30 years, and many do not get screened for iron deficiency, Yale University researcher Karen Nead wrote in the journal *Pediatrics*.

To read the complete article, go to www.nlm.nih.gov/medlineplus/news/fullstory_18782.html.www.iconcast.com/H/HealthGuide B7.6/NewsonHealth3.htm

How can someone be overweight and still suffer from a nutrient deficiency? In the United States and other developed countries, where diseases related to overconsumption are the obvious problem, we tend to forget about the dangers of nutrient deficiencies. Many of the deficiencies that were public health problems in the early part of the 20th century have been virtually eliminated by our plentiful and fortified food supply, but poor food choices can still create nutrient deficiencies even among those who are consuming more than enough calories. Several of the nutrients at risk for deficiency in the American diet are minerals. As this article illustrates, poor iron intake puts many at risk of iron deficiency anemia and despite the fact that most Americans have plenty to eat, low intakes of calcium and zinc are also a concern.

The DASH diet is a dietary pattern that may provide more health benefits than just lowering blood pressure. It is not that different from what other recommendations are advising us to eat. The Dietary Guidelines encourages the consumption of fresh fruits, vegetables, grains, meats, and dairy products. Following the Food Guide Pyramid recommendations also results in a diet similar to DASH, particularly if you aim for the high end of the recommended servings of vegetables, fruits, dairy products, and grains and frequently choose dry beans and nuts from the Meat, Poultry, Fish, Dry Beans, Eggs, & Nuts Group (see Table 9.3).

Recommendations for a healthy diet suggest a reduction in sodium consumption. You can lower your salt intake by limiting the use of salt added in cooking and at the table as well as that consumed in processed foods. Food labels can help identify low-sodium foods. All the sodium-containing additives are itemized in the ingredient list, and the total sodium content per serving is included in the Nutrition Facts section. Food labels also list the sodium content of a serving as a percent of the Daily Value. The Nutrition Facts on the label shown in Figure 9.13 tell us that a serving of spaghetti sauce contains 250 mg, or 10% of the Daily Value for sodium. Additional information can be obtained from descriptors relating to the salt or sodium content of a product (Table 9.4). Some medications can also contribute a significant amount of sodium to your diet. Drug facts labels on over-the-counter medications can help identify those that contain large amounts of sodium.

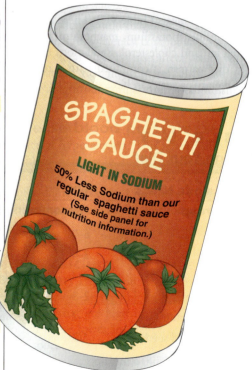

Nutrition Facts
Serving Size 1/2 cup (125g)
Servings Per Container about 3½

Amount Per Serving

Calories 50	Calories from Fat 10
	%Daily Value**
Total Fat 1g	**2%**
Saturated Fat 0g	**0%**
Cholesterol 0mg	**0%**
Sodium 250mg	**10%**
Potassium 530mg	**15%**
Total Carbohydrate 9g	**3%**
Dietary Fiber 1g	**4%**
Sugars 7g	
Protein 2g	

Vitamin A 10%	•	Vitamin C 25%
Calcium 2%	•	Iron 10%

*Percent Daily Values are based on a 2,000 calorie diet. Your daily values may be higher or lower depending on your calorie needs.

	Calories:	2,000	2,500
Total Fat	Less than	65g	80g
Sat Fat	Less than	20g	25g
Cholesterol	Less than	300mg	300mg
Sodium	Less than	2,400mg	2,400mg
Potassium		3,500mg	3,500mg
Total Carbohydrate		300g	375g
Dietary Fiber		25g	30g

Light Spaghetti Sauce, 250 milligrams (mg) per serving
Regular Spaghetti Sauce, 500mg per serving

FIGURE 9.13

Food labels help you determine how much sodium a food contributes to the diet.

TABLE 9.4
Looking for Low Sodium Food

What the Label Says	What It Means
Sodium-free	Contains less than 5 mg of sodium per serving.
Salt-free	Must meet criterion for "sodium-free."
Very low sodium	Contains 35 mg or less of sodium per serving.
Low sodium	Contains 140 mg or less of sodium per serving.
Reduced or less sodium	Contains at least 25% less sodium per serving than a reference food.
Light in sodium	Contains at least 50% less sodium per serving than the average reference amount for same food with no sodium reduction.
No salt added, without added salt, and unsalted	No salt added during processing, and the food it resembles and for which it substitutes is normally processed with salt. (If the food is not "sodium-free," the statement "not a sodium-free food" or "not for control of sodium in the diet" must appear on the same panel as the Nutrition Facts panel.)
Lightly salted	Contains at least 50% less sodium per serving than a reference amount. (If the food is not "low in sodium," the statement "not a low-sodium food" must appear on the same panel as the "Nutrition Facts" panel.)

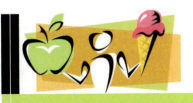

So, What Should I Eat?

To stay hydrated
- Drink before, during, and after you exercise
- Drink two extra glasses of water on hot days
- Bring a bottle of water with you on the airplane
- Keep a water bottle in your car

To reduce your salt intake
- Choose unprocessed foods—they have less sodium than processed foods
- Do not add salt to the water when cooking rice, pasta, and cereals
- Flavor foods with lemon juice, onions, garlic, pepper, curry, dill, basil, oregano, or thyme rather than salt
- Limit salty snacks like potato chips, salted nuts, salted popcorn, and crackers
- Substitute sliced roasted turkey, chicken, or beef for bologna, corned beef, hot dogs, and smoked turkey
- Watch the sauces—Worcestershire sauce, soy sauce, barbecue sauce, ketchup, and mustard add a lot of salt

To boost your potassium intake
- Double your vegetable serving at dinner
- Take two pieces of fruit for lunch
- Have orange juice instead of soda or punch

Calcium and Other Minerals Are Needed for Healthy Bones

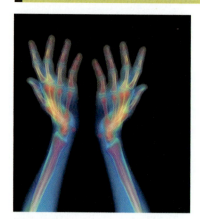

FIGURE 9.14

Our bones show up on X-rays because they are denser than the soft tissue around them, but they are not as solid as rocks. (Gusto Productions/Photo Researchers)

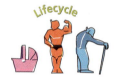

✳ Remember

The important role of vitamin C in synthesizing collagen and the importance of vitamin D for absorbing calcium from the diet are discussed in Chapter 8.

✳ Peak bone mass The maximum bone density attained at any time in life, usually occurring in young adulthood.

✳ Osteoporosis A bone disorder characterized by a reduction in bone mass, increased bone fragility, and an increased risk of fractures.

Sticks and stones can break your bones. The familiar rhyme reminds you that your bones are not as hard as rock. The reason is that bones, unlike rocks, have a protein matrix as well as hard mineral crystals (Figure 9.14). Calcium and phosphorus are the most abundant minerals in bones but magnesium, fluoride, and other trace elements are also important for bone structure. Healthy bones also depend on adequate dietary protein and vitamin C to form and maintain collagen, the most abundant protein in the bone matrix. Adequate vitamin D is needed to allow calcium absorption so appropriate levels of calcium and phosphorus are present in the blood.

Bone is a living tissue

Like other tissues in the body bone is alive and is constantly being broken down and re-formed throughout life. Most bone is formed early in life. In the growing bones of children, bone formation occurs more rapidly than breakdown so the total amount of bone increases. Even after growth stops, bone mass continues to increase into young adulthood. The greatest amount of bone that you have in your lifetime is called **peak bone mass**; peak bone mass is achieved somewhere between the ages of 16 and 30. After about age 35 to 45, the amount of bone broken down begins to exceed that which is formed, so total bone mass decreases. Over time, if enough bone is lost, the skeleton is weakened and fractures occur more easily.

Osteoporosis increases the risk of bone fractures

Osteoporosis is a loss of bone that is great enough to increase the risk of bone fractures. You can't feel your bones weakening so people with osteoporosis may not know their bone mass is dangerously low until they are in their 50's or 60's and experience a bone fracture. Osteoporosis is caused by a loss of both the protein matrix of bone and the minerals that are embedded in it (Figure 9.15). In the United States, about 28 million people have osteoporosis or are at risk due to low bone mass, and 80% of them are women.[11,12] Osteoporosis leads to 1.5 million fractures annually, which account for $10 to $15 billion per year in medical costs.[11] Your risk of osteoporosis is affected by how dense your bones are, that is, your bone mass, and how fast you lose bone. The greater a person's bone mass and the slower bone is lost, the lower the risk of osteoporosis.

Peak bone mass is determined by genetics, gender, and lifestyle
Someone who has more bone to begin with can lose more bone before being at risk for fractures. How dense your bones are is determined by your genetics, gender, and lifestyle. Some of us inherit denser bones than others. For example, African Americans have denser bones than Caucasians. Men are larger and heavier than women and therefore have a greater peak bone mass and a lower risk of fractures from osteoporosis.

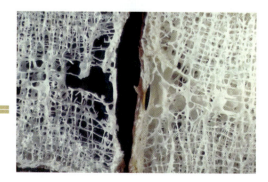

FIGURE 9.15

Osteoporosis causes a decrease in bone density and increases the risk of fractures. Normal bone (*right*). Bone weakened by osteoporosis (*left*). (Dr. Michael Klein/Peter Arnold, Inc.)

Lifestyle factors that affect bone mass include smoking, alcohol consumption, exercise, and diet. Smoking and alcohol consumption can decrease bone mass, whereas weight-bearing exercise, such as walking and jogging, increases bone mass. Having more body fat decreases the risk of osteoporosis because adipose tissue produces estrogen, which helps maintain bone mass and enhances calcium absorption. A greater body weight also increases the amount of weight-bearing exercise that an individual gets in day-to-day activities, which increases bone mass. Diet also affects bone mass. Adequate calcium intake, particularly while bone is being formed, allows greater peak bone mass.

Bone loss occurs with age and increases in women at menopause
Bone loss is a normal part of aging. Age-related bone loss occurs in both men and women, but women lose additional bone for about 5 years after menopause. This postmenopausal bone loss is related to declining estrogen levels, which affect bone cells and decrease intestinal calcium absorption. Postmenopausal bone loss is one of the reasons osteoporosis is a greater threat for women. Osteoporosis-related fractures occur in one out of every two women over age 50 and in about one in every eight men over 50 (Figure 9.16).[11] The incidence of osteoporosis in African American women is half that of Caucasian women. The reason for this difference is that African American women not only have higher peak bone mass, but also lower rates of bone loss after menopause.[13]

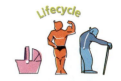

It is easier to prevent osteoporosis than to treat it

Once osteoporosis has occurred, it is difficult to restore lost bone. Therefore, the best treatment for osteoporosis is to prevent it by achieving a high peak bone mass. A low calcium intake is the most significant dietary factor contributing to osteoporosis. Low calcium intake during the years of bone formation results in a lower peak bone mass and, along with it, an increase in the risk of osteoporosis. A diet adequate in calcium and vitamin D and not excessive in phosphorus, protein, or sodium will reduce risk. Maintaining an active lifestyle that includes weight-bearing exercise and limits smoking and alcohol consumption will help to further improve bone density.

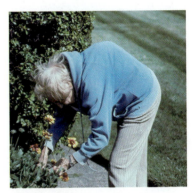

FIGURE 9.16

Bone loss due to osteoporosis can cause a stooped posture and a decrease in stature. (Larry Mulvehill/Photo Researchers)

Osteoporosis is commonly treated with estrogen to increase calcium absorption along with supplements of calcium and vitamin D and regular weight-bearing exercise. Other treatments include other hormones and drugs that increase calcium absorption or decrease bone loss; these are enhanced by calcium supplementation.[14] Increased intakes of vitamin K, magnesium, fluoride, and boron are less effective but have also been used to prevent and treat bone loss.

Calcium Is the Most Abundant Mineral in the Body

In an average person about 1.5% of body weight is calcium and 99% of this calcium is found in bone. The remaining calcium is located in body fluids where it performs other essential functions. For example, it is needed for cell communication and the regulation of body processes. Calcium helps regulate enzyme activity and is necessary for blood clotting. It is needed for the release of neurotransmitters, which allow nerve impulses to pass from one nerve to another and from nerves to other cells. Inside the muscle cells, calcium allows the two muscle proteins, actin and myosin, to interact to cause muscle contraction. Calcium also plays a role in blood pressure regulation, possibly by controlling the contraction of muscles in the blood vessel walls and signaling the secretion of substances that regulate blood pressure.

On the Web

For more information on the incidence and risks of osteoporosis, go to the National Institutes of Health Osteoporosis and Related Bone Disease National Resource Center at **www.osteo.org/**

Calcium levels are carefully regulated

The roles of calcium are so vital to survival that powerful regulatory mechanisms ensure that normal concentrations are maintained both inside and outside of cells. Slight changes in blood calcium levels trigger the release of hormones that work to keep calcium levels

PIECE IT TOGETHER

A Diet for More Than Healthy Blood Pressure

Joshua is a 41-year-old father of three children. His father died of a stroke at the age of 54 as a result of undiagnosed and untreated high blood pressure. Joshua wants to live to see his grandchildren, so he exercises as often as he can, about three times a week, has stopped smoking, and watches his diet and weight. Despite these efforts, at his recent physical his blood pressure was elevated to 138/89. Rather than start him on medication, his doctor

suggested a dietary approach first and referred him to a dietitian. A record of his diet from the previous day reveals that Joshua is maintaining a normal body weight of 175 pounds by consuming about 2500 Calories per day. After evaluating Joshua's current diet, the dietitian recommends he follow the DASH diet to reduce his blood pressure. Joshua's diet is shown here along with a modified diet that incorporates the dietitian's recommendations.

Current Diet			Modified Diet		
Breakfast			**Breakfast**		
Orange juice	3/4 cup		Orange juice	3/4 cup	
1% low-fat milk	1 cup		1% low-fat milk	1 cup	
Wheaties w/1 tsp sugar	1 cup		Wheaties w/1 tsp sugar	1 cup	
			Banana	1 medium	
Whole wheat bread w/jelly	1 slice		Whole wheat bread w/jelly	2 slices	
Margarine	1 tsp		Margarine	1 tsp	
Lunch			**Lunch**		
Tuna salad	3/4 cup		Tuna salad	3/4 cup	
Wheat bread	2 slices		Whole wheat bread	2 slices	
			Carrot sticks	1/2 cup	
			Bell pepper strips	1/2 cup	
Chips	1 oz		Fruit cocktail (light syrup)	1/2 cup	
Cola	1 can		1% low-fat milk	1 cup	
Dinner			**Dinner**		
Baked chicken	3 oz		Chicken in a stir fry with	3 oz	
			Almonds	10	
			Broccoli	1/2 cup	
			Mushrooms	1/2 cup	
Rice	1 cup		Brown rice	1 1/2 cup	
Salad	1 cup		Salad	1 cup	
Light salad dressing	1 Tbsp		Light salad dressing	1 Tbsp	
Dinner roll	1		Dinner roll	1	
Margarine	2 tsp		Margarine	2 tsp	
Cantaloupe	1/2 cup		Cantaloupe	1/2 cup	
Iced tea (sweetened)	12 oz		1% low-fat milk	1 cup	
Snacks			**Snacks**		
Cookies	2 large		Frozen yogurt	1/2 cup	
Dried apricots	5		Dried apricots	5	
Milky Way candy bar	1		Graham crackers	2	
Cola	1 can				

HOW DO JOSHUA'S CURRENT DIET AND THE MODIFIED DIET COMPARE TO THE RECOMMENDATIONS OF THE FOOD GUIDE PYRAMID?

Your answer:

HOW DO THE CHANGES IN JOSHUA'S DIET AFFECT HIS INTAKE OF SODIUM AND POTASSIUM?

His original diet was not high in sodium, containing about 2300 mg, which is slightly below the Daily Value of 2400 mg but above the DRI recommendation of 1500 mg. The changes in his diet reduce his sodium slightly but increase his potassium intake from 2870 mg to 5000 mg. The amount of magnesium is also increased slightly.

Joshua's wife Yuka is 42 years old. Although she is not concerned about her blood pressure, Yuka is concerned about osteoporosis because her mother was recently hospitalized with a hip fracture. She wants to make sure she is consuming adequate calcium. She is mildly lactose intolerant.

IF YUKA CONSUMED THE MODIFIED DIET, WOULD IT MEET HER AI FOR CALCIUM?

Yes, her AI is 1000 mg, and the modified diet contains 1320 mg of calcium.

Because of her lactose intolerance, Yuka does not drink much milk. She can tolerate a small amount on her morning cereal and can consume yogurt and cheese in moderate amounts. If the milk consumed at lunch and dinner is eliminated from her diet, she would not meet the AI.

WHAT CHANGES WOULD INCREASE THE AMOUNT OF CALCIUM FROM LOW-LACTOSE SOURCES?

To increase calcium, Yuka could substitute canned salmon for tuna in the salad at lunch. She could also include more tofu in her diet—a food she ate frequently while growing up in Japan. Including a serving of miso soup with tofu, or using tofu instead of chicken in the stir fry at dinner would increase calcium by about 130 mg. She can also replace the milk with small amounts of yogurt and low-fat cheese. She might also consider taking a calcium supplement.

Yuka only weighs 110 pounds and requires about 1800 Calories to maintain her body weight.

HOW COULD THIS DIET BE CHANGED TO REDUCE THE ENERGY CONTENT WITHOUT REDUCING THE CALCIUM?

Your answer:

★ **Parathyroid hormone (PTH)** A hormone secreted by the parathyroid gland that acts to increase blood calcium levels.

★ **Calcitonin** A hormone produced by the thyroid gland that stimulates bone mineralization and inhibits bone breakdown, thus lowering blood calcium levels.

constant. When calcium levels drop, **parathyroid hormone (PTH)** is released. PTH has multiple actions, which get more calcium into the blood and help keep it there. PTH stimulates the release of calcium from bone. It also stimulates the kidneys to activate vitamin D. Activated vitamin D increases the amount of dietary calcium absorbed from the gastrointestinal tract and acts alongside parathyroid hormone to stimulate calcium release from the bone. PTH also acts in the kidneys to reduce the amount of calcium lost in the urine, thereby conserving the calcium already present in the blood. The overall effect of PTH is to rapidly increase blood calcium levels (Figure 9.17). If blood calcium levels become too high, PTH secretion is shut off and **calcitonin** is released. Calcitonin acts primarily on bone to inhibit the release of calcium, resulting in a decrease in blood calcium levels.

Calcium absorption depends on diet, age, and life stage

Dietary calcium is absorbed from the intestine by both active transport and passive diffusion. Active transport depends on the active form of vitamin D and accounts for most absorption in a meal with low to moderate amounts of calcium. When calcium intake is high, passive transport becomes more important. The efficiency with which calcium is absorbed also depends on dietary factors that block absorption and the life stage of the individual.

Absorption can be helped or hindered by other dietary components
Because of vitamin D's role in the active transport of calcium, it is the nutrient that has the most significant impact on calcium absorption. When it is absent, less than 10% of dietary calcium may be absorbed compared to the typical 25% that is absorbed when it is present. The addition of vitamin D to milk therefore makes sure the calcium in the milk can be absorbed efficiently.

Other substances present in foods, including oxalates, fiber, phytates, and tannins, interfere with calcium absorption. For example, spinach is a high-calcium vegetable but only about 5% of the calcium is absorbed; the rest is bound by oxalates and excreted in the feces.[15] Vegetables such as kale, collard greens, turnip greens, mustard greens, and Chinese cabbage are low in oxalates so their calcium is well absorbed. Chocolate also contains oxalates, but chocolate milk is still a good source of calcium because the amount of oxalates from the chocolate added to a glass of milk is small. Fiber can also reduce calcium absorption but, with a few exceptions, the effect is small. Phytates, however, can have a significant effect on the absorption of calcium from foods such as wheat bran and pinto,

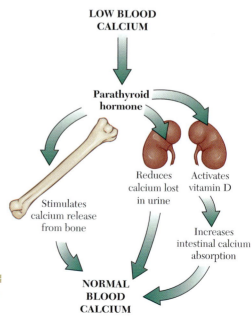

FIGURE 9.17

When blood levels of calcium drop they are quickly restored to normal by the actions of parathyroid hormone.

red, and white beans. You would need to eat almost 10 servings of red beans or 16 servings of spinach to absorb the same amount of calcium as you would from 1 cup of milk. When calcium intake is low, these dietary components may reduce absorption enough to affect calcium status, but when calcium intake is adequate, their effect is insignificant.[16]

Calcium absorption is higher when bones are growing

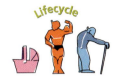

Calcium absorption is higher at times of life when the need is the greatest. During infancy, about 60% of calcium consumed is absorbed. In young adults absorption is about 25%. In older adults absorption declines in part due to a decrease in blood levels of the active form of vitamin D. An additional decrease in calcium absorption occurs in women after menopause due to the decrease in estrogen.

During pregnancy, when calcium is needed for formation of the fetal skeleton, calcium absorption increases to over 50% during the 5th or 6th month of gestation. Calcium need is also increased during lactation, but some of the calcium needed to make milk appears to come from the mother's bones. After lactation, an increase in calcium absorption and retention of calcium by the kidneys help restore bone calcium.

You need enough calcium to support bone growth and maintenance

How much calcium do you need? Early in life you need enough to support bone growth. Therefore the DRI recommendations are higher for children than adults. An intake of 1300 mg per day is recommended for growing children and adolescents when peak bone mass is being achieved; this recommendation drops to 1000 mg per day for adults age 19 through 50 years. Absorption decreases with age, so later in life the recommendation is increased again, this time to 1200 mg per day for those age 51 and older to maintain bone and prevent fractures from osteoporosis.[14]

Dairy products are the best source of calcium in the American diet The main source of calcium in the North American diet is milk, yogurt, cheese, and other dairy products. Fish such as sardines that are consumed in their entirety, including the bones, are also a good source, as are legumes and some green vegetables such as mustard greens, Chinese cabbage, kale, and broccoli (Figure 9.18). Grains are only a moderate source of calcium, but because they are consumed in such

On the Side

It is estimated that only 25% of boys and 10% of girls consume the recommended amount of calcium and only 50 to 60% of adults meet the recommendation.

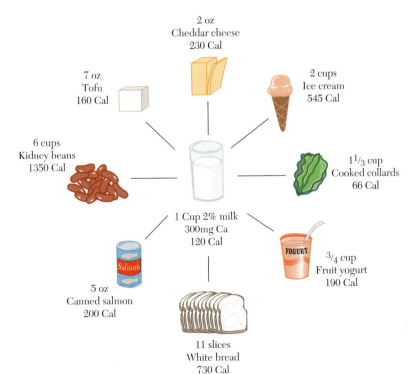

2 oz
Cheddar cheese
230 Cal

7 oz
Tofu
160 Cal

2 cups
Ice cream
545 Cal

6 cups
Kidney beans
1350 Cal

1 1/3 cup
Cooked collards
66 Cal

1 Cup 2% milk
300mg Ca
120 Cal

3/4 cup
Fruit yogurt
190 Cal

5 oz
Canned salmon
200 Cal

11 slices
White bread
730 Cal

FIGURE 9.18

This figure illustrates the amounts of various foods that you would need to eat to obtain the same amount of calcium as one cup of reduced fat milk.

TABLE 9.5
Finding Good Sources of Calcium

What the Label Says	What It Means
High-calcium, rich in calcium, excellent source of calcium	Contains 200 mg of calcium or more per serving
Good source of calcium	Contains 100 mg to 190 mg of calcium per serving
More or added calcium	Contains at least 100 mg more of calcium per serving than a reference food

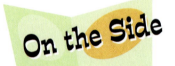

Milk may do more than add calcium for healthy bones. A recent study comparing the amount of weight lost by subjects consuming a low-calorie diet found that those who included three to four servings of dairy products daily lost more weight than those who supplemented calcium or consumed a low-dairy diet (*Obes. Res.* 12:582–590, 2004).

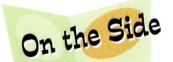

Calcium and vitamin D intakes are such a concern in the United States that some nutrition scientists have suggested that they be added to enriched grains along with B vitamins and iron.

large quantities they make a significant contribution to dietary calcium intake. Adequate calcium intake can be achieved by following the Food Guide Pyramid recommendation of two to three servings of milk, yogurt, or cheese daily plus three to five servings of vegetables a day.

Some of the calcium in our diet is added to foods during processing. For example, many baked goods such as breads, rolls, and crackers, have added nonfat dry milk powder, which provides calcium. Tortillas that are treated with lime water (calcium hydroxide) and tofu made with calcium sulfate are good sources of calcium. In addition, there are many products on the market, such as orange juice and breakfast cereals, that are fortified with calcium (Table 9.5).

Calcium supplements can help meet calcium needs Individuals who do not meet their calcium needs with diet alone can benefit from calcium supplementation. In young individuals supplemental calcium can increase peak bone mass. In postmenopausal women, calcium supplements are not effective at increasing bone mass but they can help reduce bone loss.[17] Because calcium absorption decreases when large amounts (500 mg or more) are consumed at one time, it is better to take a lower-dose calcium supplement (no more than 500 mg per dose) twice a day than to take a once-a-day supplement that provides 100% of the AI. What you take with your supplement also affects the availability of the calcium and of other minerals in the diet. Acidic foods, lactose, and fat increase calcium absorption, whereas oxalate, phytates, and fiber inhibit calcium absorption. The large amounts of calcium contained in a supplement can also interfere with the absorption of iron, zinc, magnesium, and phosphorus, so supplements should be taken with care. Very high doses can also cause kidney stone formation and kidney insufficiency. A UL of 2500 mg per day from food and supplements has been set for adults ages 19 to 70 years.

Phosphorus Is Found in Bone and Almost Everywhere Else

Buffer A substance that reacts with an acid or base to prevent changes in acidity.

Most of the phosphorus in your body is found with calcium in bones and teeth as part of the hard mineral crystals. The smaller amount of phosphorus in soft tissues has both structural and regulatory roles. It is a component of phospholipids, which form the structure of cell membranes. It is a major constituent of DNA and RNA, which orchestrate the synthesis of proteins. Phosphorus is also involved in regulating enzyme activity because the addition of phosphorus as phosphate can activate or inactivate certain enzymes. The high-energy bonds of ATP are formed between phosphate groups. Phosphorus is also part of a **buffer** that helps regulate intracellular acidity so that chemical reactions can proceed normally.

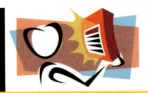

Off the Label: Counting All Your Calcium?

Do you get enough calcium? You may consume it in natural sources such as milk, yogurt, and leafy green vegetables. Or, you may choose calcium-fortified foods to help meet your needs. Perhaps you include a calcium supplement just to be sure. To find out if you get enough you need to count all your calcium sources.

You can see if a packaged food is a good source by looking at the label. All food labels list the % Daily Value for calcium in the Nutrition Facts panel. To calculate the milligrams of calcium in a food, multiply the % Daily Value by 1000 mg (the Daily Value for calcium). For example, a box of fortified breakfast cereal may show that a serving provides 25% of the Daily Value for calcium. By multiplying 25% by 1000 mg you can calculate that a serving provides 250 mg of calcium. Foods high in calcium may include a statement that they are a good source of calcium as well as the health claim that a diet high in calcium helps reduce the risk of osteoporosis.

The label on your milk carton indicates that an 8-ounce glass has 30% of your Daily Value for calcium. But, for a number of reasons, many of us don't drink milk, or drink less than we should. Teenage girls concerned about their weight will typically choose a diet soda over a glass of milk. The soda label says calorie-free, but it is also calcium-free. Twenty years ago boys and girls consumed more milk than soft drinks, but today they consume twice as much soda pop as milk. Teenage girls consume only 60% of the recommended amount of calcium, with soda drinkers consuming almost one-fifth less calcium than non-soda drinkers.[1] Many older adults do not drink milk because they are lactose intolerant, believe milk is for kids, or skimp on milk to decrease their calorie intake.

If your calcium count from food comes up short, you can add to your intake by choosing a supplement. Your multivitamin and mineral supplement will only provide a small amount of the calcium you need; each pill would have to be the size of a marble to give you enough calcium along with everything else it contains. To get a significant amount of your calcium from a supplement, choose one that contains calcium alone or calcium with vitamin D. Vitamin D is commonly included in calcium supplements because it aids calcium absorption. The Supplement Facts label will tell you how much of each nutrient is included in your supplement. If you choose a product that contains vitamin D you need to be sure to monitor the amount of vitamin D, because it can be toxic in large amounts. If you double your calcium dose, you will get twice as much vitamin D.

The form of calcium used in supplements is also important. Calcium carbonate is absorbed as well as the calcium from milk, and the other forms, including calcium citrate, calcium gluconate, calcium lactate, calcium citrate-malate, and calcium phosphate, are absorbed as well as calcium from a mixed diet.[2] Calcium preparations such as bone meal, coral calcium, powdered bone, dolomite (limestone), and oyster shell should be avoided because they may contain enough contaminants to be dangerous if consumed routinely.[3]

Some calcium supplements are also over-the-counter antacids. These will have a Drug Facts, rather than a Supplement Facts label (see Chapter 3, Antacids: Getting the Drug Facts). Some of these, such as Tums, which contains calcium carbonate, are safe, effective calcium supplements. However, antacids that contain aluminum and magnesium may actually increase calcium losses from the body.

To see if you are getting enough calcium, you need to check the labels on your foods, supplements, and drugs; consider the form of calcium in each; and watch for excesses of other nutrients and contaminants. Sound complicated? Maybe an extra glass of milk is an easier choice.

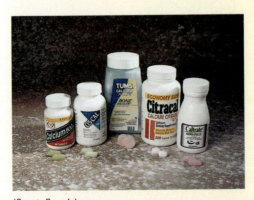

(George Semple)

References

1. Center for Science in the Public Interest. Liquid candy highlights. Available online at www.cspinet.org/sodapop/highlights.htm/Accessed August 23, 2004.
2. Mortensen, L., and Charles, P. Bioavailability of calcium supplements and the effect of vitamin D: Comparisons between milk, calcium carbonate, and calcium carbonate plus vitamin D. *Am. J. Clin. Nutr.* 63:354–357, 1996.
3. Bourgoin, B. P., Evans, D. R., Cornett, J. R., et al. Lead content in 70 brands of dietary calcium supplements. *Am. J. Public Health* 83:1155–1160, 1993.

Phosphorus levels are regulated to promote bone health

Blood levels of phosphorus are not as strictly controlled as those of calcium, but levels are maintained in a ratio with calcium that allows minerals to be deposited into bone. Phosphorous is more easily absorbed than calcium. About 60 to 70% is absorbed from a typical diet. Vitamin D enhances phosphorous absorption, but enough can be absorbed even when vitamin D is absent. The regulatory mechanisms that increase calcium absorption at the intestine and increase calcium release from bone have similar effects on phosphorus. Therefore low calcium will cause an increase in both calcium and phosphorus absorption and release both calcium and phosphorus from bone. The kidney is important for regulating phosphorus levels; when blood phosphorous levels increase the amount lost in the urine also increases to keep blood levels in the normal range.

It is not difficult to get enough phosphorus in your diet

It is easy to find good dietary sources of phosphorus. Dairy products such as milk, yogurt, and cheese, as well as meat, cereals, bran, eggs, nuts, and fish are all good sources (Figure 9.19). Food additives used in baked goods, cheese, processed meats, and soft drinks also provide phosphorus. Because phosphorus is so widely distributed in food, dietary deficiencies are rare. Most diets meet the RDA of 700 mg per day for adults.[14] Marginal phosphorus status may be caused by losses due to chronic diarrhea and overuse of aluminum-containing antacids, which prevent phosphorus absorption. Phosphorus deficiency can lead to bone loss, weakness, and loss of appetite.

Toxicity from high phosphorus intake is rare in healthy adults, but excessive intakes can lead to bone resorption. Levels of phosphorus intake typical in the United States are not believed to affect bone health as long as calcium intake is adequate. The UL for phosphorus is 4.0 grams per day for adults.[14]

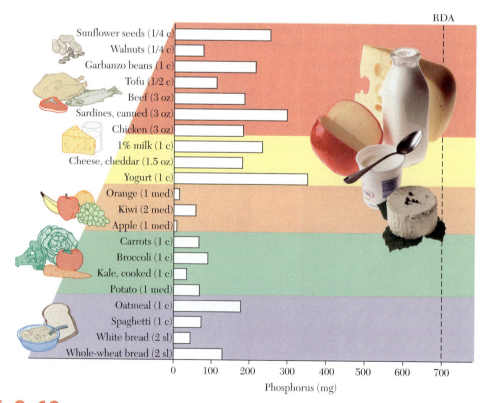

FIGURE 9.19

Phosphorus content of selections from each group of the Food Guide Pyramid. The dashed line represents the RDA for adults. As with calcium, dairy products are good sources of phosphorus. Unlike calcium, phosphorus is plentiful in a variety of other foods. (Brian Hagiwara/Food Pix)

Magnesium Is Needed in Bone and Body Fluids

Magnesium is far less abundant in the body than calcium or phosphorus, but it is still essential for healthy bones. About 50 to 60% of the magnesium in the body is in bone where it is essential for maintaining structure. The rest of the magnesium is found in cells and fluids throughout the body. The kidneys regulate blood levels of magnesium. When intake is low, excretion in the urine is decreased. As intake increases, urinary excretion increases to maintain normal blood levels.

Magnesium functions in over 300 reactions

In addition to its role in bone structure, magnesium is involved in regulating calcium homeostasis and is needed for the action of vitamin D and many hormones including PTH.[18] Magnesium is important for blood pressure regulation and may play a role in maintaining cardiovascular health. In addition, magnesium is involved in chemical reactions throughout metabolism including those necessary for the generation of energy from carbohydrate, lipid, and protein (see Table 9.1). In some of these reactions it is an enzyme activator, but it is also needed to stabilize ATP, so every reaction that generates or uses ATP requires magnesium. It is important for the functioning of the nerves and muscles because it is needed to transport sodium and potassium across cell membranes. It is needed to allow muscles to relax after a contraction. Because it is involved in DNA, RNA, and protein synthesis, magnesium is particularly important for dividing, growing cells.

We get magnesium from greens and whole grains

Magnesium is found in many foods but in small amounts, so you can't get all you need from a single food. It is found in leafy greens such as spinach and kale because it is a component of the green pigment chlorophyll. Nuts, seeds, bananas, and the germ and bran of whole grains are also good sources of magnesium (Figure 9.20). Processed

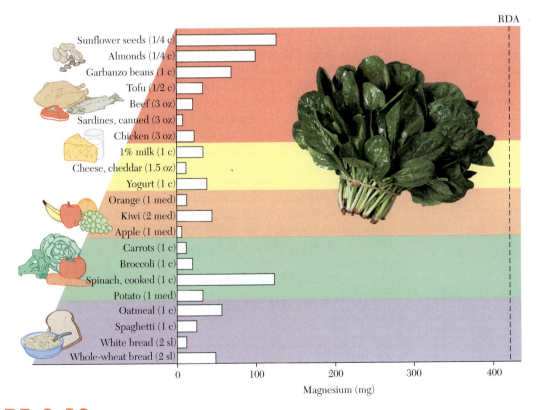

FIGURE 9.20

Magnesium content of selections from each group of the Food Guide Pyramid. The dashed line represents the RDA for adult men age 31 and older. Leafy greens such as spinach are excellent sources. (Corbis Images)

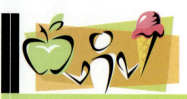

So, What Should I Eat?

To get calcium into your body and your bones

- Drink your milk!
- Have at least one serving of a leafy green vegetable a day
- Bone up on calcium by having sardines or canned salmon, which are eaten with the bones
- Taste some tofu
- Snack on yogurt; ounce for ounce it has more calcium than milk
- Walk, jog, or jump up and down—weight-bearing exercises build up bone

Don't fret about phosphorus—it's in almost everything you eat

To maximize your magnesium

- Have whole grains
- Sprinkle nuts and seeds on salads, cereals, and stir fries
- Go for the green—whenever you eat green you are eating magnesium and most greens contain calcium too

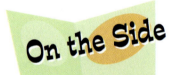

The incidence of heart attacks is lower in areas that have hard water, which is water that has a high content of minerals such as calcium and magnesium.

foods are generally poor sources. For example, removing the bran and germ of the wheat kernel reduces the magnesium content of a cup of white flour to only 28 mg, compared with the 166 mg in a cup of whole wheat flour. "Hard" water, which is high in calcium and magnesium, can be a significant source. Magnesium absorption is enhanced by the active form of vitamin D and decreased by the presence of phytates and calcium.

The RDA for magnesium is 400 mg per day for young men and 310 mg per day for young women.[14] A deficiency can cause nausea, muscle weakness and cramping, irritability, mental derangement, and changes in blood pressure and heartbeat. Low blood magnesium levels affect levels of blood calcium and potassium; therefore some of these symptoms may be due to alterations in the levels of these other minerals.

Magnesium deficiency is rare in the general population. However, it does occur in those with alcoholism, malnutrition, kidney disease, and gastrointestinal disease, as well as in those who use diuretics that increase magnesium loss in the urine. Marginal intakes of magnesium have been associated with a number of chronic diseases including osteoporosis, atherosclerosis, and high blood pressure.

No adverse effects have been observed from magnesium consumed in foods, but toxicity may occur from concentrated sources such as magnesium-containing drugs, like milk of magnesia and magnesium-containing supplements. Magnesium toxicity causes nausea, vomiting, low blood pressure, and other cardiovascular changes. The UL for adults and adolescents over 9 years of age is 350 mg of nonfood magnesium.

Iron Is Needed to Transport Oxygen to Body Tissues

▲ **Hemoglobin** An iron-containing protein in red blood cells that binds oxygen and transports it through the bloodstream to cells.

Iron is good for your blood. We have known since the 18th century that iron is a major constituent of blood. By 1832, iron tablets were used to treat young women in whom "coloring matter" was lacking in the blood. Today we know that the red color in blood is due to the iron-containing protein **hemoglobin** (Table 9.6). The hemoglobin in red blood cells transports oxygen to body cells and carries carbon dioxide away from cells for elimination by the lungs. Most of the iron in the body is part of hemoglobin but iron is also needed for the production of a number of other iron-containing proteins. It is part of myoglobin found in muscle, where it enhances the amount

TABLE 9.6
A Quick Summary of the Trace Elements

Mineral	Food Sources	Recommended Intake for Adults	Major Functions	Deficiency Symptoms	Groups at Risk of Deficiency	Toxicity and UL
Iron	Red meats, leafy greens, dried fruit, whole and enriched grains	8–18 mg/day	Part of hemoglobin, which delivers oxygen to cells, myoglobin, which holds oxygen in muscle, and compounds needed in energy production and immune function	Fatigue, weakness, small pale red blood cells, low hemoglobin (iron deficiency anemia)	Infants and preschool children, adolescents, women of childbearing age, pregnant women, athletes	Gastrointestinal upset, liver damage; UL is 45 mg
Copper	Organ meats, nuts, seeds, whole grains, seafood, cocoa	900 μg/day	A part of proteins needed for iron absorption, lipid metabolism, collagen synthesis, nerve and immune function, and antioxidant protection	Anemia, poor growth, bone abnormalities	Those who over-supplement zinc	Vomiting; UL is 10 mg
Zinc	Meat, seafood, whole grains, eggs	8–11 mg/day	Regulates protein synthesis; functions in growth, development, wound healing immunity, and antioxidant protection	Poor growth and development, skin rashes, decreased immune function	Vegetarians, low-income children, elderly	Decreased copper absorption, depressed immune function; UL is 40 mg
Selenium	Organ meats, seafood, eggs, whole grains	55 μg/day	Antioxidant protection as part of glutathione peroxidase, synthesis of thyroid hormones	Muscle pain, weakness, a form of heart disease	Populations in areas with low-selenium soil	Nausea, diarrhea, vomiting, fatigue, hair changes; UL is 400 μg
Iodine	Iodized salt, salt water fish, seafood, dairy products	150 μg/day	Needed for synthesis of thyroid hormones	Goiter, cretinism, mental retardation, growth and developmental abnormalities	Populations in areas with low-iodine soil and where iodized salt is not used	Enlarged thyroid; UL is 1110 μg
Chromium	Brewers yeast, nuts, whole grains, mushrooms	25–35 μg/day	Enhances insulin action	High blood glucose	Malnourished children	None reported; no UL
Fluoride	Fluoridated water, tea, fish, toothpaste	3–4 mg/day	Strengthens tooth enamel, enhances remineralization of tooth enamel, reduces acid production by bacteria in the mouth	Increased risk of dental caries	Populations in areas with unfluoridated water	Mottled teeth, kidney damage, bone abnormalities; UL is 10 mg

(Continued)

TABLE 9.6

A Quick Summary of the Trace Elements (*Continued*)

Mineral	Food Sources	Recommended Intake for Adults	Major Functions	Deficiency Symptoms	Groups at Risk of Deficiency	Toxicity and UL
Manganese	Nuts, legumes, whole grains, tea	1.8–2.3 mg/day	Functions in carbohydrate and lipid metabolism and antioxidant protection	Growth retardation	None	Nerve damage; UL is 11 mg
Molybdenum	Milk, organ meats, grains, legumes	45 µg/day	Aids the action of a number of enzymes	Unknown in humans	None	Arthritis and joint inflammation; UL is 2 mg

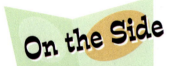

One strange symptom that is occasionally associated with iron deficiency is pica. Pica is a compulsion to eat nonfood items such as clay, ice, paste, laundry starch, paint chips, and ashes. Sometimes the things consumed contain toxic minerals, such as lead or substances that inhibit mineral absorption.

Iron deficiency anemia A condition that occurs when the oxygen-carrying capacity of the blood is decreased because there is insufficient iron to make hemoglobin. It is diagnosed in adults when hemoglobin concentration is less than 11 grams per 100 ml of blood.

Heme iron A readily absorbed form of iron found in animal products that is chemically associated with proteins such as hemoglobin and myoglobin.

of oxygen available for use in muscle contraction. It is also essential for energy production as a part of several proteins needed in aerobic metabolism. Iron-containing proteins are involved in drug metabolism and the immune system. Iron is also a component of the enzyme catalase, which protects the cell from oxidative damage.

Iron deficiency causes weakness and fatigue

When iron is deficient, hemoglobin cannot be produced. When not enough hemoglobin is available, the red blood cells that are formed are small and pale and unable to deliver adequate oxygen to the tissues. This is known as **iron deficiency anemia** (Figure 9.21a). Symptoms of iron deficiency anemia include fatigue, weakness, headache, decreased work capacity, an inability to maintain body temperature in a cold environment, changes in behavior, decreased resistance to infection, impaired development in infants, and an increased risk of lead poisoning in young children. Anemia is the last stage of iron deficiency. Earlier stages have no symptoms because they do not affect the amount of iron in red blood cells but they can be detected by blood tests that measure levels of iron in the plasma and in body stores (Figure 9.21b).

Despite the fact that iron is one of the best understood of the trace elements, iron deficiency anemia is the most common nutritional deficiency in the United States and worldwide.[19] In the United States, it affects 7.8 million adolescent girls and women of childbearing age and 700,000 children between the ages of 1 to 2 years. The incidence is greatest among low-income and minority women and children. Worldwide it is estimated that over 2 billion people suffer from iron deficiency anemia and another 3 billion have deficient iron stores.[20]

Absorption regulates how much iron is in the body

Iron is not easily eliminated from the body so iron level is regulated primarily by adjusting the amount of iron that is absorbed. How much iron reaches body cells depends on the form of iron in the diet and the body's need.

Iron from animal sources is better absorbed Iron in the diet comes from both plant and animal sources. Much of the iron in animal products is part of a chemical complex called **heme iron**, which is found in certain proteins such as myoglobin and hemoglobin. The best sources of heme iron are red meats and organ meats such as liver and kidney (Figure 9.22). Heme iron is absorbed more than twice as efficiently as nonheme iron. The iron found in plant sources such as leafy green

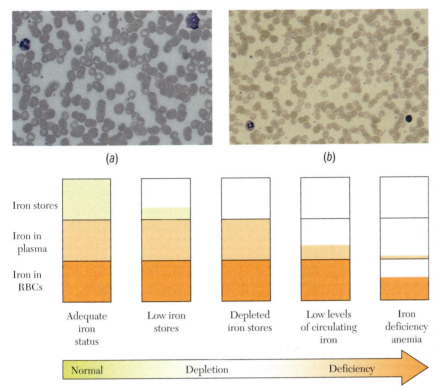

(a)   (b)

Iron stores

Iron in plasma

Iron in RBCs

| Adequate iron status | Low iron stores | Depleted iron stores | Low levels of circulating iron | Iron deficiency anemia |

Normal   Depletion   Deficiency

Iron Status

FIGURE 9.21

(a) Iron deficiency anemia occurs when there is not enough iron to synthesize adequate amounts of hemoglobin. It causes the red blood cells to become small and pale. Normal red blood cells are shown on the left and those typical of iron deficiency anemia are illustrated on the right. (b) Iron deficiency anemia is the final stage of iron deficiency. Inadequate iron first causes a decrease in the amount of stored iron, followed by low iron levels in the plasma. It is only after plasma levels drop that there is no longer enough iron available to maintain hemoglobin in red blood cells. (a: B&B Photos/Custom Medical Stock Photo, Inc.; b; Custom Medical Stock Photo, Inc.)

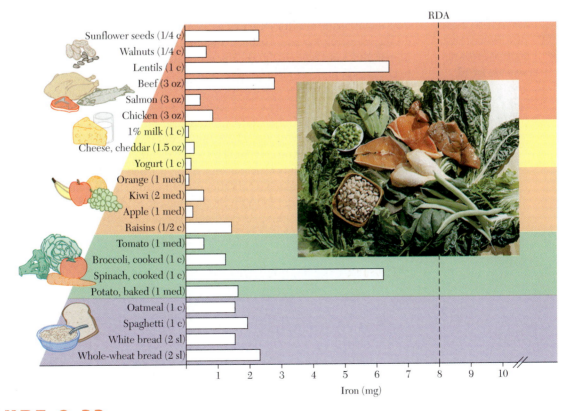

RDA

Sunflower seeds (1/4 c)
Walnuts (1/4 c)
Lentils (1 c)
Beef (3 oz)
Salmon (3 oz)
Chicken (3 oz)
1% milk (1 c)
Cheese, cheddar (1.5 oz)
Yogurt (1 c)
Orange (1 med)
Kiwi (2 med)
Apple (1 med)
Raisins (1/2 c)
Tomato (1 med)
Broccoli, cooked (1 c)
Spinach, cooked (1 c)
Potato, baked (1 med)
Oatmeal (1 c)
Spaghetti (1 c)
White bread (2 sl)
Whole-wheat bread (2 sl)

1   2   3   4   5   6   7   8   9   10

Iron (mg)

FIGURE 9.22

Iron content of selections from each group of the Food Guide Pyramid. The dashed line represents the RDA for adult men and postmenopausal women. Both plant and animal foods are good sources of iron, but the heme iron in animal foods is more readily absorbed. (Tony Freeman/PhotoEdit)

vegetables like spinach and kale, legumes, and grains is nonheme iron. Animal foods also contain nonheme iron in addition to heme iron. Nonheme iron absorption can be enhanced as much as sixfold by consuming it with foods rich in vitamin C. Consuming beef, fish, or poultry in the same meal as nonheme iron also increases absorption. For example, a small amount of hamburger in a pot of chili will enhance the body's absorption of iron from the beans. On the other hand, fiber, phytates, tannins, and oxalates prevent absorption by binding iron in the gastrointestinal tract. The presence of other minerals may also decrease iron absorption.

Iron absorption depends on iron needs

When iron is absorbed, it enters the cells of the small intestine. It can either be stored there or transported in the blood to other parts of the body. Stored iron is bound to the iron storage protein **ferritin**. Iron that is to be transported must first be bound to an iron transport protein called **transferrin**. When the iron-transferrin complex reaches body cells, it binds to a protein on the cell membrane called a transferrin receptor, which allows the iron to be taken into the cell. When iron is in short supply, the number of transferrin receptors increases. Having more transferrin receptors allows more iron to be delivered to the cells. When iron is plentiful, the number of transferrin receptors decreases so less iron is delivered to cells, while the amount of ferritin increases to enhance the ability to store iron. As a result, more iron is then left in the mucosal cells bound to ferritin and is therefore lost when the cells die and are sloughed into the intestinal lumen (Figure 9.23).

Iron is also stored as ferritin in other parts of the body, primarily the liver, spleen, and bone marrow. When ferritin concentrations in the liver become high, some is converted to an insoluble storage protein called hemosiderin. Iron can be mobilized from body stores as needed, and deficiency signs will appear only after stores are depleted (see Figure 9.21b).

Iron is lost primarily through blood loss

Iron is not readily excreted. Even when red blood cells die, the iron in their hemoglobin is not lost from the body; the iron is recycled and can be incorporated into new red blood cells. Most iron lost even in healthy individuals occurs through blood loss, including that lost during menstruation and the small amounts lost from the gastrointestinal tract. Some iron is also lost through the shedding of cells from the intestine, skin, and urinary tract.

Women require more iron than men

Iron is the only nutrient for which the recommended intake is greater for young women than it is for young men. The RDA for iron for menstruating women is 18 mg per day, but for adult men it is only 8 mg per day. The greater need is due to the iron lost in menstrual blood. Only about one-fourth of adolescent girls and women of childbearing age meet the RDA for iron through their diet.[19] After menstruation stops the need for iron decreases, so the requirement for postmenopausal women is the

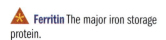

Ferritin The major iron storage protein.

Transferrin An iron transport protein in the blood.

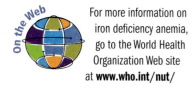

For more information on iron deficiency anemia, go to the World Health Organization Web site at **www.who.int/nut/**

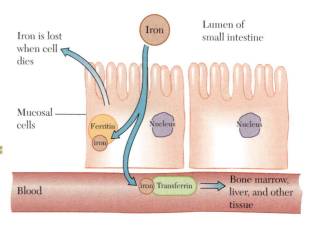

FIGURE 9.23

Iron that enters the mucosal cells of the small intestine may either be bound to ferritin or transported in the blood by the protein transferrin. Iron trapped in the mucosal cell by ferritin is lost when the cell dies. Iron transported by transferrin reaches body cells that need iron. When iron levels are high, more iron is stored as ferritin.

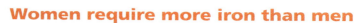

TABLE 9.7
How Much Iron Do You Need?

Gender/Life Stage	Recommended Intake
Infants	
0–6 months	0.27 mg*
7–12 months	11 mg
Children	
1–3 years	7 mg
4–8 years	10 mg
Males	
9–13 years	8 mg
14–18 years	11 mg
≥ 19 years	8 mg
Females	
9–13 years	8 mg
14–18 years	15 mg
19–50 years	18 mg
≥ 51 years	8 mg
Females taking oral contraceptives	
14–18 years	11.4 mg
19–50 years	10.9 mg
Pregnancy	
≤ 18–50 years	27 mg
Lactation	
≤ 18 years	10 mg
19–50 years	9 mg
Vegetarians	
Men ≥ 19 years	14 mg
Menstruating women	33 mg
Adolescent girls	26 mg

*This value is an AI; all other values are RDAs.

same as for adult men. The RDA for iron assumes that the diet contains both plant and animal sources of iron.[21] A separate RDA category was created for vegetarians and these recommendations are higher to account for the poorer iron absorption from plant sources (Table 9.7).

The risk of iron deficiency is increased in groups whose needs are higher. Pregnant women are at risk because the need for iron is increased due to the increase in maternal blood volume and the growth of other maternal tissues and the fetus. Iron deficiency is common among pregnant women even in industrialized countries and can lead to premature delivery and greater risk to the mother. Iron deficiency is also common in infants, children, and adolescents because their rapid growth increases iron needs. Athletes are another group susceptible to iron deficiency. The DRIs suggest that athletes' iron needs may be 30 to 70% higher than the general population (see Chapter 11).

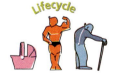

Lifecycle

To meet needs consider the amount and bioavailability of iron

Someone who consumes 2 to 3 servings of meat, fish, or poultry a day is getting about 5 to 8 mg of iron, much of which is highly absorbable heme iron. If you are not a meat eater you can meet your iron needs from plant sources. A peanut butter sandwich and a box of raisins provide 3.3 mg. The amount of iron absorbed from these foods is lower, but can be increased if you include a source of vitamin C with the meal. For example, you could add orange sections to your lunch or have strawberries for dessert. You can

PIECE IT TOGETHER

Adding to Your Iron Intake

Hanna is a 23-year-old graduate student. She has been feeling tired and run down all semester. She recently read an article about iron deficiency in young women and became concerned about her iron status. She decides to go to the health center where she has blood drawn. The results of her tests indicate that she does not have iron deficiency anemia, but her iron stores are very low.

A review of her typical diet shows that Hanna's iron intake is less than the recommended amount. She decides to try to increase the amount of iron she gets from her diet before considering iron supplements. Hanna is from South Carolina and consumes a primarily vegetarian diet. At home her mother prepared meals in iron cookware, but the pans in Hanna's college apartment are stainless steel. Her typical diet is shown below.

Typical Diet

Food	Amount	Iron (mg)
Breakfast		
Grits with	1 cup	0.5
butter	1 tsp	0
Plantain	1	0.9
Whole wheat toast	1 slice	1.2
Apple juice	3/4 cup	0.7
Tea with	1 cup	0
sugar	1 tsp	0
Lunch		
Apple	1 medium	0.2
Cornbread with	1 piece	1.5
butter	1 tsp	0
Yogurt	1 cup	0.2
Tomato	1 medium	0.5
Tea with	1 cup	0
sugar	1 tsp	0
Dinner		
Rice	1 cup	2.4
Peanuts	1/3 cup	0.9
Kale	1 cup	1.2
Yams	1 cup	1.1
Apple juice	3/4 cup	0.7
Tea with	1 cup	0
sugar	1 tsp	0
Total		12.0

DOES HANNA'S IRON INTAKE MEET THE RDA FOR A YOUNG FEMALE VEGETARIAN?

No. The RDA for a vegetarian woman who is menstruating is 33 mg. Hanna's diet only provides 12 mg.

WHAT OTHER DIETARY FACTORS COULD BE CONTRIBUTING TO HANNA'S POOR IRON STATUS?

Your answer:

HOW COULD HANNA INCREASE THE IRON CONTENT OF HER DIET?

Hanna is a vegetarian, so her iron sources are limited to plant foods, which are generally lower in iron and contain only the less-well-absorbed nonheme form of iron. There are, however, good plant sources of naturally occurring iron as well as sources fortified with iron. For instance, switching from the half cup of grits, containing about 0.5 mg of iron, to a fortified cereal will greatly increase her intake. Adding 2 tablespoons of raisins to the hot cereal contributes another 0.4 mg. Another good vegetarian source of iron is beans. A bowl of chili with beans at lunch will add 8 mg of iron. Cooking her meals in an iron skillet would add iron to foods cooked in it.

WHAT COULD HANNA DO TO INCREASE THE AMOUNT OF IRON ABSORBED FROM HER MEALS?

Your answer:

DOES HANNA'S DIET PROVIDE GOOD VEGETARIAN SOURCES OF CALCIUM? ARE THERE OTHER NUTRIENT DEFICIENCIES FOR WHICH SHE MAY BE AT RISK?

Your answer:

also use iron-fortified foods to help meet your iron needs. Food labels can help identify foods that are good sources of iron. The iron content of packaged foods must be listed on food labels as a percent of the Daily Value. A serving of enriched grains provides anywhere from 4 to 10% of the Daily Value; a serving of fortified breakfast cereal may supply 30, 40, or even 100% of the Daily Value.

Although diet is the ideal way to meet iron needs, supplements are often recommended for groups at risk for deficiency. Iron supplements typically contain nonheme iron. Therefore, to enhance absorption, iron supplements should be consumed with foods containing vitamin C, such as orange juice; taken with a meal containing meat, fish, or poultry; and not taken with dairy products or substances that bind iron. Iron supplements should not be taken at the same meal as calcium supplements, which decrease iron absorption. Large intakes of iron from supplements can interfere with the absorption of zinc and copper. They can also cause stomach upset and constipation. Taking a fiber supplement can help alleviate constipation, but be aware that the fiber will reduce iron absorption if these are taken at the same time.

Too much iron is toxic

A single, large dose as well as more moderate doses of iron consumed over a longer period of time can both cause toxicity symptoms. Acute iron toxicity from excessive consumption of iron-containing supplements is one of the most common forms of poisoning among children under age 6. Accumulation of iron in the body over time, referred to as iron overload, generally occurs only in individuals with hereditary abnormalities in iron absorption, diseases requiring frequent blood transfusions, or conditions in which red blood cell synthesis is abnormal. A UL has been set at 45 mg per day from all sources.

Even a single large dose can be life-threatening Iron poisoning may cause damage to the intestinal lining, abnormalities in body acidity, shock, and liver failure. Even a single large dose can be fatal. To protect children from accidental poisoning, iron-containing products such as drugs and supplements are required to display a warning on the label (Figure 9.24). In addition, since most cases of serious iron poisoning have occurred with products containing 30 mg or more per dose, these products are packaged in individual doses to make consumption of many pills difficult for a young child.[22] Iron-containing supplements should be taken only as suggested on the label and stored out of the reach of children or others who may consume them in excess.

Hemochromatosis is an inherited condition that leads to iron overload Hemochromatosis is a genetic disorder in which iron absorption is increased. The accumulation of excess iron that occurs in hemochromatosis causes

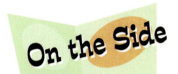

On the Side

Iron cooking utensils provide iron to the body when it leaches into food. Leaching is enhanced by acidic foods. For example, 3 ounces of spaghetti sauce cooked in a glass pan contains about 0.6 mg of iron, but the same amount of sauce cooked in an iron skillet contains about 5.7 mg, depending on how long it is cooked.

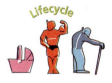

Lifecycle

Hemochromatosis An inherited condition that results in increased iron absorption.

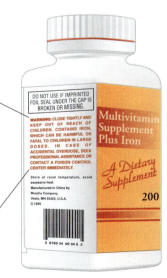

WARNING: CLOSE TIGHTLY AND KEEP OUT OF REACH OF CHILDREN. CONTAINS IRON, WHICH CAN BE HARMFUL OR FATAL TO CHILDREN IN LARGE DOSES. IN CASE OF ACCIDENTAL OVERDOSE, SEEK PROFESSIONAL ASSISTANCE OR CONTACT A POISON CONTROL CENTER IMMEDIATELY.

FIGURE 9.24

Labels on iron-containing supplements and medications must carry a toxicity warning.

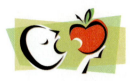

Iron supplements can be dangerous because consumption of excess iron can cause liver failure. In fact, iron supplement overdose is the leading cause of liver transplants in children.

oxidative changes resulting in heart and liver damage, diabetes, and certain types of cancer. Iron deposits also darken the skin. To have these symptoms, an individual must inherit the hemochromatosis gene from both parents. If you inherit the gene from only a single parent you won't have these serious symptoms, but you will absorb iron better than people who do not have the gene at all. The treatment for hemochromatosis is simple: regular blood withdrawal. Iron loss through blood withdrawal will prevent the complications of iron overload, but to be effective it must be initiated before organs are damaged. Therefore, genetic screening is essential to identify and treat individuals before any damage has occurred.

Copper Deficiency Can Cause Iron Deficiency Anemia

It is logical that consuming too little iron will cause iron deficiency anemia but too little copper can also cause this problem. Iron and copper status are interrelated because a copper-containing protein is needed for iron to be transported from the intestine. Even if iron intake is adequate, without copper, iron can't get to tissues and this results in iron deficiency that may lead to anemia. Copper also functions in a number of important proteins and enzymes that are involved in connective tissue synthesis, lipid metabolism, maintenance of heart muscle, and function of the immune and central nervous systems.[21] Some of these roles are also reflected in the symptoms seen with copper deficiency. When copper is deficient the protein collagen does not form normally, so changes in the skeleton occur that are similar to those seen in vitamin C deficiency. Blood cholesterol levels are elevated in copper deficiency, reflecting copper's role in cholesterol metabolism. Copper deficiency has also been associated with impaired growth, degeneration of the heart muscle, degeneration of the nervous system, and changes in hair color and structure. Because copper is needed to maintain the immune system, a diet low in copper increases the incidence of infections. Copper is also an essential component of a form of the antioxidant enzyme superoxide dismutase (SOD), so a deficiency weakens antioxidant defenses.

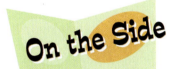

Much of what we know about copper was discovered by studying people who have a rare disorder called Menke's kinky hair syndrome in which the ability to use copper is defective.

Copper also interacts with zinc

The zinc content of the diet can have a major impact on copper absorption. When zinc intake is high, it stimulates the synthesis of a zinc-binding protein. This protein helps regulate zinc absorption; but it also binds copper, preventing it from being moved out of mucosal cells into the blood.[23] The antagonism between copper and zinc is so great that phytates, which inhibit zinc absorption, actually increase the absorption and utilization of copper. Copper absorption is also reduced by high intakes of vitamin C, iron, manganese, and molybdenum.

Most Americans consume adequate amounts of copper

The RDA for copper for adults is 900 μg per day. We consume it in seafood, nuts and seeds, whole grain breads and cereals, and chocolate; the richest dietary sources of copper are organ meats such as liver and kidney (Figure 9.25). As with many other trace elements, soil content affects the amount of copper in plant foods.

Severe copper deficiency is relatively rare, although it may occur in premature infants. Copper toxicity from dietary sources is also rare but has occurred as a result of drinking from contaminated water supplies or consuming acidic foods or beverages stored in copper containers. Toxicity is more likely to occur from copper-containing supplements. Excessive copper intake causes abdominal pain, vomiting, and diarrhea. The UL has been set at 10 mg of copper per day.

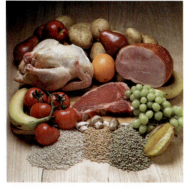

FIGURE 9.25

These foods are good sources of copper. (Charles D. Winters)

Zinc Is Needed for Enzyme, Hormone, and Vitamin Activity

Many body processes depend on zinc. It is involved in the functioning of nearly 100 different enzymes. These enzymes are needed for the synthesis of DNA and RNA, the metabolism of carbohydrate, antioxidant protection, acid-base balance, and folate absorption. Zinc also plays a role in the storage and release of insulin, the mobilization of vitamin A from the liver, and the stabilization of cell membranes. Zinc is involved in gene expression and therefore is needed for the growth and repair of tissues, the activity of the immune system, and the development of sex organs and bone. Zinc-containing proteins are needed for the activity of vitamin A, vitamin D, and a number of hormones including the thyroid hormones, estrogen, and testosterone. Without zinc, these nutrients and hormones cannot bind to DNA to increase or decrease gene expression and, hence, the synthesis of certain proteins.

A high phytate intake can cause zinc deficiency

The essentiality of zinc in the human diet was not recognized until the 1960's, when a syndrome of growth depression and delayed sexual development was seen in Iranian and Egyptian men consuming diets based on vegetable protein. Although the diet was not low in zinc, it was high in grains containing phytates, which interfered with zinc absorption, causing a deficiency.

In addition to poor growth and development, zinc deficiency causes skin rashes, diarrhea, and impaired immune function. The impact of zinc deficiency on immune function is rapid and extensive, causing a decrease in the number and function of immune cells in the blood. The drop in immune function can lead to an increased incidence of infections. Diminished immune function is a concern even for moderate zinc deficiency. Because zinc is needed for the proper functioning of vitamins A and D and the activity of numerous enzymes, deficiency symptoms can resemble deficiencies of other essential nutrients. Zinc is also needed for the thyroid hormones to function; a deficiency slows energy metabolism.

Symptomatic zinc deficiency is relatively uncommon in North America, but in developing countries it has important health and developmental consequences. Supplements have been shown to reduce the incidence of infections and diarrhea in children in developing nations.[24] The risk of zinc deficiency is greater in areas of the world where the diet is high in phytate, fiber, tannins, and oxalates, which limit zinc absorption. Groups at greatest risk of deficiency worldwide are the elderly, low-income children, and vegetarians—particularly female vegans. Groups likely to be at risk of deficiency in the United States include young children, adolescent females, and older adults.[25]

Zinc in animal foods is better absorbed than that in plant foods

The RDA for zinc is 11 mg per day for adult men and 8 mg per day for adult women. We consume it in red meat, liver, eggs, dairy products, vegetables, and some seafood (Figure 9.26). Whole grains are a good source, but refined grains are not because zinc is lost in milling and not added back in enrichment. Because plant foods are high in substances that bind zinc it is better absorbed from animal sources. Grain products leavened with yeast provide more zinc than unleavened products because the yeast leavening of breads reduces the phytate content.

Zinc absorption and excretion are regulated

Zinc consumed in the diet can be used by the cells lining the intestine, pass through these cells into the blood, or, in a manner analogous to iron, be trapped in the intestinal mucosal cells by a zinc-binding protein. When zinc intake is high more of this zinc-binding protein is made, so more zinc is held in the mucosal cells and lost into the gut

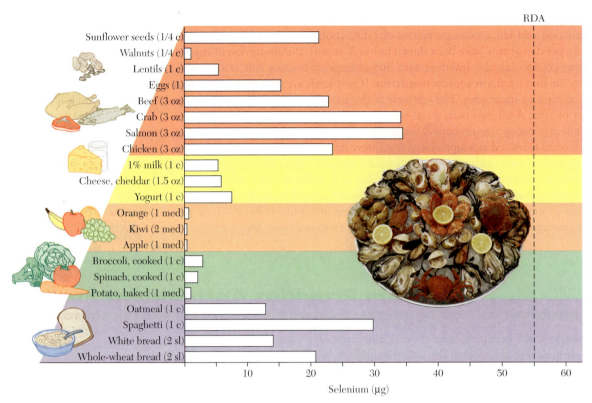

FIGURE 9.29

Selenium content of selections from each group of the Food Guide Pyramid. The dashed line represents the RDA for adults. Seafood is rich in selenium and other animal products and plant foods are also good sources. (PhotoDisc, Inc./Getty Images)

gastrointestinal upset have been reported at much lower levels. The UL for adults is 400 µg per day from diet and supplements.[21]

Selenium levels may affect cancer development

The role of selenium in cancer has been under investigation for three decades. An increased incidence of cancer has been observed in regions where selenium intake is low. In 1996 a study investigating the effect of selenium supplements on people with a history of skin cancer found that the supplement had no effect on the recurrence of skin cancer but the incidence of lung, prostate, and colon cancer all decreased in the selenium-supplemented group.[26] There was a great deal of excitement about this result. Could selenium supplements reduce cancer risk? Many were hopeful, but continued study has found that the results were not as miraculous as they originally seemed. Evidence now suggests that selenium supplements actually increase the incidence of certain types of skin cancer.[27] The reduction in the incidence of lung and prostate cancer seen in the 1996 study is believed to have occurred primarily in people who began with low levels of selenium. So, enough selenium is necessary to prevent cancer, but supplements of selenium have not been shown to be of additional benefit in the general population.

Iodine Is Needed to Synthesize Thyroid Hormones

More than half of the iodine in your body is stored in a small gland in your neck called the thyroid gland. The reason iodine is concentrated in this gland is that it is an essential component of the thyroid hormones. Thyroid hormones regulate metabolic rate, growth, and development, and promote protein synthesis. If blood levels of the thyroid hormones drop, thyroid-stimulating hormone is released. This hormone signals the thyroid gland to take up iodine and synthesize more thyroid hormones. When the supply of iodine is adequate, thyroid hormones can be made and their presence turns off the synthesis of thyroid-stimulating hormone.

Iodine deficiency causes goiter and affects growth and development

If iodine is deficient, thyroid hormones cannot be made. Without sufficient thyroid hormones metabolic rate slows, causing fatigue and weight gain. The most obvious outward sign of deficiency is an enlarged thyroid gland called a **goiter** (Figure 9.30). A goiter forms when reduced thyroid hormone levels cause thyroid-stimulating hormone to be released, stimulating the thyroid gland to make more thyroid hormones. Because iodine is unavailable, the hormones cannot be made, but the stimulation continues causing the thyroid gland to enlarge. In milder cases of goiter, treatment with iodine causes the thyroid gland to return to normal size, but it may remain enlarged in more severe cases.

Thyroid hormone is needed for growth, development, and protein synthesis, so iodine deficiency causes other problems in addition to goiter. If iodine is deficient during pregnancy, it increases the risk of stillbirth and spontaneous abortion. Deficiency also can cause a condition called **cretinism** in the offspring. Cretinism is characterized by symptoms that include mental retardation, deaf mutism, and growth failure. Iodine deficiency during childhood and adolescence can result in goiter and impaired mental function.

Iodine deficiency was common in the central United States and Canada in the early 1900's, but today it is rare in this part of the world due to the addition of iodine to table salt. Iodized salt was first used in Switzerland in the 1920's as a way to combat iodine deficiency. Salt iodinization and other forms of iodine supplementation, such as injections or oral doses of iodized oil, are now used in most countries with an iodine deficiency disease problem of public health significance. Despite these efforts iodine deficiency remains a world health problem. Worldwide, 600 million people have goiter and 1.5 billion people are at risk for iodine deficiency.[28]

Iodine comes from the sea and is added to our salt

The iodine content of foods varies depending on the soil where plants are grown or where animals graze. Iodine is found in sea water so seafood and plants grown near the sea are high in iodine. Plants grown inland have lesser amounts, depending on the iodine content of the soil. In some plant foods substances called goitrogens increase the risk of iodine deficiency by interfering with the utilization of iodine or with thyroid function. Goitrogens are found in turnips, rutabaga, cabbage, cassava, and millet. When these foods are boiled, the goitrogen content is reduced because some of these compounds leach into the cooking water. They are primarily a problem in African countries where cassava is a dietary staple. In the American diet goitrogens are not a problem because they are present in foods that are not consumed to any large extent in the typical diet.

Since the iodinization of salt began in the early 1900's, the typical iodine intake in North America has met or exceeded the RDA of 150 μg per day for adult men and women. Iodized salt is commonplace in the United States, and only iodized salt is sold in Canada. It takes only about half a teaspoon of iodized salt to meet recommendations. We also get iodine from contaminants and other additives in foods. Iodine-containing additives used in cattle feed and disinfectants used on milking machines and storage tanks increase the iodine content of dairy products. Iodine-containing sterilizing agents are also used in fast-food restaurants, and iodine is used in dough conditioners and some food colorings.

Despite our intake of iodine from iodized salt and contaminants, toxicity is rare. Chronically high intakes of iodine can cause an enlargement of the thyroid gland

Goiter An enlargement of the thyroid gland caused by a deficiency of iodine.

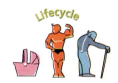

Cretinism A condition resulting from poor maternal iodine intake during pregnancy that causes stunted growth and poor mental development in offspring.

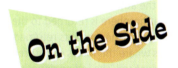

On the Side

Although the seas provide much of our iodine, sea salt is a poor source because the iodine is lost in the drying process.

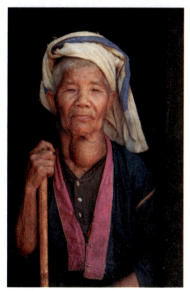

FIGURE 9.30

Iodine deficiency causes enlargement of the thyroid gland, a condition called goiter. (Alison Wright/Corbis)

Sulfur is a part of proteins and other molecules

Sulfur is one of the major minerals; over 100 mg is present in our bodies. Sulfur is found in sulfur-containing amino acids in proteins, the sulfur-containing vitamins, and a few other molecules. The sulfur-containing amino acids methionine and cysteine are needed for protein synthesis. Cysteine is also part of the compound glutathione, which is important in detoxifying drugs and protecting cells from oxidative damage. Thiamin and biotin are sulfur-containing vitamins that are essential for energy production. We consume sulfur in proteins and in food preservatives such as sulfur dioxide, sodium sulfite, and sodium and potassium bisulfite, which are used as antioxidants. There is no recommended intake for sulfur, and no deficiencies are known when protein needs are met (see Table 9.1).

Other minerals may be important for health

There is evidence that arsenic, boron, nickel, silicon, and vanadium play a role in human health. The need for and functions of these minerals have been reviewed by the DRI committee but there was not sufficient data to establish a recommended intake for any of these elements. ULs have been set for boron, nickel, and vanadium. Other trace elements that play a physiological role include aluminum, bromine, cadmium, germanium, lead, lithium, rubidium, and tin. The specific functions of these have not been defined, and they have not been evaluated by the DRI committee. All the minerals, both those known to be essential and those that are still being assessed for their role in human health, can be obtained by choosing a variety of foods from each of the groups of the Food Guide Pyramid.

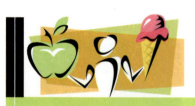

So, What Should I Eat?

To add more high iron foods
- Eat red meat, poultry, or fish—they are all good sources of heme iron
- Add raisins to your oatmeal
- Have a fortified breakfast by eating iron-fortified cereal
- Dust off the iron skillet
- Have some beans—they are a good vegetarian source of iron

To increase your iron absorption
- Have orange juice with your iron-fortified cereal
- Don't take your calcium supplement with your iron sources

Think zinc
- Scramble some eggs
- Beef up your zinc by having a few ounces of meat
- Eat whole grains but make sure they are yeast leavened

Trace down your minerals
- Check to see if your water is fluoridated
- See if your salt is iodized
- Replace refined grains with whole grains to increase your chromium intake
- Have some seafood to add selenium to your diet

THINKING FOR YOURSELF

1. How does your diet compare to the DASH diet?
   a. Use 1 day of the food record you kept in Chapter 2 to compare the number of servings you ate from each of the food groups to the number of servings recommended by the DASH diet for your energy intake as shown in Table 9.3.
   b. Suggest modifications to your diet that would allow it to meet DASH guidelines.
   c. What difficulties or inconveniences do you see with following this dietary pattern?
   d. What other dietary or lifestyle changes might you make if you are at high risk of hypertension?

2. Do you drink enough fluid?
   a. Keep a log of all the fluids you consume in 1 day. Calculate your fluid intake by totaling the volume of water, beverages, and foods that are liquid at room temperature.
   b. How does your intake on this day compare with your estimated requirement? How about if you added an hour of jogging or basketball to your day?

3. How much sodium do processed foods add to your diet?
   a. Use food labels to estimate the amount of sodium you consume from processed foods each day.
   b. Make a list of processed foods you commonly eat that contain more than 10% of the Daily Value for sodium per serving.
   c. What less-processed choices could you substitute for these?

4. Do you get enough calcium?
   a. Using the food record you kept in Chapter 2, calculate your average calcium intake.
   b. How does your intake compare with the AI for calcium for someone of your age and sex?
   c. If your calcium intake is below the AI, modify your diet to increase your calcium consumption without significantly increasing your energy intake.

5. Are you at risk for iron deficiency?
   a. Using the 3-day food intake record you kept in Chapter 2, calculate your average daily intake of iron.
   b. How does your iron intake compare with the recommendation for someone of your age and sex?
   c. If your intake is low, suggest modifications to your diet to meet the RDA for iron for someone your age and sex.
   d. If your diet already meets the recommendations for iron, make a list of foods you like that are good sources of iron.
   e. Identify the major food sources of iron in your current diet and indicate whether they contribute heme iron.

SUMMARY

1. Minerals are elements needed by the body to regulate chemical reactions and provide structure. Their bioavailability is affected by their food sources, the body's need, and interactions with other minerals, vitamins, and other dietary components such as fiber, phytates, oxylates, and tannins.

2. Water is an essential nutrient that accounts for about 60% of adult body weight. Since water isn't stored in the body, intake from water, other fluids, and foods must replace losses in urine, feces, and sweat, and from evaporation. Water provides transport, protection, lubrication, and temperature regulation in the body. Water balance is controlled by stimulating intake with thirst and regulating the amount lost in the urine. The recommended intake of water is 2.7 liters per day for women and 3.7 liters per day for men; needs vary depending on environmental conditions and activity level. Dehydration can occur if water intake is too low or output is excessive.

3. The minerals sodium, chloride, and potassium are electrolytes important in the maintenance of fluid balance and the functioning of nerves and muscles. The North American diet is abundant in sodium and chloride from processed foods and table salt but generally low in potassium, which is high in unprocessed foods such as fresh fruits and vegetables. Recommendations for health suggest that we should eat more potassium and less salt.

4. Electrolyte and fluid balance is regulated primarily by the kidneys. Failure of these regulatory mechanisms may be a cause of hypertension. Diet affects the risk of hypertension: a high sodium intake increases risk; a low potassium, magnesium, and calcium intake also increases risk.

5. Bone is a living tissue that is constantly being broken down and reformed. Peak bone mass occurs in young adulthood. As adults age more bone is broken down than is made, causing a decrease in overall bone mass.

This bone loss is accelerated in women for about 5 years after menopause. A low bone mass causes osteoporosis, a condition that increases the risk of bone fractures.

6. Most of the calcium in the body is found in bone, but calcium is also essential for nerve transmission, muscle contraction, blood clotting, and blood pressure regulation. Blood levels of calcium are tightly regulated by the hormones PTH and calcitonin, which affect the amount of calcium excreted in the urine, absorbed from the diet, and released from bone. Good sources of calcium in the American diet include dairy products, fish consumed with bones, and leafy green vegetables.

7. Phosphorus is widely distributed in foods. It has an important structural role in bones and teeth. Phosphorus is also part of a buffer system that helps prevent changes in acidity and is an essential component of phospholipids, ATP, and DNA.

8. Magnesium is important for bone health and it is needed as a cofactor for numerous reactions throughout the body as well as to stabilize ATP. It is important for blood pressure regulation and is essential for nerve and muscle conductivity. The best dietary sources are whole grains and green vegetables.

9. Iron functions as part of hemoglobin, which transports oxygen in the blood. Iron deficiency anemia is the most common nutritional deficiency worldwide. The amount of iron absorbed depends on other foods in the diet as well as the type of iron. Heme iron, found in meats, is more absorbable than nonheme iron, found in meat and plant foods. If iron stores are low, more iron is transported from the intestinal cells to body cells. When body stores are adequate, less iron is transported. If too much iron is absorbed, the heart and liver can be damaged and diabetes and cancer are more likely. A single large dose of iron is toxic and can be fatal.

10. Copper functions in a number of proteins that affect iron and lipid metabolism, synthesis of connective tissue, and antioxidant protection. A copper-containing protein is needed for iron transport. High levels of zinc can cause a copper deficiency. A copper deficiency can result in anemia and bone abnormalities. Seafood, nuts, seeds, and whole grain breads and cereals are good sources of copper.

11. Zinc is needed for the activity of many enzymes, and zinc-containing proteins are needed for the activity of vitamins A and D and a number of hormones. Zinc absorption is regulated by a protein that binds zinc in the mucosal cells and limits how much can enter the blood. High levels of phytate interfere with zinc absorption. Zinc deficiency depresses immunity but too much can have the same effect; zinc deficiency also contributes to copper and iron deficiency. Good sources of zinc include red meats, eggs, dairy products, and whole grains.

12. Selenium is part of the enzyme glutathione peroxidase, which protects against oxidative damage by preventing free radical formation. Adequate dietary selenium spares some of the need for vitamin E. Dietary sources include seafood, eggs, organ meats, and plant foods grown in selenium-rich soils. In China, selenium deficiency is associated with a heart condition known as Keshan disease. Low selenium intake has been linked to increased cancer risk.

13. Iodine is an essential component of thyroid hormones, which control basal metabolic rate, growth, and development. When iodine is deficient, the thyroid gland enlarges, forming a goiter. Iodine deficiency also affects growth and development. The use of iodized salt has virtually eliminated iodine deficiency in North America, but it remains a world health problem. The best sources of iodine in the diet are seafood, foods grown near the sea, and iodized salt.

14. Chromium is needed for normal insulin action and glucose utilization. It is found in liver, brewer's yeast, nuts, and whole grains.

15. Fluoride is necessary for the maintenance of bones and teeth and prevention of dental caries. Most of the fluoride in the diet in the United States comes from fluoridated drinking water and toothpaste.

16. Manganese and molybdenum are both cofactors needed for the activity of a number of enzymes. Sulfur is a major mineral found in sulfur-containing amino acids, the sulfur-containing vitamins, and a few other molecules; it is part of a buffer that helps regulate acid-base balance. Boron, arsenic, nickel, silicon, and vanadium may be essential in small amounts but can be toxic if consumed in excess.

R E V I E W   Q U E S T I O N S

1. How is the amount of water in the body regulated?
2. Describe the functions of water in the body.
3. List three factors that increase water needs.
4. What is the role of the electrolytes (sodium, potassium, and chloride) in the body?
5. What types of foods contribute the most sodium to the North American diet?
6. What types of foods are good sources of potassium?
7. What is the DASH diet, and how does it affect blood pressure?

8. What is the major source of calcium in the North American diet?
9. When blood calcium levels drop too low, how does the body return levels to normal?
10. Why might low calcium intake during childhood increase the risk of osteoporosis?
11. Why are women more likely than men to develop osteoporosis?
12. Name four structures or molecules that contain phosphorus.

13. What is the function of magnesium in the body?
14. Why does iron deficiency cause red blood cells to be small and pale?
15. List several good sources of iron in the diet and indicate if they contain heme iron.
16. Discuss three factors that affect iron absorption.
17. What is hemochromatosis?
18. Explain why a deficiency of copper can contribute to anemia.

19. How does zinc affect the synthesis of proteins?
20. Why does excess zinc cause a deficiency of copper?
21. What is the role of selenium in the body?
22. What is a goiter and what causes it?
23. What is the role of chromium in the body?
24. How does fluoride function in dental health?

REFERENCES

1. Askew, E.W. Nutrition and performance in hot, cold, and high-altitude environments. In *Nutrition in Exercise and Sport*, 3rd ed. Wolinsky, I., ed. Boca Raton, Fla: CRC Press, 1998: 597–619.

2. Shen, H-P. Body fluids and water balance. In *Biochemical and Physiological Aspects of Human Nutrition*. Stipanuk, M. ed. Philadelphia: W. B. Saunders, 2000: 843–865.

3. Institute of Medicine, Food and Nutrition Board. *Dietary Reference Intakes for Water, Salt and Potassium*. Washington, DC: National Academy Press, 2004.

4. Oppliger, R. A., Case, H. S., Horswill, C. A., et al. American College of Sports Medicine position statement: Weight loss in wrestlers. *Med. Sci. Sports Exerc.* 28:ix–xii, 1996.

5. Chobanian, A. V., Bakris, G. L., Black, H. R., et al. Seventh report of the Joint National Committee on Prevention, Detection, Evaluation, and Treatment of High Blood Pressure. Joint National Committee on Prevention, Detection, Evaluation, and Treatment of High Blood Pressure. National Heart, Lung, and Blood Institute. *Hypertension* 42:1206–1252, 2003.

6. American Heart Association. Factors that contribute to high blood pressure. Available online at www.americanheart.org/presenter.jhtml?identifier-4650/Accessed August 31, 2004.

7. Sacks, F. M., Svetkey, L. P., Vollmer, W. M., et al. Effects on blood pressure of reduced dietary sodium and the Dietary Approaches to Stop Hypertension (DASH) diet. DASH-Sodium Collaborative Research Group. *N. Engl. J. Med.* 344:3–10, 2001.

8. Jee, S. H., Miller, E. R., 3rd, Guallar, E., et al. The effect of magnesium supplementation on blood pressure: A meta-analysis of randomized clinical trials. *Am. J. Hypertens.* 15:691–696, 2002.

9. Allender, P. S., Cutler, J. A., Follmann, D., et al. Dietary calcium and blood pressure: A meta-analysis of randomized clinical trials. *Ann. Intern. Med.* 124:825–831, 1996.

10. Greenland, P. Beating high blood pressure with low sodium DASH. *N. Engl. J. Med.* 344:53–55, 2001.

11. National Institutes of Health. Consensus Development Conference Statement: Osteoporosis Prevention, Diagnosis, and Therapy, March 27–29, 2000. Available online at consensus.nih.gov/cons/111/111_statement.htm/Accessed August 31, 2004.

12. Osteoporosis overview. Osteoporosis and related bone diseases. National Resource Center. Available online at www.osteo.org/osteo.html/Accessed August 23, 2004.

13. Bohannon, A. D. Osteoporosis and African American women. *J. Womens Health Gend. Based Med.* 8:609–615, 1999.

14. Institute of Medicine, Food and Nutrition Board. *Dietary Reference Intakes for Calcium, Phosphorus, Magnesium, Vitamin D, and Fluoride*. Washington, DC: National Academy Press, 1997.

15. Heaney, R. P., Weaver, C. M., and Recker, R. R. Calcium absorption from spinach. *Am. J. Clin. Nutr.* 47:707–709, 1988.

16. Bronner, F., and Pansu, D. Nutritional aspects of calcium absorption. *J. Nutr.* 129:9–12, 1999.

17. Riggs, B. L., O'Fallon, W. M., Muhs, J., et al. Long-term effects of calcium supplementation on serum parathyroid hormone level, bone turnover, and bone loss in elderly women. *J. Bone Miner. Res.* 13:168–174, 1998.

18. Sojka, J. E., and Weaver, C. M. Magnesium supplementation and osteoporosis. *Nutr. Rev.* 53:71–74, 1995.

19. Centers for Disease Control and Prevention. Recommendations to prevent and control iron deficiency in the United States. *Morb. Mortal. Wkly. Rep.* 47:1–29, 1998. Available online at www.cdc.gov/mmwr/preview/mmwrhtml/00051880.htm/ Accessed August 23, 2004.

20. World Health Organization. Micronutrient deficiencies, battling iron deficiency anemia. The challenge, updated September 3, 2003. Available online at www.who.int/nut/ida.htm/Accessed August 23, 2004.

21. Food and Nutrition Board, Institute of Medicine. *Dietary Reference Intakes: Vitamin A, Vitamin K, Arsenic, Boron, Chromium, Copper, Iodine, Iron, Manganese, Molybdenum, Nickel, Silicon, Vanadium, and Zinc*. Washington, DC: National Academy Press, 2001.

22. Iron-containing supplements and drugs: Label warning statements and unit-dose packaging requirements. *Federal Register*, January 1997.

23. Turnlund, J. R. Copper. In *Modern Nutrition in Health and Disease*, 9th ed. Shils, M. E., Olson, J. A., Shike, M., and Ross, A. C., eds. Baltimore: Williams & Wilkins, 1999: 241–252.

24. Fraker, P. J., King, L. E., Laakko, T., and Vollmer, T. L. The dynamic link between the integrity of the immune system and zinc status. *J. Nutr.* 130:1399S–1406S, 2000.

25. Briefel, R. R., Bialostosky, K., Kennedy-Stephenson, J., et al. Zinc intake of the U.S. population: Findings from the Third National Health and Nutrition Examination Survey, 1988–1994. *J. Nutr.* 130:1367S–1373S, 2000.

26. Clark, L. C., Combs, G. F., Jr., Turnbull, B. W., et al. Effect of selenium supplementation for cancer prevention in patients with carcinoma of the skin. *JAMA* 276:1957–1968, 1996.

27. Duffield-Lillico, A. J., Slate, E. H., Reid, M. E., et. al. Selenium supplementation and secondary prevention of nonmelanoma skin cancer in a randomized trial. *J. Natl. Cancer Inst.* 95:1477–1481, 2003.

28. World Health Organization. Eliminating iodine deficiency disorders. Available online at www.who.int/nut/idd.htm/Accessed August 23, 2004.

29. Vincent, J. B. The biochemistry of chromium. *J. Nutr.* 130:715–718, 2000.

30. Anderson, R. A. Chromium as an essential nutrient for humans. *Regul. Toxicol. Pharmacol.* 26:S35–S41, 1997.

31. Lukaski, H. C. Chromium as a supplement. *Ann. Rev. Nutr.* 19:279–301, 1999.

32. Pak, C. Y., Sakhaee, K., and Zerwekh, J. E. Sustained-release sodium fluoride in the management of established menopausal osteoporosis. *Am. J. Med. Sci.* 313:23–32, 1997.

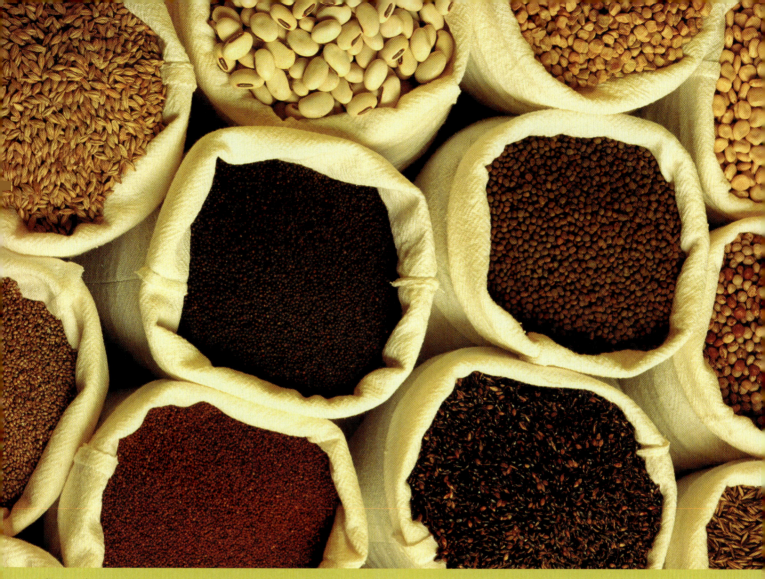

(Fernando Bueno/The Image Bank/Getty Images)

CHAPTER 10 CONCEPTS

- We consume nutrients found naturally in foods, those added in fortification, and those contained in supplements.
- A well-chosen diet can provide all of the nutrients needed by most healthy people.
- Food contains substances such as phytochemicals that are not nutrients but can be beneficial to our health.
- Functional foods are foods that provide benefits beyond those supplied by the nutrients they contain.
- Fortified foods are foods with added nutrients.
- Dietary supplements are a source of nutrients; many also provide substances that are not classified as nutrients.
- There are no mandatory standards for the manufacture of dietary supplements, the FDA regulates their labeling and monitors them for safety once they are on the market.
- Supplemental nutrients are recommended for nutritionally vulnerable groups.
- Dietary supplements must be chosen carefully to assure that needs are met without toxicity.

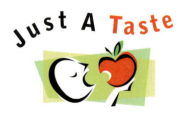

Just A Taste

Can a well-planned diet meet your nutrient needs?

Is the safety of dietary supplements regulated by the government?

Can you assume herbs are safe because they are natural?

Meeting Our Needs: Food, Fortified Food, and Supplements

10

INTRODUCTION

Reuters

Fortified Foods Could Spread Fish Oil's Benefits

Dec. 2003—Adding fish oil to a range of commercial foods, from margarine to lunch meats, could get more of the heart-healthy fats into the Western diet, according to Australian researchers.

Their study of 16 men found that foods rich in omega-3 fatty acids—including products fortified with fish oil—boosted blood levels of the fats, which are believed to help ward off heart disease.

Participants' menus included offerings of fresh and canned fish, canola oil and flaxseed, which are all naturally high in omega-3. The men were also offered fish oil-enriched versions of foods that do not normally provide omega-3: margarine, lunch meat, sausage, French onion dip and shelf-stored milk. . . . "Incorporating fish oil into a range of novel commercial foods," they write, "provides the opportunity for wider public consumption of omega-3 fatty acids with their associated health benefits."

To read the complete article go to www.danhosp.org/healthnews/reuters/20040102elin013.htm.

D

o you want fish oil spread on your toast? How about added to your breakfast sausage? It doesn't sound very appetizing. Why not simply eat more fish? The reason is that telling people to eat more fish doesn't make them do it, but adding one of the health-promoting substances in fish to something they are going to eat anyway may get it into their diet where it hopefully will benefit their health. This approach is analogous to hiding a child's medicine in a spoonful of applesauce. Researchers are literally designing foods to treat the chronic diseases that plague us. These foods can be beneficial but they don't come with a prescription. Should you be choosing these or sticking to plain old unadulterated foods like fish, asparagus, and honeydew? Shouldn't we be able to meet our nutrient needs by simply eating food? Is adding health-promoting substances to our foods the answer to good health, or does it introduce an element of risk?

There Are Many Ways to Meet Your Nutrient Needs

On the Side

Eggs may be high in cholesterol, but they can also be a source of heart healthy omega-3 fatty acids, depending on what the chickens eat. Including flaxseed in the feed of lying hens increases the omega-3 fatty acid content of the egg yolk. The resulting designer eggs provide a convenient way for people to boost omega-3 intake.

⚠ **Dietary supplements** Products sold to supplement the diet; they may include vitamins; minerals; herbs, botanicals, or other plant-derived substances; amino acids; enzymes; concentrates or extracts.

In the past, the human diet was limited to what we could grow or collect from the lands and waters around us and then store for the winter. Today we can harvest a variety of foods from the grocery store shelves year round. We choose from a huge assortment of fresh, packaged, canned, and frozen foods. Some of our foods are grown locally and others are shipped across countries, continents, and oceans. In the depths of winter we can buy fresh produce grown in parts of the world where the summer sun is shining. For example, grapes are shipped from Peru to supply grocery stores on the snow swept prairies of Wyoming. If the California strawberry crop fails, we import them from Mexico. Our diet today is no longer dependent on the local economy or climate.

In addition to this plentiful supply of naturally nutritious foods the modern marketplace provides other options for meeting our nutrient needs (Figure 10.1). Our food supply includes thousands of foods fortified with added nutrients. Almost all the milk sold in the United States is fortified with vitamins A and D; refined grains have added thiamin, niacin, riboflavin, folic acid, and iron. You can buy orange juice fortified with calcium, eggs fortified with fish oils, and even water containing added B vitamins. If you are still worried about meeting your nutrient needs you can take a **dietary supplement** to boost your intake.

Fortified foods and supplements provide additional nutrients

The development and proliferation of nutrient-fortified foods and dietary supplements emerged from the realization that many people do not or cannot always consume a nutritionally adequate diet. These foods and supplements do help many people meet their nutrient needs. For example, older adults may have difficulty meeting their vitamin B_{12} needs without fortified foods or supplements because absorption of this vitamin may decrease with age. Young women may benefit from the addition of folic acid to foods because it can be difficult to consume enough natural sources of this vitamin to ensure a healthy pregnancy. Women may need a supplement during pregnancy to supply enough iron to support the high demands of growing a baby. The fact that there are some circumstances under which supplemental sources of nutrients are necessary has been recognized by the recommendations of the Dietary Reference Intakes (DRIs) and addressed by government food fortification programs.

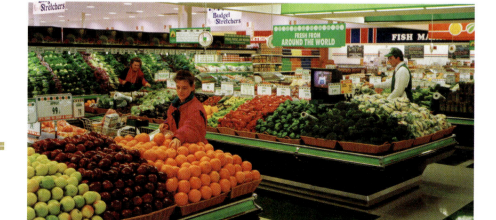

FIGURE 10.1

Modern supermarkets provide consumers with a cornucopia of fresh foods from around the world as well as a variety of fortified foods and dietary supplements. (Mark Segal/Stone/Getty Images)

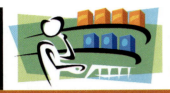

Your Choice: Fresh, Frozen, or Canned

Fresh fruits and vegetables seem the healthiest, but can be expensive and are not always available in the winter. Frozen are appealing if you have a freezer in which to store them, but canned fruits and vegetables are the cheapest. Does it matter which you choose?

Heat, light, air, and the passage of time all cause the loss of nutrients from food. Therefore, it is important to consider how a food has been handled when you are trying to make the most nutritious choice. Fresh produce would seem to be the best, but if the "fresh" vegetable has actually spent a week in a truck traveling to your store, several days on the shelf, and then another week in your refrigerator, is it really the most nutritious choice?

A frozen version of your vegetable may actually supply more vitamins. Manufacturers of frozen vegetables often freeze their produce in the fields where it is grown. Although freezing itself can cause some losses, by freezing right in the field, the produce does not lose any nutrients due to time and exposure after it is picked.

What about canned vegetables or fruits? The processing and high temperature used in canning reduces nutrient content; however, because canned foods keep for a long time, do not require refrigeration, and are often less expensive than fresh or frozen, they provide an available, affordable source of nutrients, which may be the best choice in some situations.

Whichever packaging you choose, how you handle your produce at home can also affect its nutrient content. Remembering that exposure to oxygen, light, and heat can destroy vitamins can help you to store, prepare, and cook foods in ways that minimize losses. It is best to store food away from heat and light and begin preparation as close to serving time as possible. Cutting vegetables and fruits

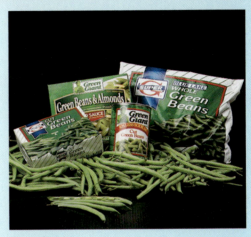

(George Semple)

increases the exposure to light, so don't cut up your fruit salad or chop your stir fry veggies until the last minute. When cooking, the higher the temperature and the longer the heat is applied, the greater the vitamin losses. Pressure cookers and microwaves, which cook foods quickly, can reduce nutrient losses. Water-soluble vitamins can be washed away in cooking water; to avoid this try roasting, grilling, stir-frying, or baking. If foods are cooked in water, use the cooking water to make soups and sauces so you retrieve some of the nutrients.

So, which should you choose? You should choose whichever helps you get your recommended intake of three or more vegetables and two or more fruits daily. Choose what works for your lifestyle—even a vegetable that has lost some of its vitamins still provides nutrients as well as fiber and phytochemicals.

The popularity of fortified foods and supplements has continued to grow because people believe that they provide benefits beyond meeting nutrient needs. Americans consume these products not only to ensure that their nutrient needs are met but also to protect themselves from diseases such as cardiovascular disease, cancer, and osteoporosis; to boost their energy levels; help them lose weight and build muscle; and to slow aging. The diverse functions of the vitamins and minerals and their importance in the promotion of health and the prevention of disease has motivated the manufacturers of dietary supplements to offer an overwhelming variety of supplemental options.

For more information on meeting your vitamin needs, go to the USDA Center for Nutrition Policy and Promotion at **www.usda.gov/cnpp/** or the National Cancer Institute's 5-a-Day program at **www.5aday.gov/**

What you choose to eat is still key to your nutritional health

Advances in our knowledge about nutrient structures, functions, and interactions have helped us understand our nutrient needs—but they don't always help us meet them. Choosing a diet that contains too little or too much energy or nutrients can lead to debilitating deficiency diseases, cause toxic reactions, and in some cases increase the risk of chronic disease. Meeting needs requires that we choose appropriate combinations of available foods in the proper proportions. The many options available today for meeting nutrient needs have made selecting a healthy diet both easier and more complicated. We have to decide not only what foods to choose, but whether these foods should contain added nutrients or if we need to take dietary supplements. Because we do not yet know all there is to know about essential nutrients and other biologically active components in foods and supplements, consumers must be aware of the importance of wise food choices and the risks of over-supplementation.

You Can Get It All from Food

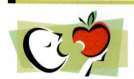

Most people don't need supplements to meet their nutrient requirements. A diet that includes a variety of nutrient-dense foods provides all the essential nutrients and other substances needed to promote health and prevent disease.

✳ Remember
The Food Guide Pyramid provides selection tips to promote healthy, nutrient-dense, and varied choices from within and among the different food groups (see Table 2.1).

Most people can get all the nutrients they need from food, without relying on supplements. But to do so, you have to choose what you eat wisely so your diet includes a variety of nutrient-dense foods. Many of the choices you make should be less processed foods, such as fresh fruits and vegetables and whole grains; these are good sources of a multitude of nutrients and other health-promoting substances. Some choices may also be foods fortified with nutrients. This dietary pattern provides the nutrients you need to meet your needs as well as other substances found in foods that promote health.

A healthy diet includes a variety of nutrient-dense foods

A healthy diet provides the right amounts of energy and nutrients to keep you alive and well. You don't need to consume the exact requirement for each nutrient every day in order to meet your needs. It is the total diet, consisting of the average intake consumed over a period of days or weeks, that is important. This diet must include a wide variety of foods because each food choice provides some vitamins and minerals and other essential substances, but none provides them all. Grains are good sources of iron and zinc and most of the B vitamins, including folate; leafy green vegetables provide iron, calcium, magnesium, vitamin A, folate, vitamin E, and vitamin K; fruits provide potassium, vitamin A, and vitamin C; meat provides iron, zinc, thiamin, and vitamin B_6 and B_{12}; milk contains calcium, phosphorus, riboflavin, vitamin A, and vitamin D; and oils contain vitamin E (Figure 10.2).

A variety of different choices from within each food group provides different amounts and types of nutrients. Variety is also important because nutrients and other food components interact. Interactions may be positive, enhancing nutrient utilization, or negative, inhibiting nutrient use. Variety averages out these interactions.

Nutrient density is important to assure that you meet your nutrient needs without excessive calories. Nutrient-dense choices provide more nutrients per calorie. For example, a baked potato contains more nutrients per calorie than potato chips so it is a more nutrient-dense food. Whole wheat toast is more nutrient dense than a Danish, skim milk is more nutrient dense than ice cream, and roasted chicken is more nutrient dense than fried chicken. The degree of refinement, the amount of added sugar and fat, and the way the food is cooked can all affect nutrient density.

Food provides health benefits beyond basic nutrition

Food provides an unlimited variety of tastes, textures, smells, and nutrient combinations. In addition to nutrients and gastronomic delight, food contains factors that affect absorption and nutrient utilization and offers disease protection. Foods that provide health benefits beyond basic nutrition have been termed **functional foods**.

🔶 **Functional foods** Foods that provide a health benefit beyond that provided by the nutrients they contain.

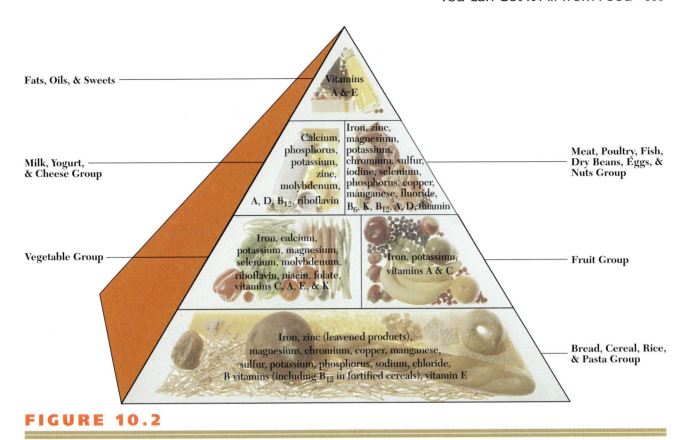

FIGURE 10.2

Each food group of the Food Guide Pyramid provides sources of vitamins and minerals, but no one group can meet all micronutrient needs. (Michael Malyszko/Taxi/ Getty Images)

Although the term is relatively new, interest in the health-promoting properties of foods is not new. Eastern cultures have long used foods for their medicinal benefits and early medicine relied on many food prescriptions to treat disease. Until recently most of these treatments were based on cultural beliefs and tradition rather than scientific evidence. During the last decade, however, many studies have examined the relationships among the consumption of specific foods, typical dietary patterns, and health.

Almost all foods can be considered functional In the broadest interpretation of the definition, almost any food can be considered a functional food. The simplest functional foods are unmodified whole foods that naturally contain substances that provide a health benefit beyond that provided by the nutrients they contain.[1] Many fruits and vegetables fit into this category. For instance, broccoli and other **cruciferous** vegetables have been associated with a decreased cancer risk. Further research into these relationships has shown that these vegetables contain a number of **phytochemicals** that have anticancer properties. There are also animal products that can be considered functional foods; the chemicals that provide health benefits in animal foods are called **zoochemicals**. For example, fish is functional; consumption of a diet high in fish has been related to a reduced risk of heart attacks.[2] This is believed to be due to the omega-3 fatty acids in fish. Functional foods also include foods fortified with nutrients or enhanced with phytochemicals or other substances. For example, special margarines contain added plant sterols to help lower blood cholesterol (two such products currently on the market are Benecol and Take Control) and some brands of orange juice have added calcium to help prevent osteoporosis. Fruit punch with added ginseng and St. John's wort also fall within the realm of functional foods. These modified foods have also been called designer foods or nutraceuticals. Table 10.1 lists some examples of foods that can be considered functional foods.

On the Web To read more about functional foods go to the American Dietetic Association at **www.eatright.org/Public** and click on Position Papers to read the paper on functional foods and look for the nutrition fact sheet on vitamins, minerals, and functional foods.

Cruciferous A group of vegetables (also called crucifers) named for the cross shape of their four-petal flowers. They include broccoli, Brussels sprouts, cabbage, cauliflower, kale, kohlrabi, mustard greens, rutabagas, and turnips. Their consumption is linked with lower rates of cancer.

Phytochemicals Substances found in plant foods (*phyto* means plant) that are not essential nutrients but may have health-promoting properties.

Zoochemicals Substances found in animal foods (*zoo* means animal) that are not essential nutrients but may have health-promoting properties.

TABLE 10.1

Functional Foods Provide Benefits Beyond Nutrients

Functional Food	What It Contains	What It Does
Whole grain products	Fiber	Reduces the risk of cancer and heart disease
Oatmeal	β-glucan, soluble fiber	Reduces blood cholesterol
Grape juice	Phenols	Improves cardiovascular health
Green or black tea	Tannins, catechins	Reduces the risk of certain types of cancer
Fatty fish	Omega-3 fatty acids	Reduces heart disease risk
Soy	Phytoestrogens, soy protein	Reduces the risk of cancer and heart disease, reduces menopausal symptoms
Garlic	Organic sulfur compounds	Reduces the risk of cancer and heart disease
Spinach, kale, collard greens	Lutein, zeaxanthin	Reduces the risk of age-related blindness (macular degeneration)
Tree nuts	Monounsaturated fatty acids	Reduces the risk of heart disease
Foods containing sugar alcohols	Sugar alcohols	Reduces the risk of tooth decay
Cereal fortified with folic acid	Folic acid	Reduces the risk of neural tube defects
Juice fortified with calcium	Calcium	Reduces the risk of osteoporosis
Modified margarine	Plant sterols, plant stanol	Reduces blood cholesterol levels

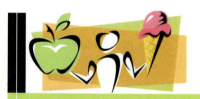

So, What Should I Eat?

Choose a variety of nutrient-dense foods
- Add extras to your sandwich—extra lettuce, extra tomatoes, extra onions
- Try a new type of whole grain bread
- Eat fish for dinner twice a week
- Have whole fruit instead of juice drinks
- Don't forget beans as a protein source

Preserve the nutrients in your produce
- Wrap refrigerated produce
- Chop vegetables just before serving
- Don't soak vegetables before cooking
- Cook frozen vegetables without thawing them
- Don't make your veggies mush—stop cooking them when they are still slightly crisp
- Use less cooking water by steaming, microwaving, roasting, grilling, or stir-frying

If you choose functional or fortified foods
- Read the label so you know what has been added to your food
- Don't pay for what you don't need—if you have healthy cholesterol, pass on the Benecol spread
- Look beyond the banner that says "Contains Fruit Juice"
- Don't pick high sugar snack foods just because they are fortified with nutrients

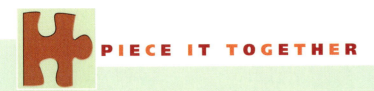

PIECE IT TOGETHER

The Nutrient Density Game

Max is doing his student teaching in the local middle school. In the cafeteria, he can't help but notice how much junk food the kids bring in their lunches. He decides he will use this as an opportunity to teach the concept of nutrient density. He begins by making some posters for the cafeteria that offer suggestions for more nutrient-dense choices.

HERE ARE A FEW OF MAX'S SUGGESTIONS. DID HE GIVE GOOD ADVICE OR WERE SOME OF HIS SUGGESTIONS NO MORE NUTRIENT DENSE THAN THE ORIGINAL ITEM?

Food	Max's Suggestions	Does It Increase Nutrient Density? Why or Why Not?
Peanut butter and marshmallow on white bread	Use whole wheat bread and substitute sliced bananas or raisins for the marshmallow	Yes. The whole wheat bread adds fiber and some vitamins and minerals and the fruit adds vitamins, minerals, and fiber without the added sugar in the marshmallow.
Pudding cups	Yogurt cups	Yes. Although both are high in added sugar, the yogurt provides more calcium than the pudding.
Boxed juice drinks	Boxed fruit juice	*Your answer:*
Chocolate chip cookies	Sugar cookies	*Your answer:*
Fruit roll-ups	Fresh fruit	*Your answer:*
Chocolate snack cakes	Granola bar	*Your answer:*

ALMOST ALL THE KIDS BROUGHT SOME TYPE OF SNACK CHIP. WHAT WOULD BE A MORE NUTRIENT-DENSE FOOD TO SUBSTITUTE FOR THESE?

One option would be carrot sticks but substituting popcorn or a baked corn chip would also provide a more nutrient-dense choice.

Some of the choices offered by the school lunch program are not much better than the foods brought in bag lunches.

MAKE SOME NUTRIENT-DENSE SUGGESTIONS FOR THESE LUNCH MENU ITEMS THAT ARE FOODS 10- TO 13-YEAR-OLDS WOULD ENJOY EATING.

Food	More Nutrient-Dense Suggestions	Why Does It Increase Nutrient Density?
Breaded chicken nuggets	Grilled chicken sandwich on whole grain roll	Grilling reduces the amount of fat and the whole grain roll adds fiber and other nutrients.
Grilled cheese sandwich on white bread	Toasted cheese and tomato sandwich on whole grain bread	*Your answer:*
Pepperoni pizza	*Your answer:*	*Your answer:*

Labeling claims can help identify functional foods Although food labels generally do not use the term "functional food," labels can be helpful in determining the health-related functions that foods provide. Functional foods that contain nutrients or other substances that have been demonstrated by careful research to affect a disease or health-related condition may carry a health claim on their labels (see Chapter 2). For example, oats contain a soluble fiber that helps lower cholesterol. The evidence supporting this effect is strong enough for the FDA to permit foods containing oats to claim that they help reduce blood cholesterol and the risk of heart disease. Foods contain many substances that have been associated with health benefits.

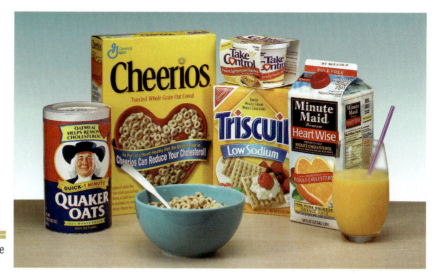

FIGURE 10.3

Health claims on food labels help identify foods that have health benefits. (Andy Washnik)

It has not been possible to isolate each of these substances and accumulate enough evidence for a specific health claim, but health claims recognize the importance of many types of foods in disease prevention (Figure 10.3). For example, health claims can be used to point out the role of fruits and vegetables and whole grains in reducing the risk of both cancer and heart disease.

Phytochemicals Promote Health

The term phytochemical refers to the hundreds, perhaps thousands, of biologically active nonnutritive chemicals found in plants. In the plants where they are found, phytochemicals serve functions that are beneficial to the plants. For example, compounds in onions and garlic are natural pesticides that protect plants from insects. Gardeners often grow these near other vulnerable plants to protect them from insect infestation. When we consume these plant chemicals most have no effect on our health, some promote health, while a few can be toxic. An example of toxic chemicals are those found in some wild mushrooms, which can cause symptoms ranging from stomach upset, dizziness, and hallucinations to liver and kidney failure, coma, and death.

Despite the variety of effects these chemicals can have, we generally use the term "phytochemical" to refer to those substances found in plants that have health-promoting properties. Many research studies have shown that diets high in certain foods lower the incidence of chronic disease. For instance diets high in garlic, soybeans, cruciferous vegetables, legumes, onions, citrus fruits, tomatoes, whole grains, and a variety of herbs have been found to be associated with a lower risk of cancer.[3] Some of the health-promoting phytochemicals in these foods and others have been identified. However, often studies that set out to determine the benefits of a specific nutrient or phytochemical find that the health-promoting effects are associated with a combination of nutrients and phytochemicals rather than a single substance. Therefore, obtaining these substances from whole foods will likely provide more benefit than supplementing them individually.

Phytochemicals have many effects in the body

The phytochemicals in our food protect our health in a variety of ways. Some, such as carotenoids, are antioxidants. Others provide benefits because they mimic the structure or function of natural substances in the body. Phytoestrogens, for instance, have structures similar to hormones and affect us by blocking or mimicking hormone action. Phytosterols resemble cholesterol in structure and thus compete with cholesterol for absorption from the gastrointestinal tract. This reduces cholesterol absorption and

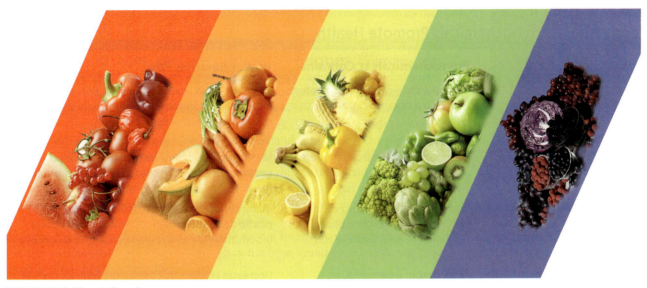

FIGURE 10.4

The best way to ensure you are getting a variety of phytochemicals is to choose foods with every color of the rainbow. (*red, orange, yellow,* and *green*: A. J. J. Estudi/ Age Fotostock America; *blue* and *violet*: Andy Washnik)

helps lower blood cholesterol—a major risk factor for cardiovascular disease. Some phytochemicals stimulate the body's natural defenses; sulfides and isothiocyanates stimulate the activity of enzymes that help deactivate **carcinogens**. Other phytochemicals protect against cancer by altering the way in which cells communicate and influencing other cellular processes.[4]

The chemical names of the phytochemicals can be confusing and hard to pronounce but their food sources are easy to remember; they are plentiful in the fruits, vegetables, and whole grains. When you choose a colorful varied diet, you will be consuming a diet high in phytochemicals (Figure 10.4). Table 10.2 provides a quick reference for some of the phytochemicals in foods and their benefits.

Yellow-orange foods are loaded with carotenoids
Carrots, sweet potatoes, acorn squash, apricots, and mangoes have something in common—their yellow-orange color. Their color comes from the carotenoids, a group of more than 600 yellow, orange, and red compounds found in living organisms. Carotenoids are also found in some green vegetables but their color is masked by the green of the chlorophyll pigment these vegetables contain. Carotenoids have antioxidant properties and some also have vitamin A activity. The major sources of carotenoids in the diet are fruits and vegetables. Because of this, people who eat more fruits and vegetables have higher blood carotenoid levels. A high intake of carotenoid-containing fruits and vegetables has been associated with a reduced risk of certain cancers, cardiovascular disease, and age-related eye diseases such as cataracts and **macular degeneration**.[5]

The most prevalent carotenoids in the North American diet include β-carotene, α-carotene, β-cryptoxanthin, lycopene, lutein, and zeaxanthin. β-carotene is the best known and it provides the most vitamin A activity, but it may be a less effective antioxidant than some of the others. Lycopene, the carotenoid that gives tomatoes their red color, is a more potent antioxidant than other dietary carotenoids.[6] The carotenoids lutein and zeaxanthin accumulate in the macula, which is the central portion of the retina of the eye. High intakes of these are associated with reduced risk of macular degeneration, the leading cause of blindness in older adults.

Flavonoids paint our produce with purples, reds, and pale yellows
Like carotenoids, flavonoids are plant pigments that add color to your plate. They are found in fruits, vegetables, wine, grape juice, and tea. One of the most abundant types of flavonoids is the anthocyanins, which give the blue and red colors to

Carcinogens Substances that promote the development of cancer.

Macular degeneration An incurable eye disorder that is caused by a deterioration of the central portion of the retina. It is the leading cause of blindness in adults over the age of 55 years.

simplifies the message by encouraging us to eat at least 5 fruit and vegetable servings daily. If these vegetables include dark green-colored vegetables as well as yellow-orange, pale yellow, and deep red and purple fruits and vegetables you are getting an abundance of phytochemicals.

Unfortunately we are still not doing what we were told as children. Recent surveys of the typical American diet suggest that although our fruit and vegetable intake has increased, only 24% of those surveyed met their recommended intake for fruit and for vegetables.[12] White potatoes represent a disproportionately large share of our total vegetable intake, while phytochemical- and nutrient-rich dark green and deep yellow vegetables account for a disproportionately small share.[13]

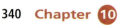
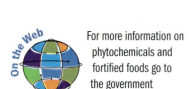

For more information on phytochemicals and fortified foods go to the government nutrition Web site at **www.nutrition.gov/**

Fortified Foods Can Increase Your Intake of Specific Nutrients

You don't have to look very hard to find fortified foods in the grocery store. In fact it might be harder to find a food that hasn't had something added to it to either boost its vitamin or mineral content or endow it with some other healthful properties. Fortified foods by definition are foods to which one or more nutrients have been added. The added nutrients may or may not have been present in the original food.

Fortification is an effective way to increase nutrient intake and reduce deficiency diseases in a population. Recently, however, fortification has also become a marketing tool. People associate vitamins and minerals with health so they assume that a food with these added must be a healthy choice. As consumers have become more and more aware of the benefits of a nutritious diet, food manufacturers have capitalized on this and the number of fortified foods has skyrocketed. The increase in the sales of fortified foods confirms their appeal. The market for fortified food tripled between 1997 and 2001, when sales reached almost $18 billion. Projections for coming years anticipate that this trend will continue, with retail sales forecast to reach $28.6 billion by 2006.[14]

Fortification is used to prevent deficiency diseases

The fortification of foods in the United States has a long history. One of the earliest successful fortification efforts was the fortification of salt with iodine. This program was initiated in 1924 to prevent goiter, cretinism, and other iodine-deficiency disorders. In the early 1930's vitamin D was added to cow's milk to enhance calcium absorption and prevent rickets. In 1938 voluntary enrichment of flours and breads with thiamin, niacin, riboflavin, and iron was motivated by the widespread deficiency of these nutrients in the diet. By 1943 most flour and bread products were enriched with these nutrients in order to improve the nutritional status of the population. This enrichment program required the addition of many but not all of the nutrients lost in the milling of grain for the purpose of restoring them to the same or a higher level than originally present. Thiamin was added to prevent beriberi, niacin to prevent pellagra, riboflavin because it is needed for proper functioning of vitamin B_6 and niacin, and iron was added to prevent iron-deficiency anemia. The fortification of margarine with vitamin A began when margarine replaced butter in many diets. Butter is naturally high in vitamin A so the vitamin was added to margarine, which replaced butter but contained no vitamin A. Similarly, vitamin A is added to low-fat and nonfat cow's milk because vitamin A is lost when the fat is removed from whole milk. The most recent fortification program in the Untied States, begun in 1998, is the fortification of grain products with folic acid to reduce the incidence of neural tube birth defects (Figure 10.6). Fortification programs are used throughout the world to increase the intake of nutrients likely to be deficient in the diet of local populations (see Chapter 15).

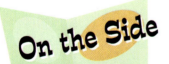

On the Side

University of Wisconsin biochemistry professor Harry Steenbock demonstrated in 1923 that irradiation of food with ultraviolet light increased the vitamin D content. This technique was originally used to fortify milk with vitamin D but was replaced in the 1940's by the simpler technique of adding vitamin D concentrate to milk.

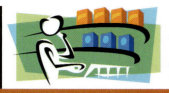

Your Choice: Are They Foods? Should You Choose Them?

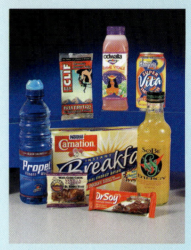

(Andy Washnik)

An energy bar that contains soy protein and 23 vitamins and minerals; a canned soft drink with echinacea and 100% of the Daily Value for most of the B vitamins; a fruit juice designed for women that provides 600% of the Daily Value for thiamin, riboflavin, vitamin B_6, and vitamin B_{12} along with guarana and Dong Quai; bottled water with 100% of the Daily Value for vitamin C—are these foods?

As food manufacturers cash in on the concept that "health sells," the line between what is a supplement and what is a food has become blurred. Claims that a product provides nutrients or other substances that will promote health, reduce disease risk, or enhance athletic performance do sell products. But do these products provide the benefits they claim, and are these benefits ones you need? Should they be part of your diet? Are they safe? As with dietary supplements, it is important to know what you are choosing and to consider the risks and benefits of the product before you consume it.

One of the first things to consider when selecting a fortified product is what nutrients it provides. These products must all carry either a Nutrition Facts or Supplement Facts label. If you are looking for a way to ensure that you get enough vitamins, you may choose a breakfast cereal or beverage that provides close to 100% of your vitamin needs. These products can provide this insurance and give you an alternative to a multivitamin pill. If you are looking for a source of phytochemicals or herbs, you may be disappointed. A close look at the label will probably reveal that the amounts of these substances added are quite small.

If the product provides nutrients or other substances you want to add to your diet, it is then important to consider whether it also contains things you don't want to supplement. For example, an energy bar with added soy may help you increase your intake of soy protein. But if it also includes more calories and other added nutrients than you want, you may do better getting your soy protein from tofu. Likewise, fortified fruit juice may seem like a good way to get your vitamins, but if the juice also includes one or more herbs that you don't want, a glass of orange juice with a vitamin pill might be a better choice.

Finally, what are the risks of the product? When you add this food to your overall diet, are you exceeding the recommended intakes for any nutrients? We are used to consuming foods in amounts that satisfy our sensory desires, fill our stomach, and quench our thirst. In contrast, we dole out vitamin pills in accordance with the recommended dose.

Too much of a supplement can be toxic, but it is almost impossible to consume harmful amounts of nutrients in unfortified foods. However, when faced with a product that tastes like a food but has the nutrients of a supplement, we may consume it with the abandon of a food but be exposed to the risks of a supplement. For example, adults need to consume about 3 liters of fluid per day. If this fluid is water-fortified with vitamin C, niacin, vitamin E, and vitamins B_6 and B_{12} the risk of toxicity increases with every glass. If it is a hot day and you drink an extra bottle you may be consuming these nutrients well in excess of your needs and be increasing your risk of a toxic dose. What if these products also contain herbs? Is it an herb that you have researched and determined will be a healthy addition to your diet? There are no Daily Values or ULs for herbs, so you may not be able to tell if you are getting a dose that is too low to have any effect or perhaps high enough to cause an adverse reaction.

There are many products on the market—promoted to enhance your health and nutrition—that lie somewhere between foods and supplements. These products may have enticing claims, but their contents should be carefully considered before adding them to your diet on a regular basis. Do you really need water that is fortified with vitamins? Are the benefits worth the extra cost? Does the juice with St. John's wort help you? Or can it hurt you? Consumers today enjoy a great variety of choices, but they need to choose wisely to be sure they are getting health benefits, not health risks.

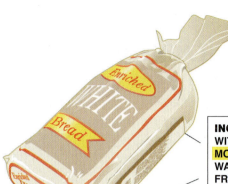

INGREDIENTS: WHEAT FLOUR (ENRICHED WITH BARLEY MALT, NIACIN, IRON, THIAMINE MONONITRATE, RIBOFLAVIN, FOLIC ACID), WATER, SOYBEAN AND/OR CANOLA OIL, HIGH FRUCTOSE CORN SYRUP, YEAST, SUGAR, SKIM MILK, BUTTER. CONTAINS 2% OR LESS OF EACH OF THE FOLLOWING: SOY LECITHIN, SOYA FLOUR, MALTODEXTRIN, DEXTROSE, MALT, CORN STARCH, WHEAT GLUTEN, SALT, HONEY, CALCIUM PEROXIDE, CALCIUM SULFATE, CALCIUM PROPIONATE (TO RETARD SPOILAGE), DOUGH CONDITIONERS (MONO & DIGLYCERIDES, ETHOXYLATED MONO & DIGLYCERIDES), VINEGAR.

FIGURE 10.6

The ingredient list from this bread label shows the nutrients that are currently added to enriched flour.

Government-supported fortification programs are developed to improve public health. The fortified foods increase the intake of nutrients that are deficient in the population's diet without relying on consumers to make the recommended choices or to take nutrient supplements. What foods are to be fortified and how much of the nutrient or nutrients should be added are carefully considered. Dietary staples are typically selected for fortification because they are consistently consumed by the majority of the population. The level of fortification is chosen based on an amount that is high enough to benefit those who need to increase their intake but not so high as to increase the risk of excessive intakes in others. For example, the level of folic acid used in fortification was determined by evaluating the average grain consumption by various groups in the United States and then choosing a fortification level that would benefit the majority of the population but not be toxic to any subgroup of the population. The level of folic acid currently added to grain products is not high enough for women of childbearing age to meet the recommendation of 400 μg from these products alone; if it was high enough to satisfy this need it would have also been high enough to mask vitamin B_{12} deficiency.

Fortification is used as a sales tool

Fortification today extends beyond government-monitored programs. Manufacturers are now voluntarily fortifying their products with a variety of nutrients. Many of the added nutrients are ones that are of public health concern. For example, public health messages tell us to consume adequate calcium to avoid osteoporosis. As a result, there has been a boom in the number of calcium-fortified foods. People who don't drink milk can now get calcium in fortified orange juice, fortified breakfast cereal, or fortified cheese. Other nutrients that are commonly added are those that are easy and inexpensive to add to a food and may help to promote sales as well as promote your health. For instance, a bowl Cheerios has over ten vitamins and minerals added to it in addition to what it naturally contains. Not all of these added nutrients are ones that are deficient in the American diet.

When fortification is voluntary both the level of fortification and the foods and beverages fortified is somewhat arbitrary. For example, some calcium-fortified foods may contain levels equivalent to those in a glass of milk whereas others may contain only a small fraction of this. Therefore it is important to pay attention to the actual nutrient contribution, not just the fact that the banner on the label says it is fortified. Also, just because a food is fortified does not mean that it is a nutritious choice.

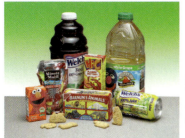

For example a fruit roll-up that has added vitamin C is still a food that is high in added sugars and low in most nutrients that would be consumed in a piece of fruit (Figure 10.7).

Indiscriminant fortification increases the risk of toxicity

Fortification can be beneficial, but it can also result in toxicities and nutrient imbalances. The purpose of consuming fortified foods is to meet nutrient needs. However, because of the plethora of products currently available, the risk of exceeding the Tolerable Upper Intake Levels (ULs) of some vitamins and minerals is increased. For example, almost all breakfast cereals contain a complement of B vitamins as well as iron and calcium (Figure 10.8). When these are consumed in addition to a multivitamin, it would be easy to consume more than the recommended amounts for some vitamins. For example, a growing teen who takes a multivitamin supplement and consumes three cups of breakfast cereal each morning is exceeding the RDA for many nutrients. National food survey data indicate that 20 to 30% of young children may exceed the UL for folic acid because of the frequent use of fortified breakfast cereals and supplements in addition to fortified grain products.[15] Over half of infants and children 3 years of age and under have zinc intakes that exceed the UL.[16] Extensive fortification in the breakfast cereal industry has also made it difficult for those who must limit iron intake to find breakfast cereals that are not fortified with iron.

Because of the potential for over and under fortification and nutrient imbalances, the FDA cautions against the indiscriminant addition of nutrients to foods and the fortification of snack foods and candy.[17] To meet nutrient needs but not risk nutrient excesses, consumers must be aware of what has been added to the foods they are choosing and consider all the sources of nutrients: foods, fortified foods, and supplements.

Fortified Breakfast Cereal

Nutrition Facts

Serving Size 1 Cup (50g/1.8 oz.)
Servings per Container About 10

Amount Per Serving	Cereal	Cereal with 1/2 Cup Vitamins A&D Fat Free Milk
Calories	180	220
Calories from Fat	5	5

	% Daily Value**	
Total Fat 0.5g*	1%	1%
Saturated Fat 0g	0%	0%
Cholesterol 0mg	0%	0%
Sodium 280mg	12%	14%
Potassium 100mg	3%	9%
Total Carbohydrate 35g	12%	14%
Dietary Fiber 2g	9%	9%
Sugars 7g		
Other Carbohydrate 26g		
Protein 3g		

Vitamin A	15%	20%
Vitamin C	25%	25%
Calcium	0%	15%
Iron	100%	100%
Vitamin D	10%	25%
Vitamin E	100%	100%
Thiamin	100%	100%
Riboflavin	100%	110%
Niacin	100%	100%
Vitamin B$_6$	100%	100%
Folic Acid	100%	100%
Vitamin B$_{12}$	100%	110%
Pantothenate	100%	100%
Phosphorus	10%	20%
Magnesium	8%	10%
Zinc	100%	100%
Copper	4%	6%

FIGURE 10.8

The amount and variety of nutrients added to fortified breakfast cereals is almost as great as that contained in multivitamin supplements.

Dietary Supplements Can Help Meet Needs but Also Carry Risks

About half of the adults in the United States take some kind of dietary supplement.[18] Some of these contain vitamins and minerals, some contain herbs and other plant-derived substances, and some contain compounds found in the body but not essential in the diet (Figure 10.9).[19]

Supplements are available everywhere—from health food stores, grocery stores, drug stores, convenience stores, mail-order catalogs, TV advertisements, and the Internet. People take them for a variety of reasons—to energize themselves, to protect themselves from disease, to cure their illnesses, to lose weight, to enhance what they eat in food, and simply to ensure against deficiencies. These products may be beneficial and even necessary under some circumstances for some individuals, but they also have the potential to cause harm.

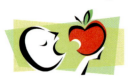

Don't assume that the government has checked out the safety of a dietary supplement before it hits the shelves. The FDA can take a product off the market if there is evidence that it is dangerous, but it is the manufacturers that have the job of testing a supplement for safety before it is sold. FDA approval is not needed to sell supplements. This doesn't mean that products aren't safe but it does mean that consumers need to choose wisely to be safe.

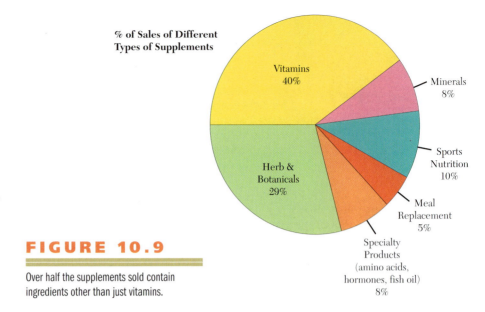

% of Sales of Different Types of Supplements

Vitamins 40%

Minerals 8%

Sports Nutrition 10%

Meal Replacement 5%

Specialty Products (amino acids, hormones, fish oil) 8%

Herb & Botanicals 29%

FIGURE 10.9

Over half the supplements sold contain ingredients other than just vitamins.

In order to help consumers choose supplements wisely, the Dietary Supplement Health and Education Act (DSHEA) was passed in 1994. This law defined dietary supplements and created standards for labeling these products but left most of the responsibility for manufacturing practices and safety in the hands of the manufacturers.

The FDA mandates labeling standards for supplements

Dietary supplements by definition include products intended for ingestion as supplements to the diet. They may contain vitamins; minerals; herbs, botanicals, or other plant-derived substances; amino acids; enzymes; concentrates; or extracts. These products must include the words "dietary supplement" on the label and carry a standard label similar to the Nutrition Facts label on foods. Using the Supplement Facts panel, it is easy to see if any nutrients are present in amounts that exceed 100% of the Daily Value. For any nutrients that are present at more than 100% of the Daily Value, you can check to see if the amount exceeds the UL (see inside cover). Taking any nutrient in amounts that exceed the UL significantly increases the risk of potentially serious toxicity symptoms. Dietary supplement labels may also include claims describing the effects of the supplement on normal function of the body. These structure function claims don't have to be approved by the FDA. This is discussed further in Off the Label: What's on Your Supplement Label.

Manufacturers and the FDA are responsible for supplement safety

According to the DSHEA, supplement manufacturers are responsible for ensuring their products are safe before they are sold. The regulations for supplement safety give the FDA authority to collect information on supplement safety once a supplement is on the market and to remove it from the market if it can prove that the product carries significant risk. The FDA exercised its authority to remove a product from the marketplace once, with products containing ephedra. Ephedra contains ephedrine, a stimulant that mimics the effects of epinephrine in the body. It speeds the heart rate and constricts blood vessels, causing an increase in blood pressure. Supplements containing ephedrine were shown to promote weight loss when compared to placebo.[20] They were also shown to provide a modest improvement in athletic performance when taken with caffeine. However, they were taken off the market due to their side

On the Side

The risks of ephedra were dramatically demonstrated in February 2003 when 23-year-old baseball pitcher Steve Belcher died of heat stroke while taking an ephedra-containing supplement to lose weight. He collapsed during a training session in the hot, humid Florida weather and died the next day when his body temperature reached 108° F. There are many factors that contributed to the heat stroke, but the fact that Belcher was taking ephedra is believed to have played a role because it constricts blood vessels in the skin and raises body temperature.

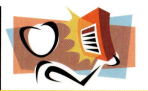

Off the Label: What's on Your Supplement Label?

Products ranging from multivitamin pills to high-protein powders and herbal elixirs all meet the definition of a dietary supplement. They must follow the regulations for labeling and advertising established by the Dietary Supplement Health and Education Act (DSHEA) of 1994.

Supplement labels must include the words "dietary supplement" and carry a "Supplement Facts" panel similar to the "Nutrition Facts" panel found on food labels. The Supplement Facts panel lists the recommended serving size and the name and quantity of each ingredient per serving. The source of the ingredient may be given with its name in the "Supplement Facts" panel or in the ingredient list below the panel. The nutrients for which Daily Values have been established are listed first followed by other dietary ingredients for which no Daily Values have been established.[1]

Supplements may also include a number of different claims on their labels.[2] One type describes the amount of a nutrient in a supplement. For example, a product that claims to be an excellent source of a nutrient must contain at least 20% of the Daily Value for that nutrient per serving. "High potency" means that a serving provides 100% or more of the Daily Value for the nutrient it contains. For multinutrient products, high potency means that a serving provides more than 100% of the Daily Value for two-thirds of the vitamins and minerals present.

Supplement label claims that point out a link between a supplement and a disease or health-related condition must be approved by the FDA before they are permitted on the labels. However, there are other types of claims that need not be approved by the FDA. These include those that point out the link between a nutrient and a deficiency disease that can result if the nutrient is lacking in the diet. For example, a vitamin C supplement could state that "vitamin C prevents scurvy." Other claims refer to the effect of a supplement on maintaining the normal structure or function of the body. For example, a calcium supplement may claim that "calcium builds strong bones." The ginseng supplement shown here claims that ginseng improves performance by stating that "when you need to perform your best, take ginseng." These structure/function claims are based on the manufacturer's review and interpretation of the scientific literature and must not be untrue or misleading. Any product that includes this type of claim must also include the disclaimer "This statement has not been evaluated by the Food and Drug Administration. This product is not intended to diagnose, treat, cure, or prevent any disease."

Although supplement labels provide important information about the contents of dietary supplements, they are not a reliable guide for supplement use. Before purchasing a supplement, you should know what you are purchasing and why. When consuming supplements, follow dosage recommendations and, when available, refer to the ULs (see inside cover) to avoid toxicities.

References
1. New FDA labeling rules for dietary supplements. *FDA Consumer* 32:2, Jan./Feb., 1998.
2. Kurtzweil, P. An FDA guide to dietary supplements. *FDA Consumer* 32:28–35, Sept./Oct., 1998.

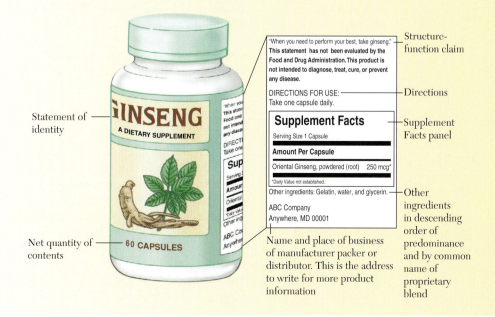

Statement of identity

Net quantity of contents

"When you need to perform your best, take ginseng." This statement has not been evaluated by the Food and Drug Administration. This product is not intended to diagnose, treat, cure, or prevent any disease.

DIRECTIONS FOR USE: Take one capsule daily.

Supplement Facts
Serving Size 1 Capsule

Amount Per Capsule

Oriental Ginseng, powdered (root)   250 mcg*

*Daily Value not established.

Other ingredients: Gelatin, water, and glycerin.

ABC Company
Anywhere, MD 00001

Structure-function claim

Directions

Supplement Facts panel

Other ingredients in descending order of predominance and by common name of proprietary blend

Name and place of business of manufacturer packer or distributor. This is the address to write for more product information

effects, which include nervousness, headaches, nausea, hypertension, cardiac arrhythmias, heart attack, stroke, and even death. After their use was linked to 155 deaths and dozens of heart attacks and strokes, the sale of ephedra-containing supplements was banned by the FDA. In other instances when the FDA believed an ingredient was hazardous it has asked that these ingredients be voluntarily removed. In 2000 the FDA requested that firms marketing products containing the stimulant phenyl-propanolamine, used in decongestants and weight loss products, voluntarily discontinue them. More recently the FDA sent letters to companies suggesting they stop distributing products containing the anabolic steroid androstenedione (Andro) (see Chapter 11).

Manufacturers are responsible for product consistency

There are no mandatory standards in supplement manufacturing, therefore the amount of an ingredient in a dietary supplement and how well it is absorbed by the body may vary from dose to dose. To address this problem, the United States Pharmacopoeia (USP) Convention, which sets the standards for drug manufacture, has developed the USP Dietary Supplement Verification Program (DSVP).[21] This program evaluates and confirms the contents of dietary supplements, manufacturing processes, and compliance with standards of purity. A dietary supplement company that wishes to participate in the program must submit its products to the USP, which then inspects manufacturing facilities, reviews manufacturing procedures, analyzes samples of the product, and evaluates the manufacturer's quality control systems. Products that have been reviewed and meet USP criteria can use the DSVP verification mark on the label or the statement "made to U.S. Pharmacopoeia (USP) quality, purity, and potency standards" (Figure 10.10). Consumers can be assured that products that have been USP verified contain the ingredients in the amounts as listed on the label, will disintegrate or dissolve effectively to release ingredients for absorption into your body, meet requirements for limits on contaminants, and comply with good manufacturing practices. Once a product has been verified by the USP, it will be routinely surveyed to ensure that it continues to meet USP criteria.

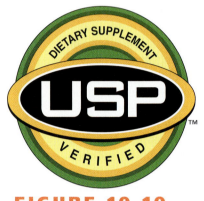

FIGURE 10.10

This Dietary Supplement Verification Program mark indicates that the supplement has been manufactured according to quality, purity, and potency standards set by the U.S. Pharmacopoeia (USP) Convention.

Do You Need a Vitamin/Mineral Supplement?

How can you be sure that you are meeting your needs with food or if you should take a supplement? Your diet probably contains some processed foods from which nutrients have been lost, but it also likely contains some foods that are naturally high in nutrients and many that are fortified with nutrients. Is this enough to meet your needs? Should you take a supplement, or will it increase your risk of vitamin and mineral toxicity?

Most people don't need vitamin/mineral supplements but some do

Eating a variety of foods is the best way to meet nutrient needs, and most healthy adults who consume a reasonably good diet do not need supplements. In fact, an argument against the use of supplements is that it gives people a false sense of security, causing them to pay less attention to the nutrient content of the foods they choose. However, although there is little evidence that the average person benefits from a low-dose multivitamin or multivitamin-mineral supplement that does not exceed 100% of the RDA, there is also little evidence of harm. And, for some people, supplements may be the only way to meet needs because they have low intakes, increased needs, or excess losses. Groups for whom vitamin and mineral supplements are typically recommended include dieters, vegans, pregnant women and women of childbearing age,

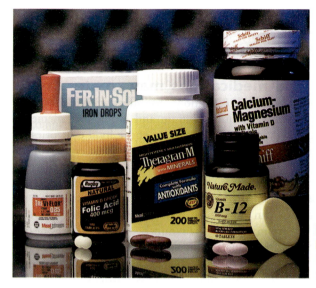

FIGURE 10.11

Many vitamin and mineral supplements target groups with increased needs for certain nutrients. (George Semple)

older adults, individuals suffering from chronic disease, and others who are nutritionally vulnerable because of the use of cigarettes or alcohol (Figure 10.11).

Dieters may not consume enough food to meet micronutrient needs Individuals dieting to lose weight restrict their food intake and consequently reduce their intake of micronutrients. It is difficult to consume the recommended amounts of all vitamins and minerals if your intake is less than 1200 Calories per day, no matter how well planned the diet is. Therefore, it is important to supplement diets that contain fewer than 1200 Calories with a multivitamin-mineral supplement that meets the DRI recommendations (see Chapter 7).

Vegan diets should be supplemented with vitamin B$_{12}$ Although vegetarian diets are generally high in micronutrients, a vegan diet, which excludes all animal food products, will be deficient in vitamin B$_{12}$. Vegans therefore need to obtain vitamin B$_{12}$ from fortified foods or from supplements (see Chapters 6 and 8).

Folate and iron supplements may be needed by young women Women of childbearing age, whether or not they are pregnant, may need supplements to meet their micronutrient needs. Research demonstrating that the risk of bearing children with neural tube defects is reduced by folic acid supplementation has led to the recommendation that women capable of becoming pregnant consume 400 µg of synthetic folic acid daily from either fortified foods or supplements, in addition to consuming food folate from a varied diet (see Chapters 8 and 12). Once a woman becomes pregnant, the need for folate remains high and iron requirements increase. Although a well-planned diet can meet the needs of pregnant women, supplements of iron and folate are recommended, and multivitamin and mineral supplements are usually prescribed (Figure 10.12).

Older adults may need to supplement vitamin B$_{12}$, calcium, and vitamin D Micronutrient supplements may also benefit older adults because the capacity to absorb or utilize vitamins may decrease with aging. For example, 10 to 30% of individuals over 50 have a condition called atrophic gastritis, which reduces the ability to absorb vitamin B$_{12}$ bound to food components. The vitamin B$_{12}$ in fortified foods and supplements is more available so B$_{12}$ from these sources is recommended for this age group (see Chapters 8 and 13).[22] Meeting the AI

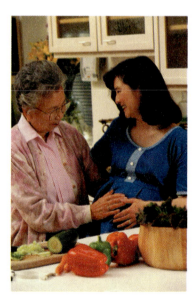

FIGURE 10.12

Pregnant women and older adults are life-stage groups that may benefit from micronutrient supplements. (Larry Dale Gordon/The Image Bank)

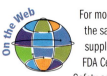

For more information on the safety of dietary supplements go to the FDA Center for Food Safety and Applied Nutrition at **www.cfsan.fda.gov/** and click on dietary supplements, or go to the NIH Office of Dietary Supplements at **www.dietary-supplements.info.nih.gov/**

reported to improve reproductive performance in rats fed a diet deficient in vitamin E, but there is no evidence that it is needed in the diet of healthy humans.

Glucosamine, chondroitin, and SAMe are taken for joint health Glucosamine, chondroitin, and SAMe are needed for the maintenance of healthy joints and are sold to alleviate the pain and progression of arthritis.[27] Glucosamine and chondroitin are molecules found in and around the cells of cartilage, the type of connective tissue that cushions our joints. They are made in the body and consumed in the diet in meat. Supplements of both glucosamine and chondroitin are said to reduce arthritis pain, stop cartilage degeneration, and possibly stimulate the repair of damaged joint cartilage. Supplements of these may be beneficial in relieving the symptoms of arthritis in some people.[28]

SAMe, chemically known as S-adenosyl-methionine, is present in the body normally as an intermediate in the metabolism of methionine. SAMe promotes the production of cartilage and is also marketed for the treatment of arthritis. It is also claimed to be effective for treating depression and liver disease. Although there is preliminary evidence that SAMe may be somewhat beneficial in individuals with depression and arthritis, the results of large, well-controlled studies are not yet available and the risks of taking this supplement have not been adequately assessed.[29]

Carnitine and creatine are taken to enhance athletic performance Carnitine and creatine are both involved in supplying energy to muscle cells. Carnitine is a molecule that is needed to transport fatty acids into the mitochondria where they are broken down by aerobic metabolism to produce energy. Supplements are marketed to improve the use of fat as an energy source during exercise. Despite its role in transporting fatty acids, carnitine supplements have not been shown to improve athletic performance. Creatine is a small molecule used to make a high-energy molecule, called creatine phosphate, that provides energy to the muscle for short bursts of activity. Creatine supplements have been shown to benefit some athletes by enhancing strength, performance, and recovery from high-intensity exercise. They do not improve endurance (see Chapter 11).

Some supplements contain phytochemicals

A diet rich in fruits and vegetables has been shown to reduce the risk of heart disease and cancer; some of this benefit may be due to the phytochemicals contained in these foods. Although we have not yet isolated and identified all of these substances, some have been extracted, purified, and pressed into pills or capsules. These are advertised as having health-promoting properties but it is unclear whether they are as beneficial as the whole foods that are rich sources of these as well as a host of other phytochemicals and nutrients.

Lutein and zeaxanthin are carotenoids that are good for your eyes Lutein and zeaxanthin are carotenoids found in leafy green vegetables. They do not have vitamin A activity but are concentrated in the macula of the eye, where they protect against oxidative damage. Diets high in these carotenoids have been associated with a reduced incidence of age-related eye disorders, such as macular degeneration. Even though the same effect has not been demonstrated with supplements, lutein supplements are still often taken to promote healthy vision.[30]

Many carotenoids are strong antioxidants, but their importance in antioxidant protection in the body is still unclear.[24] The most available carotenoid supplement is β-carotene, which is marketed for its antioxidant properties, but under some circumstances it may promote rather than prevent oxidative damage. For example, some studies show that when β-carotene is added to a vitamin E-deficient diet, it promotes oxidation.[31] But in the presence of vitamin E, β-carotene acts as an antioxidant. One explanation for the increase in the incidence of lung cancer among smokers supplemented with β-carotene is that pro-oxidant activity prevails over antioxidant activity. Supplements don't provide the same balance of antioxidants and other substances found in foods so their effect is sometimes unpredictable.

Rutin, hesperidin, and pycnogenol are flavonoids Like carotenoids, flavonoids, which are often called bioflavonoids, are antioxidants. Supplements containing categories of flavonoids, such as rutin and hesperidin and the flavonoid complex pycnogenol, are advertised as cures for arthritis, heart disease, high blood pressure, and colds. Hesperidin is often called vitamin P but it does not meet the definition of a vitamin because it has not been shown to be essential in the diet. The flavonoids are often included in supplements containing vitamin C because they are purported to promote the action of this vitamin. Although the foods containing these phytochemicals have been shown to have health-promoting properties, supplements have not been shown to have the same health effects.

Some supplements contain herbs

Technically an herb is a non-woody, seed-producing plant that dies at the end of the growing season. However, the term herb is generally used to refer to any botanical or plant-derived substance. Throughout human history herbs have been used as medicine. For example, the herb lobelia, also called Indian tobacco, was smoked by Native Americans to treat asthma. Today herbal supplements are offered to improve general well-being as well as for their specific medicinal functions. They are taken to cure a variety of ailments such as colds, arthritis, depression, and menopausal symptoms as well as to slow aging and improve memory. For some herbs scientific research has confirmed that they have an effect on human physiology, but for others suggested benefits are based on their history of use in traditional medicine.

Herbal supplements that are currently popular include garlic, ginseng, gingko biloba, St. John's wort, and echinacea. Because they are "natural" herbs are often viewed as harmless. Natural, however, is no guarantee of safety.

Garlic and ginseng have been used medicinally for centuries Throughout history garlic has been used for a lot more than to keep vampires away. Hippocrates, who is considered the father of Western medicine, recommended garlic to treat pneumonia and other infections, as well as cancer and digestive disorders. Although it is no longer recommended for these purposes, recent research has shown that it may lower blood cholesterol. Eating enough garlic to lower cholesterol will probably keep your friends and family away as well as the vampires so supplement manufacturers have provided a way to increase intake without eating this odiferous food at every meal; some preparations contain a deodorized form. Ginseng also has a long history. It has been used in Asia for centuries for its energizing, stress-reducing, and aphrodisiac properties. It has a short-term stimulatory effect but in high doses may cause nervousness and heart palpitations.

Ginkgo biloba, St John's wort, and echinacea are flowers Gingko biloba, also called "maiden hair," is an herb that has been used to enhance memory and to treat a variety of circulatory ailments. Consumption of the leaves may cause side effects such as headaches, gastrointestinal upset, and dizziness. Consumption of other parts of the plant can cause allergic skin reactions.

St. John's wort is an herb taken to promote mental well-being. Analysis reveals that it contains low doses of the chemical found in the antidepressant drug fluoxetine (Prozac). Individuals taking antidepressant drugs should not take St. John's wort.

Petals of the echinacea plant were used by Native Americans as a treatment for colds, flu, and infections. Today it is a popular herbal cold remedy. Studies have documented that it is an immune system stimulant. Although side effects have not been reported, allergies are possible (Figure 10.13).[32]

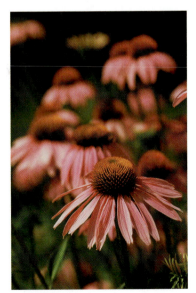

FIGURE 10.13

Echinacea is also known as purple coneflower, but just because it is natural doesn't mean it is safe for everyone at any dose. (Linda Lewis/ Botanica/PictureArts Corp.)

TABLE 10.4
Potential Benefits and Side Effects of Common Herbal Ingredients

Product	Suggested Benefit	Side Effects
Astralagus (Huang ch')	Immune stimulant	Low blood pressure, dizziness, fatigue
Cat's Claw (uña de gato)	Relieves arthritis and indigestion, immune stimulant	Should not be taken by individuals with thrombocytopenia (a blood disorder)
Chamomile[a]	Aids indigestion, promotes relaxation	Allergy possible
Chaparral[b,c*]	Cancer cure, acne treatment, antioxidant	Liver damage, possibly irreversible
Comfrey (borage, coltsfoot)[b,c*]	As a poultice for wounds and sore joints; as a tea for digestive disorders	Do not take orally, even as a tea; obstruction of blood flow to liver resulting in liver failure and possibly death
Dong Quai[a]	Increases energy	May cause birth defects
Echinacea (purple coneflower, snake root, Indian head)[b,d]	Topically for wound healing, internally as an immune stimulant, cold remedy	Allergy possible, adverse effects in pregnant women and people with autoimmune disorders
Ephedra (Ma Huang, Chinese ephedra, epitonin)[b,c*]	Relieves cold symptoms, weight loss	High blood pressure, irregular heartbeat, heart attack, stroke, death; banned by the FDA
Ginger[a]	Relieves motion sickness and nausea	Irregular heartbeat with large doses
Gingko biloba[b] (maiden hair, kew tree, Pak ko)	Improved memory and mental function, improved circulation	GI distress, headache, allergic skin reactions
Ginseng[b]	Enhanced immunity, improved sexual function	High blood pressure
Germander[c]	Weight loss, increased energy	Liver disease, possibly death
Kombochu tea[b] (mushroom tea, kvass tea, kwassan, kargasck)	General well-being	GI upset, liver damage, possibly death
Lobelia[b,c*] (Indian tobacco)	Relaxation, respiratory remedy	Breathing problems, rapid heartbeat, low blood pressure, convulsions, coma, death
Milk thistle[a]	Protects against liver disease	May decrease effectiveness of some medications
Saw palmetto[b]	Improves urinary flow with enlarged prostate	Stomach upset
St. John's wort[b] (hypericum)	Promotes mental well-being	Contains similar ingredients as the antidepressant drug fluoxetine (Prozac) and should not be used by people taking antidepressants
Stephania[b,c*] (magnolia)	Weight loss	Kidney damage, including kidney failure resulting in transplant or dialysis
Valerian[b]	Mild sedative	GI upset, headache, restlessness
Willow bark[b,c*]	Pain and fever relief	Reye's syndrome, allergies
Wormwood[c*]	Relieves digestive ailments	Numbness or paralysis of legs, delirium, paralysis
Yohimbe[b]	Aphrodisiac	Tremors, anxiety, high blood pressure, rapid heart beat, psychosis, paralysis

*Has been shown to have serious side effects and should be avoided.
[a]Mayo Clinic, Blurbs on Herbs. Available online at www.mayohealth.org/mayo/9703/htm/herb_b.htm Accessed May 15, 2000.
[b]Mayo Clinic. Herbs can have many health effects—some beneficial, some dangerous. Available online at www.mayohealth.org/mayo/0707/htm/me_6sb.htm Accessed Apr. 1, 2000.
[c]Kurtzweil, P. An FDA guide to dietary supplements. *FDA Consumer* 32:28–35, Sept./Oct., 1998.
[d]Bartels, C. L., and Miller, S. J. Herbal and related remedies, *NCP* 13:5–14, 1998.

TABLE 10.5
Guidelines to Keep Herbal Supplements Safe

- If you are ill or taking medications, consult your physician before taking herbs.
- Do not take herbs if you are pregnant.
- Do not give herbs to children.
- Do not assume herbal products are safe.
- Do not take herbs with known toxicities.
- Read label ingredients and the list of precautions.
- Start with low doses, and stop taking any product that causes side effects.
- Do not take combinations of herbs.
- Do not use herbs for long periods.

Herbal supplements are not always safe or the best choice

Herbal supplements are readily available and relatively inexpensive. They can be purchased without a trip to the doctor or a prescription. Although consumers who want to manage their own health may view this as beneficial, it can also cause problems. When a drug is prescribed by a physician, we assume that it will have a beneficial effect, that each dose will contain the same amount of drug, that the physician or pharmacist has considered other medications we are taking and other medical conditions that may alter the effectiveness of the drug, and that the drug itself will not cause a severe side effect. These assumptions cannot be made with herbs. Some herbs may be toxic either alone or in combination with other drugs and herbs being consumed. Some may contain bacteria or other contaminants. It is difficult to know what dose of an herb you are taking because even those pressed and packaged into pills may not provide a consistent dose. Also, because consumers decide what to treat, herbal remedies can be used inappropriately or can be used instead of necessary medical intervention.

For some herbs, the risks outweigh the benefits. Serious side effects from excessive doses or unusual combinations of herbs and medications are not uncommon (Table 10.4). The use of herbal supplements also may be inappropriate at certain times. For example, St. John's wort can prolong and intensify the effects of narcotic drugs and anesthetic agents, so it should not be taken before surgery. It is recommended that herbal products not be used for 2 to 3 weeks prior to surgery (Table 10.5).

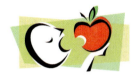

Chaparral and comfrey can cause liver damage, lobelia can cause a drop in blood pressure, and wormwood can cause paralysis. These are all natural herbs, but they are anything but safe. Just because a substance is produced naturally by a plant does not make it either safe or beneficial. Many of the drugs we use today are derived from plants, but you wouldn't take them without first consulting a physician.

Choose Supplements with Care

The FDA estimates that there are 29,000 different products available as dietary supplements[19] (Figure 10.14). You can purchase almost any nutrient as an individual supplement or you can choose from a surfeit of combinations of nutrients, herbs, and other components. Formulations of B vitamins are marketed to boost your energy, a complex of B vitamins and C offers stress reduction, antioxidant mixes are sold to protect you from cancer and heart disease, and herbal products advertise to relax you and promote mental well-being. Special mixes target women, men, seniors, and vegetarians. Some claim to be "all natural", others add herbal ingredients that promise everything from a better memory to a reduced risk of cancer. They entice you with terms like "mega", "advanced formula", "high potency", and "ultra". If you choose to take a dietary supplement, whether to ensure an adequate nutrient intake, prevent disease, or optimize health, products must be chosen with care to assure that nutrient needs are met and the risk of toxicity is minimal. Choosing a supplement can be confusing.

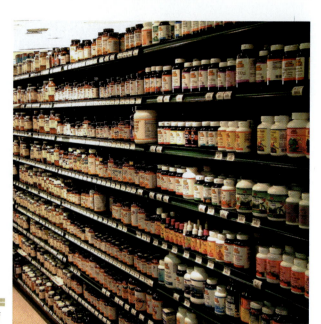

FIGURE 10.14

There are thousands of different types of dietary supplements available on the shelves of health food stores, drug stores, and grocery stores. (Tom Carter/PhotoEdit)

Make sure your supplement provides what you want and won't harm you

If you choose to take a supplement, it is important to be sure that the product provides all the nutrients you need to satisfy your individual concerns, but does not contain ingredients or amounts that could cause adverse effects. Label claims on the supplement bottle will try to convince you that the product is the one you need. But does it really provide what you want (Table 10.6)?

TABLE 10.6
Think Before You Supplement

- Why do you want a supplement? If you are taking it to ensure better health, does it provide both vitamins and minerals? If you want to supplement specific nutrients, are they contained in the product?
- Does it contain potentially toxic levels of any nutrient? Check the % DV. For any nutrients that exceed 100%, check to see if they exceed the UL (see inside cover).
- Does it contain any nonvitamin/nonmineral ingredients? If so, have any been shown to be toxic to someone like you?
- Do you have a medical condition that recommends against certain nutrients or other ingredients? Are you a smoker? (Smoking increases the need for vitamin C, but also increases the risks associated with taking β-carotene.)
- Are you taking prescription medication with which an ingredient in the supplement may interact? Check with your physician, dietitian, or pharmacist to help identify these interactions.
- Compare product costs before you buy. Just as more isn't always better, more expensive is not always better either.
- Make sure you are getting what you pay for. Check the expiration date. Some nutrients degrade over time so expired products will have less than is on the label. Look for the DSVP mark that tells you the product has met industry quality, purity, and potency standards.

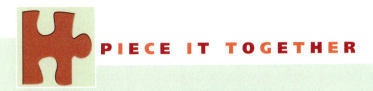

PIECE IT TOGETHER

Supplemental Choices

Hazel is suffering through her third cold of the winter. She is tired of being sick! When she complains at a local health food store, the clerk recommends several supplements to keep her healthy. These include a vitamin C supplement, a stress formula B vitamin supplement called B₅₀, and another supplement called Prevention Plus. When she gets home with her new supplements, her friend who is a nutrition student questions whether Hazel needs all of these products.

WHAT ARE HAZEL'S NUTRIENT NEEDS?

Hazel is a generally healthy 22-year-old. Her Body Mass Index (BMI) is in the healthy range. She exercises a couple of days each week. Therefore, Hazel's needs should be met by the recommendations for someone of her age and sex.

HOW HEALTHY IS HAZEL'S TYPICAL DIET?

Hazel tries to eat well. Comparing her diet to the Food Guide Pyramid reveals that she meets all of the serving recommendations except for dairy products and fruits.

Using information from each product's Supplement Facts label, Hazel compiles a list of the amounts and % Daily Values of each ingredient in her supplements.

WILL HAZEL'S INTAKE EXCEED THE UL FOR ANY NUTRIENTS IF SHE TAKES THESE PRODUCTS?

- Vitamin C: Her total intake from all of these at the recommended frequency would be 2500 mg per day, which exceeds the UL of 2000 mg per day.
- Niacin: Three tablets of B₅₀ provide 150 mg per day. This is well in excess of the UL of 35 mg per day.
- Vitamin B_6: *Your answer:*
- In addition, although there are no ULs for the other B vitamins, Hazel's intake for many is well above 100% of the Daily Value.

WHAT ABOUT FORTIFIED FOODS?

In searching for nutritious foods, Hazel selected a highly fortified breakfast cereal. A look at the label reveals that if she eats this cereal every day she will be consuming an additional 20 mg of niacin and 2 mg of vitamin B_6 as well as at least another 50% of the Daily Value for the other B vitamins. This will further increase her risk of an adverse effect from excess intakes.

WHAT WOULD YOU RECOMMEND TO HAZEL?

Your answer:

Supplement	Ingredient	Dose	%DV/ Dose	Frequency	Total Amount (% DV)
Vitamin C	Vitamin C	500 mg	833%	3/day	1500 mg (2500%)
B₅₀	Thiamin	50 mg	3333%	3/day	150 mg (10,000%)
	Niacin	50 mg	250%		150 mg (750%)
	Vitamin B_6	50 mg	2500%		150 mg (7500%)
	Riboflavin	50 mg	2941%		150 mg (8823%)
	Biotin	50 mg	16.66%		150 mg (50%)
	Pantothenic acid	50 mg	500%		150 mg (1500%)
	Folic acid	50 mg	12.5%		150 mg (38%)
	Vitamin B_{12}	50 mg	833%		150 mg (2500%)
Prevention Plus	Vitamin C	1000 mg	1667%	1/day	1000 mg (1667%)
	Zinc	15 mg	100%		15 mg (100%)

If you are looking for a vitamin/mineral supplement make sure the product you choose provides minerals as well as vitamins. If you want to increase your calcium intake, check to see if the supplement provides the amount of calcium that you want. If you are anemic, does it provide iron? Does it provide enough vitamin B_{12} to meet your needs if you are over 50 or eat a vegan diet? If you are a woman of childbearing age, you might want to ensure that you supplement your diet with 400 μg of folic acid. Special formulas for men, seniors, or women may not necessarily provide what you need even if you fit into a specific target group. These claims are not regulated so it is up to the company to decide what each special group needs.

Be sure to consider your medical condition and the medications you are taking that may interact with supplements. For example, individuals taking anticoagulant medications should not take supplements containing vitamin E. People who tend to develop kidney stones should avoid vitamin C supplements. Those with iron storage disorders should not take iron supplements. Dietary supplements are easily obtained without a prescription. If they are used to treat illnesses that require medical attention, they may delay conventional therapy causing additional harm. Check with your physician, dietitian, or pharmacist to help identify these interactions.

Consider the dose

The doses of nutrients contained in supplements vary from those that contain less than or equal to 100% of the Daily Value to those providing two, three, or ten times the Daily Value. High doses of individual nutrients or combinations of several different nutrients or other substances can lead to nutrient imbalances or toxicities. For years it was thought that only the fat-soluble vitamins could build up to toxic levels in the body and excesses of water-soluble vitamins were merely excreted in the urine and could not reach toxic levels. However, as use of nutrient supplements became more popular, reports of toxicities of water-soluble vitamins, such as niacin and vitamin B_6, began to appear. If the popularity of fortified foods and supplements continues, toxicity symptoms are likely to become more common.

More is not always better when it comes to supplements. When considering a product, first compare the dose to the UL (see inside cover); ULs are the suggested maximum level above which symptoms of toxicity are likely to occur. Once you have determined that the amounts in your supplement do not exceed the UL, make sure you follow the dosage recommendations. If the label says two tablets provide 100% of the Daily Value, you don't need to take four tablets a day. One nutrient to be particularly careful of is vitamin A; too much increases the risk of bone fractures.[33] To minimize your risk, do not take supplements of preformed vitamin A and if you take a multivitamin look for one that contains vitamin A as β-carotene.

The ULs are a good guide, but are not always available and don't always tell the whole story. For example, there are no ULs or Daily Values for herbs, carotenoids, flavonoids, isoflavones, and other phytochemicals, so it is difficult to assess whether the amount in a supplement is high or low and whether that amount could be harmful. Even when ULs are available they don't consider combinations of nutrients. For instance, excess folic acid can be dangerous for those with marginal vitamin B_{12} intake because the supplemental folic acid can mask the symptoms used to diagnose the B_{12} deficiency. They also don't consider specific individual conditions or circumstances. For instance, β-carotene supplements may increase the risk of lung cancer among smokers, but supplements don't provide this information. Iron can be a more serious toxicity concern in those with the inherited condition hemochromatosis, in which regulation of iron absorption is abnormal.

Don't believe everything you hear

Product labels and literature often make fabulous claims about the physiological benefits of dietary supplements. Unfortunately you can't believe everything you hear or read. To help distinguish fact from fallacy you can use the suggestions for judging nutrient claims discussed in Chapter 1 (see Table 1.4). For example, if you are considering taking echinacea, an herbal immune enhancer often taken to prevent or treat cold symptoms, start by thinking about whether the claims made for the herb make sense. The claim that it may help prevent or reduce cold symptoms is reasonable but what is the source of this claim? It turns out that much of the information available on echinacea is anecdotal—that is, it comes from personal testimonies, but there are some good research studies in humans that support the claim that this herb enhances the immune response. Next consider the cost. Some dietary supplements are very expensive, but echinacea is not prohibitively so. A bottle of echinacea capsules costs about $5.00—similar to the cost of other over-the-counter cold medications. You should also check out the product's safety record, particularly for people of your life stage and with similar health conditions. Research has shown echinacea to be relatively nontoxic in healthy adults. However, individuals with the disease lupus, in which the immune system attacks body tissues, should not take this supplement because echinacea can worsen symptoms of the disease. So for most people the risks of echinacea are small and the herb may have some benefits. However, this conclusion is not valid for all herbal products. Some are associated with significant risks, so before choosing an herbal supplement consider its risks and evaluate claims about its benefits.

Report problems

If you suffer a harmful effect or illness that you think is related to the use of a supplement, seek medical attention and report the incident to FDA MedWatch by calling 1-800-FDA-1088 or going into the MedWatch Web site at www.fda.gov/medwatch.

Supplements Can't Provide the Benefits of a Healthy Diet

Despite the appeal of supplements, consumers should not rely heavily on these to meet their dietary or health needs. Epidemiological research has shown that supplements do not provide all the benefits that foods do. Studies show that people who eat more fruits and vegetables have a lower incidence of a host of chronic diseases. These same benefits are not duplicated by taking supplements of nutrients found in these foods. In addition to nutrients, foods contain phytochemicals and other substances that are not nutrients but that have health-promoting properties. Scientists have not yet identified all the substances contained in foods, nor have they determined all of their effects on human health. What is clear is that a wholesome, varied diet is important for optimal health.

If you choose to use dietary supplements remember, that they, like functional and fortified foods, are only one part of your overall diet. Diet in turn is only one aspect of a comprehensive lifestyle approach to good health. A healthy lifestyle should include regular exercise, tobacco avoidance, maintenance of a healthy body weight, stress reduction, and other positive health practices as well as a healthy diet. Supplements, fortified foods, and functional foods can be part of an effective strategy to promote good health, but they should never be considered a substitute for other good health habits and they should never be used instead of medical therapy to treat a health problem. The only way to tell for sure if you need a dietary supplement is to have a complete nutritional assessment that analyzes both your individual nutrient needs and your typical dietary intake.

THINKING FOR YOURSELF

1. Are the doses of supplements sold always safe?
   a. Using the Internet, find a Web site for a nutritional supplement manufacturer.
   b. What is the highest dose of vitamin B$_6$ (pyridoxine) that you see included in one of its products? Is this a safe dose?
   c. What advertising promises are included with supplements containing pyridoxine? Evaluate these claims for accuracy.
   d. What forms of niacin are in supplements marketed by this company?
   e. How much niacin is included per dose? What are the risks and benefits associated with this dose?

2. What supplements are your friends taking? Are they safe?
   a. Do a supplement survey of ten people. Record all of the dietary supplements they take including the number of doses taken per day as well as the reason they chose to take each supplement.

   b. Tabulate the total amount of each vitamin, mineral, or other component.
   c. Are there any nutrients consumed in excess of the recommendation (RDA or AI)?
   d. Are any consumed in excess of the UL?
   e. Do you think these supplements will fulfill the expectations of the consumers? Why or why not?

3. What nutrients are added to your breakfast cereal?
   a. Make a table listing the micronutrient content of three varieties of breakfast cereal.
   b. Is the amount of iron the same in each? What is the range of % Daily Values of iron?
   c. Is the amount of folic acid the same in each? What is the range of % Daily Values of folic acid?
   d. How many servings of this cereal would you need to eat to meet your calcium needs?
   e. Find a cereal that would be safe to consume if you must limit your iron intake.

SUMMARY

1. A wholesome varied diet is important for optimal health. Dietary supplements and fortified foods may be needed by some groups to meet nutrient needs.

2. Our needs for vitamins and minerals can be met by a carefully selected diet that follows the recommendations of the Food Guide Pyramid. Choose a variety of nutrient-dense foods from each food group.

3. Foods containing substances that provide physiological benefits beyond that of simply meeting nutrient needs are termed functional foods. These may contain phytochemicals, which are health-promoting substances in plant foods, or zoochemcials, which are found in animal foods.

4. Diets high in phytochemicals have been associated with reductions in the risk of cancer and other degenerative diseases. Some phytochemicals act as antioxidants, some affect the activity of enzymes or hormones, and others work by different mechanisms. A diet rich in plant foods is rich in phytochemicals.

5. Fortified foods provide supplemental nutrients—some foods are fortified with nutrients according government guidelines to promote public health. Others are fortified according to manufacturers' perceptions of what will sell in the marketplace.

6. About half the adult population in the United States takes some type of dietary supplement. Dietary supplements may contain vitamins; minerals; herbs, botanicals, or other plant-derived substances; amino acids; enzymes; concentrates; or extracts. Manufacturers are responsible for the consistency and safety of supplements before they are marketed. The FDA regulates dietary supplement labeling and can monitor their safety once they are being sold.

7. Vitamin and mineral supplements are recommended for some groups of individuals such as dieters, vegetarians, pregnant women and women of childbearing age, older adults, and other nutritionally vulnerable groups.

8. Supplemental sources of nutrients—either from fortified foods or supplements—must be used carefully to avoid toxicity.

9. Many substances that are not nutrients are available as supplements. Some dietary supplements contain compounds that are already present in the body but are not essential in the diet. Others contain plant extracts and herbs. These products may have beneficial physiological actions, but they can also have dangerous side effects.

10. When choosing a dietary supplement, it is important to carefully consider both the potential risks and benefits of the product.

REVIEW QUESTIONS

1. Can everyone meet all his or her nutrient needs with foods? Why or why not?
2. Define functional food and give three examples of foods that you consider functional and why.
3. Why is it important for the diet to include a variety of foods from each group of the Food Guide Pyramid?
4. What are phytochemicals?
5. List three types of phytochemicals and their suggested health benefits.
6. What are zoochemicals?
7. How can you ensure that your diet is plentiful in phytochemicals?
8. Who determines which nutrients are added to fortified foods?
9. Are fortified foods beneficial for everyone?
10. List three groups for whom supplemental nutrients are recommended.
11. Can the label on a dietary supplement tell you if the dose of an herbal ingredient is safe? Why or why not?
12. Who tests dietary supplements for safety before they are marketed?
13. Discuss the process recommended for deciding whether or not to take a dietary supplement.

REFERENCES

1. American Dietetic Association. Position of the American Dietetic Association: Functional foods. *J. Am. Diet. Assoc.* 104:814–826, 2004.
2. Richter, W. O. Long-chain omega-3 fatty acids from fish reduce sudden cardiac death in patients with coronary heart disease. *Eur. J. Med. Res.* 8:332–336, 2003.
3. Fund, W. C. R. *Food, Nutrition, and the Prevention of Cancer: A Global Perspective.* Washington, D.C.: American Institute for Cancer Research, 1997.
4. Surh, Y. J. Cancer chemoprevention with dietary phytochemicals. *Nat. Rev. Cancer* 3:768–780, 2003.
5. Cooper, D. A., Eldridge, A. L., and Peters, J. P. Dietary carotenoids and certain cancers, heart disease, and age-related macular degeneration: a review of recent research. *Nutr. Rev.* 57:201–214, 2000.
6. Miller, N., Sampson, J., Candeias, L. P., et al. Antioxidant activities of carotenes and xanthophylls. *FEBS Lett.* 384:240–246, 1996.
7. Silalahi, J. Anticancer and health protective properties of citrus fruit components. *Asia Pac. J. Clin. Nutr.* 11:79–84, 2002.
8. Fehey, J. W., Zhang, Y., and Talalay, P. Broccoli sprouts: an exceptionally rich source of inducers of enzymes that protect against carcinogens. *Proc. Natl. Acad. Sci. USA* 94:10367–10372, 1997.
9. Duncan, A. M., Phipps, W. R., and Kurzer, M. S. Phyto-oestrogens. *Best Pract. Res. Clin. Endocrinol. Metab.* 17:253–271, 2003.
10. Vincent, A., and Fitzpatrick, L. A. Soy isoflavones: are they useful in menopause? *Mayo Clin. Proc.* 75:1174–1184, 2000.
11. McCann, S. E., Muti, P., Vito, D., et al. Dietary lignan intakes and risk of pre- and post-menopausal breast cancer. *Int. J. Cancer* 111:440–443, 2004.
12. Cleveland, L. E., Cook, A. J., Wilson, J. W., et al. Pyramid Servings Data Results from the USDA's CSFII, ARS Food Surveys Research Group. Available online at www.barc.usda.gov/bhnrc/foodsurvey/home/htm/Accessed March 13, 2004.
13. Krebs-Smith, A. M., and Kantor, L. S. Choose a variety of fruits and vegetables daily: understanding the complexities. *J. Nutr.* 131:487S–501S, 2001.
14. The U.S. Market for Fortified Foods and Drinks: Expanding the Boundaries, April, 2002, Packaged Facts a division of MarketResearch.com
15. Lewis, C. J., Crane, N. T., Wilson, D. B., and Yetley, E. A. Estimated folate intakes: data updated to reflect food fortification, increase bioavailability, and dietary supplement use. *Am. J. Clin. Nutr.* 70:198–207, 1999.
16. Arsenault, J. E,. and Brown, K. H. Zinc intake of US preschool children exceeds new dietary reference intakes. *Am. J. Clin. Nutr.* 78:1011–1017, 2003.
17. Institute of Medicine, Food and Nutrition Board. *Dietary Reference Intakes: Guiding Principles for Nutrition Labeling and Fortification.* Washington D.C.: National Academy Press, 2003.
18. Millen, A., Dodd, K., and Subar, A. Use of vitamin, mineral, nonvitamin and nonmineral supplements in the United States: the 1987, 1992, and 2000 National Healthy Interview Survey results. *J. Am. Diet. Assoc.* 104:942–951, 2004.
19. Sarubin, A. *The Health Professional's Guide to Popular Dietary Supplements.* Chicago: American Dietetic Association, 2000.
20. U.S. Food and Drug Administration. Evidence Report/Technology Assessment No. 76. Ephedra and Ephedrine for Weight Loss and Athletic Performance Enhancement: Clinical Efficacy and Side Effects. Available online at www.fda.gov/bbs/topics/NEWS/ephedra/summary.html/ Accessed April 24, 2004.
21. USP Dietary Supplement Verification Program. Available online at www.uspverified.org/ Accessed January 16, 2004.
22. Institute of Medicine, Food and Nutrition Board. *Dietary Reference Intakes for Thiamin, Riboflavin, Niacin, Vitamin B$_6$, Folate, Vitamin B$_{12}$, Pantothenic Acid, Biotin, and Choline.* Washington D.C.: National Academy Press, 1998.
23. Institute of Medicine, Food and Nutrition Board. *Dietary Reference Intakes for Calcium, Phosphorus, Magnesium, Vitamin D, and Fluoride.* Washington, D.C.: National Academy Press, 1997.
24. Institute of Medicine. Food and Nutrition Board. *Dietary Reference Intakes for Vitamin C, Vitamin E, Selenium, and Carotenoids.* Washington, D.C.: National Academy Press, 2000.
25. American Dietetic Association. Position of the American Dietetic Association: Food fortification and dietary supplements. *J. Am. Diet. Assoc.* 101:115–125, 2001.
26. Radimer, K. L., Subar, A. F., and Thompson, F. E. Nonvitamin, nonmineral dietary supplements: Issues and findings from NHANES III. *J. Am. Diet. Assoc.* 100:447–454, 2000.
27. Kelly, G. S. The role of glucosamine sulfate and chondroitin sulfates in the treatment of degenerative joint disease. *Altern. Med. Rev.* 3:27–39, 1998.
28. Brief, A. A., Maurer, S. G., and Di Cesare, P. E. Use of glucosamine and chondroitin sulfate in the management of osteoarthritis. *J. Am. Acad. Orthop. Surg.* 9:71–78, 2001.
29. Ramos, L. Beyond the headlines: SAMe as a supplement. *J. Am. Diet. Assoc.* 100:414, 2000.
30. Mares-Perlman, J. A., and Erdman, J. W. Can lutein protect against chronic disease. *Symp. J. Nutr.* 132:517s–540s, 2002.
31. Palozza, P. Prooxidant actions of carotenoids in biologic systems. *Nutr. Rev.* 56:257–265, 1998.
32. Mullins, R. J., and Heddle, R. Adverse reactions associated with echinacea: The Australian experience. *Ann. Allergy Asthma Immunol.* 88:7–9, 2002.
33. Michaelsson, K., Lithell, H., Vessby, B., and Melhus, H. Serum retinol levels and the risk of fracture. *N. Engl. J. Med.* 348:287–294, 2003.

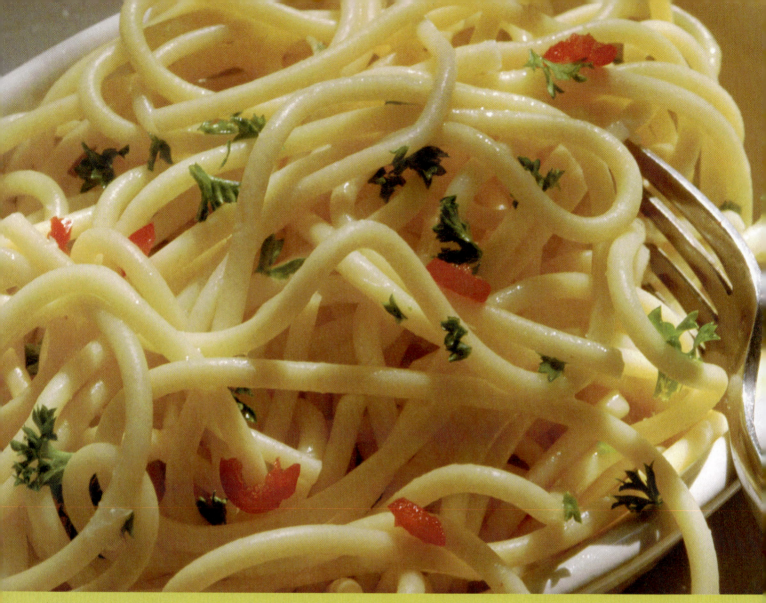

(Claver Carroll/Age Fotostock America, Inc.)

- The combination of good nutrition and regular exercise works together to promote fitness.
- Activity requires ATP generated from carbohydrate, fat, and protein in the diet and body stores.
- The ability of the heart and lungs to provide oxygen to tissues affects which nutrients can be used to produce ATP and how much is produced.
- Physically active individuals need extra energy to fuel their activity but the recommended proportions of carbohydrate, fat, and protein are the same as for the general population.
- Exercise increases the amount of water needed to transport nutrients, eliminate wastes, and cool the body.
- Appropriate food choices before, during, and after competition can help optimize athletic performance.
- Performance-enhancing (ergogenic) supplements are popular among athletes; before they are used, the risks should be weighed against the benefits.

Just A Taste

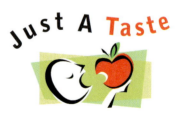

How much exercise is enough?

Does exercise increase protein needs?

Is it better to drink water or a sports drink?

Can dietary supplements enhance athletic performance?

Nutrition, Fitness, and Physical Activity

11

INTRODUCTION

CNN Headline News

A Few Extra Steps a Day, May Keep Extra Pounds Away

By *Kat Carney*

Friday, Apr. 16, 2004—Remember the phrase, "Walk a mile in my shoes?"

Unfortunately, some Americans aren't walking a mile in anyone's shoes, and a mile, you may be interested to know is just over 2,000 steps for the average person.

Coincidentally, 2,000 steps is the goal of America On the Move, a national walking program aimed at slowing down the country's rising obesity problem.

You may be surprised to find out that most people don't walk as much as they think they do. In fact, they only average between 3,000 and 6,000 steps a day, which is far short of a fitness goal of 10,000 steps.

But the America On the Move program says by adding just 2,000 additional steps to our daily routines or, by eating 100 fewer calories daily, most of us will stop gaining weight.

To read this entire article go to www.cnn.com/2004/HEALTH/04/16/walking/.

How active are you? Do you walk 10,000 steps or incorporate some other kind of exercise into your daily routine? If you are a typical American you probably don't. There are lots of excuses: too tired, too busy, too hot, too rainy. Does it really matter how much exercise you get? Public health recommendations tell us that it does. The amount of exercise you get affects your nutritional status and overall health. In turn, diet and nutritional status affect exercise performance.

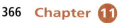

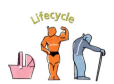

Lifecycle

Regular exercise makes it easier to keep body fat at a healthy level If you exercise you build muscle. Individuals who are physically fit have a greater proportion of muscle and a smaller proportion of fat than unfit individuals of the same body weight. Not everyone who is fit is thin, but in a fit person who carries extra pounds, more of the weight is from muscle than in an unfit person weighing the same. How much body fat we have is also affected by gender and age. In general, women have more stored body fat than men. For young adult women, the desirable percent of body fat is 21 to 33% of total weight; in adult men, the desirable percent is about 8 to 20%.[1] With aging, lean body mass decreases in both men and women, and there is an increase in the percentage of body fat even if body weight remains the same. Some of this change may be prevented by physical activity (see Chapter 13).

Exercise reduces the risk of chronic disease

In addition to making the tasks of everyday life easier, maintaining fitness through regular activity offers many health benefits. A regular exercise program can help to maintain a healthy body weight and prevent or delay the onset of cardiovascular disease, hypertension, diabetes, osteoporosis, and colon cancer. It can also prevent depression and improve mood, sleep patterns, and overall outlook on life.

Exercise reduces the risk of obesity If you exercise regularly, you are less likely to become obese. Exercise increases energy needs as well as lean body mass. During exercise, energy expenditure can rise well above the resting rate and some of this increase persists for many hours after activity slows.[2] Exercise increases lean body mass and because, even at rest, lean tissue uses more energy than fat tissue, this increases basal energy needs. The combination of increased energy output during exercise, the rise in expenditure that persists after exercise, and the increase in basal needs can have a major impact on total energy expenditure. The more energy you expend, the more food you can consume while maintaining a healthy weight. Exercise is also an essential component of any weight-reduction program. It can increase energy needs, promote the loss of body fat, and slow the loss of lean tissue that occurs with energy restriction.

Exercise reduces the risk of cardiovascular disease Exercise is good for your heart. As previously discussed aerobic exercise strengthens the heart muscle, thereby reducing resting heart rate and decreasing the heart's workload. The changes that occur with exercise also help to lower blood pressure and increase HDL (good) cholesterol levels in the blood. All of these effects help to reduce the risk of cardiovascular diseases such as heart attack and stroke.

Exercise helps to prevent and treat diabetes People with excess body fat are more likely to develop diabetes. By keeping body fat within the normal range, regular exercise can decrease one's risk of developing type 2 diabetes. Physical activity that includes both aerobic exercise and strength training is also important in the treatment of diabetes because it can increase the sensitivity of tissues to insulin.[3] Exercise can reduce or eliminate the need for medication to maintain normal blood glucose levels. People with diabetes need to develop exercise programs with the help of physicians and dietitians, because exercise can affect dietary and medication requirements.

Weight-bearing exercise helps strengthen bones and reduces arthritis Just as lifting weights helps maintain muscle size and strength, weight-bearing exercise stimulates bones to become denser and stronger. One of the causes of bone loss, like muscle loss, is lack of use; therefore, weight-bearing exercise such as walking, running, and aerobic dance can increase peak bone mass, prevent bone loss, and therefore reduce the risk of osteoporosis. Exercise can also benefit individuals with arthritis because the strength and flexibility promoted by exercise help arthritic joints move more easily.

Exercise may reduce cancer risk Individuals who exercise regularly may be reducing their cancer risk.[4] There is evidence that exercise reduces breast cancer risk; the risk reduction is related to exercise intensity, duration, and the age at which the exercise is performed. The evidence that exercise reduces colon cancer risk is stronger; active individuals are less likely to develop colon cancer than their sedentary counterparts.[5] When evaluating the impact of exercise on cancer risk, diet and other lifestyle factors also must be considered. It is possible that some of the effect is due to the fact that people who exercise regularly are more likely to have healthier overall diets and lifestyles.

Exercise makes you feel better When you exercise you feel better. Physical activity increases your energy level and self-esteem.[6] It has been shown to improve symptoms of depression, anxiety, and panic disorders. The exact mechanisms involved are not clear but one hypothesis has to do with the production of **endorphins**. Exercise stimulates the release of these chemicals, which are thought to be natural tranquilizers that play a role in triggering what athletes describe as an "exercise high." In addition to causing this state of exercise euphoria, endorphins are thought to aid in relaxation, pain tolerance, and appetite control.

Endorphins Compounds that act as natural euphorics and reduce the perception of pain under certain stressful conditions.

Everyone Should Get an Hour of Exercise Daily

Most Americans do not exercise regularly; 25% of American adults get no physical activity at all during their leisure time.[7] Because of the health benefits, public health guidelines recommend that Americans increase their activity level[8,9] (Figure 11.4). The most recent recommendations, made by the DRIs, advise Americans to engage in 60 minutes of moderate exercise every day.[2] This is an increase from previous recommendations of 30 minutes of moderate-intensity exercise on most days of the week. The recommendation was changed because this higher level of activity is associated with maintaining weight in the healthy range and maximizing the other health benefits of exercise.

To get your hour of exercise, you don't need to start running 10-kilometer races or training for a triathalon. But you do need to do something active every day; a brisk walk or a game of Frisbee will do the trick. The DRIs define moderate activity as the equivalent of walking or jogging at a rate of 3 to 4 mph, cycling leisurely, or swimming slowly. If you engage in 60 minutes of moderate exercise each day, in addition to the activities of daily living, you are considered to have an "active" physical activity level (see Chapter 7, Tables 7.5 and 7.6). This is the level that is recommended for optimal health. An "active" level can be achieved with less than 60 minutes of exercise if the exercise is more intense, for example, jogging at 6 mph or greater or swimming at a moderate to fast pace.

People who exercise moderately for more than 2.5 hours per day or more intensely for more than 1 hour per day are categorized as "very active." This higher activity level increases energy needs but does not necessarily enhance other health benefits. Individuals who perform no exercise other than the activities of daily living are considered "sedentary," and those who perform less than an hour of moderate activity fit into the "low active" category. This amount of exercise is not enough to promote the maintenance of a healthy body weight or fully reduce chronic disease risk. This doesn't mean you should give up if you can't find the time or motivation to meet exercise goals. Even a small amount of exercise is better than none, and, within reason, more exercise is better than less.

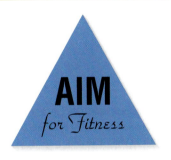

AIM for Fitness

▲ Be physically active each day

FIGURE 11.4

The Dietary Guidelines, 2000, recommends that Americans "Be physically active each day."

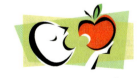

The equivalent of an hour of moderate-intensity exercise per day is recommended to optimize your health. But if you can't get this amount, do what you can. Any amount of exercise is better than none.

Exercise should include aerobic activities, stretching, and strength training

To improve your fitness level you need to engage in aerobic activities, which raise your heart rate and therefore improve cardiorespiratory fitness; stretching, which promotes and maintains flexibility; and strength training, which increases the strength and endurance of

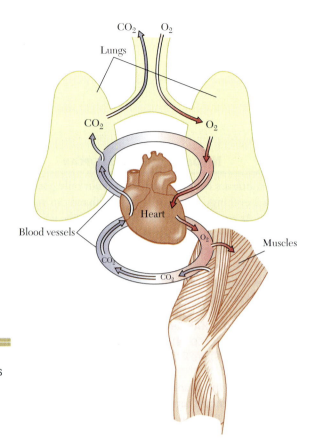

FIGURE 11.8

The oxygen you breathe into your lungs is picked up by the blood. Your heart pumps this oxygen-rich blood throughout the body. Oxygen is taken up by the muscles and other tissues and used to generate ATP, producing carbon dioxide as a waste product. Carbon dioxide is removed by your blood and exhaled through your lungs. When you exercise your muscles demand more oxygen. You respond by increasing your heart rate and breathing faster and deeper to take in and deliver more oxygen.

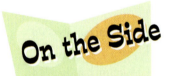

To increase the delivery of oxygen to muscles during exercise blood vessels in active muscles dilate to increase blood flow, while the blood vessels that supply organs such as the kidneys, liver, pancreas, and gastrointestinal tract constrict, decreasing blood flow.

⚠ **Creatine phosphate** A compound found in muscle that can be broken down quickly to make ATP.

The source of ATP depends on how long you have been exercising

While at rest, your muscles do not need much energy. Your heart and lungs are able to deliver enough oxygen to meet energy needs using aerobic metabolism (Figure 11.8). To increase the amount of energy produced by aerobic metabolism you must increase the amount of oxygen available at the muscle. To do this your breathing and heart rate must increase, but this takes time. When you first begin to exercise your breathing and heart rate have not yet had enough time to increase the amount of oxygen available at the muscle.

Stored ATP and creatine phosphate provide immediate energy What fuels your muscles when you jump up to answer the phone or take the first steps of your morning jog? You are asking your muscles to increase their activity but your heart and lungs have not had time to step up oxygen delivery to them. Despite this they find the energy to do their job. They get this instant energy from small amounts of ATP that are stored in resting muscle. This is enough to sustain activity for a few seconds. As the ATP in muscle is used, enzymes break down another high-energy compound, called **creatine phosphate**, to replenish the ATP supply and allow your activity to continue. But, like ATP, the amount of creatine phosphate stored in the muscle at any time is small. It will allow you to use your muscles for about an additional 8 to 10 seconds before it too is used up. So, during the first 10 to 15 seconds of exercise, the muscles must rely on energy from the ATP and creatine phosphate that is stored there (Figure 11.9).

Anaerobic metabolism uses glucose for fast energy As you continue to exercise the ATP and creatine phosphate in your muscles are used up. This occurs after only about 15 seconds so your heart and lungs have still not been able to get more oxygen to your muscles. To get energy your muscles must produce

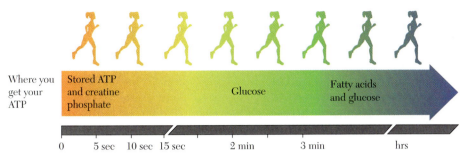

Where you get your ATP

| Stored ATP and creatine phosphate | Glucose | Fatty acids and glucose |

0   5 sec   10 sec   15 sec   2 min   3 min   hrs

Exercise duration

FIGURE 11.9

When exercise begins, ATP and creatine phosphate stored in muscles provide ATP for muscle contraction. As creatine phosphate stores are depleted, anaerobic metabolism, which breaks down glucose from the blood or from muscle glycogen, becomes the predominant source of ATP. After about 3 minutes, aerobic metabolism, which uses fatty acids and glucose to produce ATP, takes over as the predominant source.

▲ **Lactic acid** A compound produced from the breakdown of glucose in the absence of oxygen.

ATP without oxygen. This anaerobic metabolism involves glycolysis, which breaks glucose into the 3-carbon molecule pyruvate and produces ATP that can be used for muscle contraction. When oxygen is absent, the pyruvate produced by anaerobic metabolism is converted to **lactic acid**. The lactic acid is transported out of the muscle for use in other tissues. For example, it can be used by the liver to make glucose.

Anaerobic metabolism can produce ATP very rapidly, but can only use glucose as a fuel (Figure 11.10). This glucose may come from the breakdown of glycogen inside the muscle or from glucose delivered via the bloodstream. The glucose delivered in the blood comes from that released by the breakdown of liver glycogen, the synthesis of glucose by the liver, or carbohydrate consumed during exercise. Anaerobic metabolism predominates during the first few minutes of exercise and, as will be discussed, is also important during periods of intense exercise, because oxygen cannot be delivered to the cells quickly enough to meet energy demands. The amount of glucose available for anaerobic metabolism is limited, so if activity is to continue the body must use its glucose more efficiently and find a more plentiful fuel source.

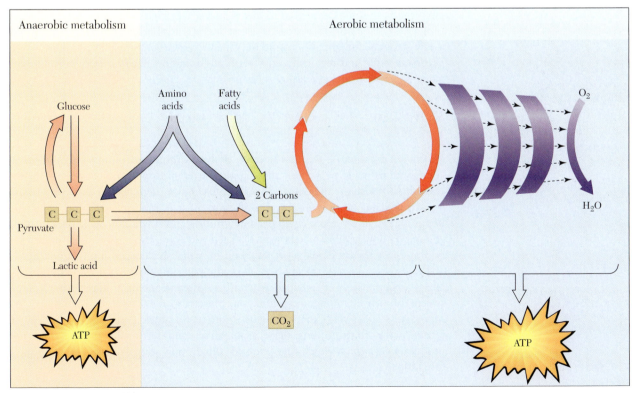

FIGURE 11.10

In the absence of oxygen, ATP is produced by the anaerobic metabolism of glucose and lactic acid is generated. When oxygen is present, ATP is produced by the aerobic metabolism of glucose, fatty acids, and amino acids. More ATP is produced and no lactic acid accumulates.

Aerobic metabolism uses fat to fuel your long runs, bikes, and swims

Once you have been exercising for 2 to 3 minutes your breathing and heart rate have increased to supply more oxygen to your muscles. When oxygen is available, ATP can be produced by aerobic metabolism. The reactions of aerobic metabolism take place in the mitochondria. When glucose is broken down by aerobic metabolism, the pyruvate produced by glycolysis is converted to a 2-carbon molecule and lactic acid is not formed. This 2-carbon molecule is further broken down, yielding more ATP along with carbon dioxide and water (see Figure 11.10).

Aerobic metabolism produces ATP at a slower rate than anaerobic metabolism but is much more efficient, producing about 18 times more ATP for each molecule of glucose. In addition, aerobic metabolism can use fatty acids, and sometimes amino acids from protein, as well as glucose, to generate ATP. About 90% of the stored energy in a typical adult is fat. It provides a lightweight, energy-dense fuel supply. Fatty acids to fuel muscle contraction can come from triglycerides stored in adipose tissue as well as small amounts stored in the muscle itself. When fatty acids are used as an energy source, the fatty acid chain is first broken into the same 2-carbon units that are produced from pyruvate and thus follow the same path to generate ATP by aerobic metabolism. If you continue to exercise at a low to moderate intensity, aerobic metabolism predominates and fat becomes the main fuel source for your exercising muscles. If you pick up the pace, the proportion of anaerobic and aerobic metabolism and the fuels you burn will change.

Protein is not a major fuel for exercise

Although protein is not considered a major energy source for the body, even at rest your body uses small amounts of amino acids for energy. The amount increases if your diet does not provide enough total energy to meet needs, if you consume more protein than you need, and if you are involved in certain types of exercise. The amino acids available to the body come from the digestion of dietary proteins and from the breakdown of body proteins. When the nitrogen-containing amino group is removed from an amino acid, the remaining carbon compound can be broken down to produce ATP by aerobic metabolism or, in some cases, used to make glucose (see Figure 11.10). Exercise that continues for many hours increases the use of amino acids both as an energy source and as a raw material for glucose synthesis. When exercise is completed, amino acids are needed to build and repair muscle. The need for amino acids for muscle building and repair is greater in strength athletes because they are actively trying to build muscle tissue.

Whether an activity is aerobic depends how intense it is

When you exercise, ATP is produced by both anaerobic and aerobic metabolism. The contributions made by each of these systems overlap to ensure that your muscles get enough ATP to meet the demand you are placing on them. The relative contribution of each depends on how intense your activity is. If it is very intense the delivery and use of oxygen at the muscle will become limiting and it will not be possible to supply enough ATP by aerobic metabolism. To keep you going the muscle gets the additional ATP it needs by using anaerobic metabolism, which breaks down only glucose. Generally, the more intense the exercise, the more your muscles rely on glucose to provide energy (Figure 11.11). When the exercise is lower in intensity, the cardiorespiratory system can deliver enough oxygen to your muscles to allow aerobic metabolism to predominate, so fatty acids and some glucose are used as fuel. Thus, exercise intensity determines the contributions that carbohydrate and fat make as fuels for energy production. In turn, which fuels are used affects how long exercise can continue before **fatigue** sets in.

Anaerobic metabolism causes fatigue sooner

If you run faster, you tire sooner. This is because more intense exercise relies more on anaerobic metabolism. Anaerobic metabolism uses glucose more rapidly than aerobic metabolism and produces lactic acid. Exercise fatigue is strongly influenced by the depletion of liver and muscle glycogen and the accumulation of lactic acid.

On the Side

Both endurance exercise and high intensity exercise can deplete glycogen stores. For example, 2 to 3 hours of cycling or running will deplete glycogen as will 15 to 60 minutes of high intensity exercise that occurs intermittently, such as tennis or basketball or soccer.

Fatigue The inability to continue an activity at an optimal level.

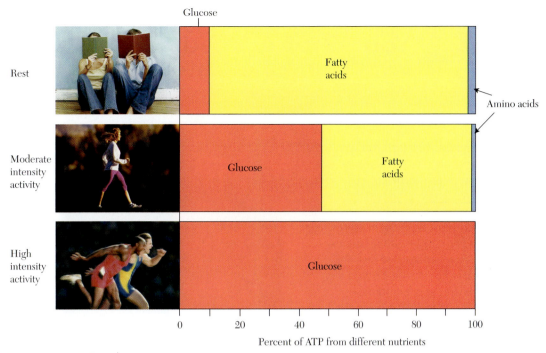

Glucose

Amino acids

Percent of ATP from different nutrients

FIGURE 11.11

As exercise intensity increases, the proportion of energy supplied by carbohydrate also increases. Remember that during exercise the total amount of energy expended is greater than at rest. (Adapted from Horton, E. S. Effects of low-energy diets on work performance. *Am. J. Clin. Nutr.* 35:1228–1233, 1982.) (*top*: PhotoDisc, Inc./Getty Images; *center*: Hughes Martin/Corbis Images; *bottom*: Jim Cummins/Taxi/Getty Images)

When athletes run out of glycogen, they experience a feeling of overwhelming fatigue that is sometimes referred to as "hitting the wall" or "bonking." Glycogen depletion is a concern for athletes because the amount of stored glycogen available to produce glucose during exercise is limited. There are between 60 and 120 grams of glycogen stored in your liver; stores are highest just after a meal. Liver glycogen is used to maintain blood glucose between meals and during the night. Eating a good breakfast will replenish the liver glycogen you used while you slept. There are about 200 to 500 grams of glycogen in the muscles of a 70-kg person. The glycogen in a muscle is used to fuel the activity of that muscle. Muscle glycogen levels can be increased by systematically consuming high-carbohydrate meals after depleting glycogen stores with exercise (see Your Choice: Loading Up with Carbohydrate).

Small amounts of lactic acid produced by anaerobic metabolism can be carried away from the muscle and used by other tissues. But if the amount of lactic acid produced exceeds the amount that can be used by other tissues it begins to build up in the muscle and subsequently the blood. This acid buildup causes an increase in the acidity of the muscle and contributes to fatigue and muscle pain. When exercise stops and oxygen is available again, lactic acid can be either carried away by the blood to other tissues to be broken down or metabolized aerobically in the muscle. After intense exercise, a mild cool-down, such as walking, may allow enough blood flow to the muscle to remove built-up lactic acid and prevent cramping.

Low-intensity exercise can continue longer You can continue lower-intensity exercise for longer periods because it relies on aerobic metabolism, which is more efficient than anaerobic metabolism and uses both glucose and fatty acids for energy. The body's fat reserves are almost unlimited so, if fat is the fuel, exercise can theoretically continue for a very long time. For example, it is estimated that a 130-pound woman has enough energy stored as body fat to run 1000 miles.[12] However, even aerobic activity uses some glucose, so if exercise continues long enough, glycogen stores will eventually be depleted causing fatigue.

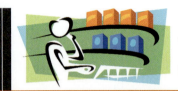

Your Choice: Loading Up with Carbohydrate

Glycogen stored in muscles provides fuel for exercise. The more glycogen you have and the more slowly you use it, the longer you can exercise before you run out. Some athletes try to load up their carbohydrate stores before a big event. This regimen, known as glycogen supercompensation or carbohydrate loading, is designed to overfill muscle glycogen stores. This is accomplished by first depleting muscle glycogen with exercise and then loading it up by cutting back the exercise and eating a very high carbohydrate diet. The process takes a total of 6 days. For the first 3 days, a diet containing about 50% of energy as carbohydrate is consumed. This is then increased to 70% carbohydrate for the last 3 days. The workout on the first day should last about 90 minutes and then workouts should be gradually tapered down—day 6, the day before competition, is a rest day. This regimen will increase the amount of muscle glycogen from about 1.7 grams of glycogen per 100 grams of muscle to 4 to 5 grams per 100 grams.[1]

Glycogen supercompensation is beneficial to endurance athletes, but it may not be the best choice for you. If your athletic activities last less than an hour, this regimen will provide no benefit and even has some disadvantages. For every gram of glycogen in your muscle, almost 3 grams of water are also deposited. The amount of water added with the extra glycogen will result in a 2- to 7-pound weight gain and may cause some muscle stiffness. As glycogen is used, the water is released. Although this can be an advantage when exercising in hot weather, carrying the extra weight may cancel out any potential benefits from the extra water or increased energy stores, especially for short duration events.

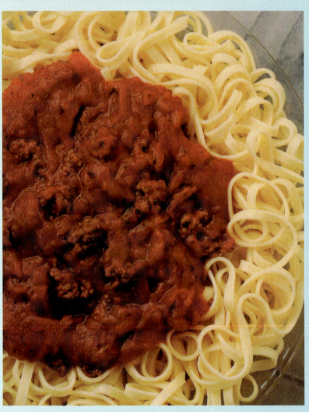

(Ross M. Horowitz/The Image Bank/Getty Images)

Reference
1. McArdle, W. D., Katch, F. I., and Katch, V. L. *Exercise Physiology: Energy, Nutrition and Human Performance*, 5th ed. Philadelphia: Lippincott Williams & Wilkins, 2001: 578.

Exercise training allows you to perform more intense activity without fatigue

Training with repeated bouts of aerobic exercise causes physiological changes that increase the amount of oxygen that can be delivered to and used by the muscle cells. The heart becomes larger and stronger so that the amount of blood pumped with each beat is increased. The number of capillary blood vessels in the muscles increases so that blood is delivered to muscles more efficiently. The total blood volume and number of red blood cells expands, increasing the amount of hemoglobin so more oxygen can be transported to the cells. Training also causes changes at the cellular level that affect the ability of cells to use different types of fuel to produce ATP. There is an increase in the ability to store glycogen, and there is an increase in the number and size of muscle-cell mitochondria. Because aerobic metabolism occurs in the mitochondria, this increases the cell's capacity to burn fatty acids to produce ATP. The use of fatty acids spares glycogen, which delays the onset of fatigue. Because trained athletes store more glycogen and use it more slowly, they can sustain aerobic exercise for longer periods at higher intensities than can untrained individuals. A conditioned athlete can also exercise at a higher percentage of his or her aerobic capacity before lactic acid begins to accumulate (Figure 11.12).

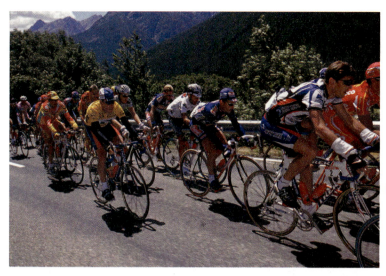

FIGURE 11.12

Riding a bicycle over the Alps would cause most of us to use anaerobic metabolism to produce ATP and we would fatigue quickly. Highly trained cyclists can perform at this intense level of activity for long periods of time using predominantly aerobic metabolism. (Doug Pensinger/Getty Images News and Sport Services)

Good Nutrition Is Essential for Optimal Performance

Whether you are a marathon runner or a mall walker, your body needs adequate nutrition in order to fuel working muscles. For every exerciser, the food consumed must provide sufficient energy from the appropriate sources to fuel activity, protein to maintain muscle mass, micronutrients to allow utilization of the energy-yielding nutrients, and water to transport nutrients and cool the body.

Athletes have higher energy needs

When you expend more energy you need to eat more. How much more depends on how intense the activity is and how often and how long you exercise. More intense activity requires more energy per unit of time (Calories per minute), but the longer an activity continues, the more energy it consumes (see Table 11.4 and Appendix J). Therefore, although weight lifting may require more calories per minute, a distance cyclist will expend more energy during his workout because cyclists continue their activity for many hours. For a casual exerciser, the energy needed for activity may increase energy expenditure by a few hundred Calories a day. For an endurance athlete, such as a marathon runner, the energy needed for training may increase expenditure by 2000 to 3000 Calories per day.

The amount of energy expended for various activities is also affected by body weight. Moving a heavier body requires more energy than moving a lighter one. Therefore, it requires less energy for a 120-pound woman to walk for 30 minutes than it does for a 250-pound woman.

As discussed in Chapter 7, the DRIs have developed equations to estimate energy requirements based on an individual's age, gender, size, and activity levels (Chapter 7 and inside cover). Calculating your estimated energy requirement (EER) can demonstrate the dramatic impact activity can have on energy needs. For example, the EER for a 25-year-old sedentary, 5 foot 11 inch tall, 154-pound man is about 2500 Calories. If this same person becomes a runner and trains several hours per day, his energy needs may increase to 3500 Calories per day or more (Figure 11.13).

The right mix of carbohydrate, fat, and protein fuels exercise

The source of energy in the diet is often as important as the amount of energy. In general, the diets of physically active individuals should contain the same proportion of carbohydrate, fat, and protein as is recommended to the general public—about 45 to 65% of total energy as carbohydrate, 20 to 35% of energy as fat, and 10 to 35% of energy as protein.[2]

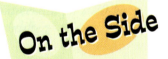

On the Side

Living and working at high altitudes, where the atmosphere contains less oxygen, causes adaptations that improve the capacity of the cardiorespiratory system to deliver oxygen. Therefore, endurance athletes often train at high altitudes to enhance their aerobic capacity.

and transmission of nerve signals. Iron is important for exercise because it is required for the formation of hemoglobin and myoglobin. A number of iron-containing proteins are also essential for production of energy by aerobic metabolism. Zinc is important during exercise because of its role in growth, synthesis and repair of muscle tissue, and energy production.

It has been suggested that exercise increases the need for vitamins and minerals because losses are increased, more nutrients are used in metabolism during exercise, and more are needed to repair tissue damage after exercise. Although these factors may affect vitamin use, most athletes can meet their needs by consuming the amounts of vitamins and minerals recommended for the general population. In addition, because athletes need to eat more food to fuel their activity, they also consume more vitamins and minerals. Athletes who restrict their intake to maintain a low body weight may be at risk for vitamin or mineral deficiencies.

Some nutritional problems are more common among athletes

Sometimes, in an effort to improve performance or achieve unrealistic goals, athletes consume unhealthy diets or push their bodies too hard. The consequences may end up hurting rather then helping performance.

Weight loss diets can impair performance and health

Body weight and composition can affect exercise performance in many sports. Athletes involved in activities where small, light bodies offer an advantage—for instance, ballet, gymnastics, and certain running events—may restrict energy intake to maintain a low body weight. While a slightly leaner physique may be beneficial, dieting to maintain an unrealistically low weight may threaten health and performance. An athlete who needs to lose weight should do so in advance of the competitive season to prevent the restricted diet from affecting performance. The general guidelines for healthy weight loss should be followed—reduce energy intake, increase activity, and change the behaviors that led to weight gain (see Chapter 7). To preserve lean body mass and enhance fat loss, weight loss should be at a rate of about 0.5 to 2 pounds per week. This can be accomplished by a combination of a reduced energy intake and an increased exercise expenditure that totals 200 to 500 Calories per day.

Athletes involved in sports with weight classes, such as wrestling and boxing, sometimes go to unhealthy extremes to lose weight before a competition so they can compete in lower weight classes. Competing at the high end of a weight class is thought to give an advantage over smaller opponents. To lose weight rapidly these athletes may use sporadic diets that severely restrict energy intake or dehydrate themselves through such practices as vigorous exercise, fluid restriction, wearing vapor-impermeable suits, and using hot environments such as saunas and steam rooms. They may also experiment with even more extreme measures, such as self-induced vomiting and the use of diuretics and laxatives. These practices can be dangerous and even fatal. They may impair performance and can adversely affect heart and kidney function, temperature regulation, and electrolyte balance (fluid needs are discussed in the section "Adequate Water Is Essential for Health and Performance" later in the chapter).

Pressure to perform optimally can lead to eating disorders
Athletes are under extreme pressure to achieve and maintain a body weight that optimizes their performance. Failure to meet weight loss goals may have serious consequences such as being cut from the team or restricted from competition. This pressure may cause athletes to use strict diets and maintain body weights that are not healthy. This combined with the self-motivation and discipline that characterizes successful athletes makes them vulnerable to eating disorders. Bulimia may begin because an athlete is unable to stick with a restrictive diet or the hunger associated with a very low-calorie diet leads to bingeing. In athletes who develop anorexia, the continued starvation leads to a decline in athletic performance because the lack of food means that there is not enough energy and nutrients to support activity and growth. Over

On the Side

In 1997 three young wrestlers died while trying to "make weight." They were exercising while wearing rubber suits to sweat off enough water to qualify for a lighter weight class. As a result of these deaths, wrestling weight classes were altered to eliminate the lightest weight class, plastic sweat suits were banned, wrestling room temperatures could be no warmer than 75°F, weigh-ins were moved to 1 hour before competition, and mandatory weight loss rules have been put in place restricting the amount of weight that can be lost prior to competition. There are minimum limits for percent body fat of 5% for college wrestlers and 7% for high school wrestlers.

time serious health problems occur, such as abnormal heart rhythms, low blood pressure, and atrophy of the heart muscle.

Some athletes use compulsive exercise to control their weight. This is also considered an eating disorder; compulsive exercisers use extreme training as a means of purging calories. This behavior is easy to justify because it is a common belief that serious athletes can never work too hard or too long and pain is accepted as an indicator of achievement. Compulsive exercisers will force themselves to exercise even when they don't feel well and may miss social events in order to fulfill their exercise quota. They often calculate exercise goals based on how much they eat. They believe that any break in the training schedule will cause them to gain weight and their performance will suffer. Compulsive exercise can lead to more serious eating disorders such as anorexia and bulimia and can lead to serious health problems including kidney failure, heart attack, and death.

Eating disorders and hormonal abnormalities combine to put bones at risk

In general, exercise is good for your bones. Weight-bearing exercise increases bone density, thereby reducing the risk of osteoporosis. However, too much exercise and too little food intake can cause hormonal abnormalities that put bone health at risk. Female athletes who exercise excessively or restrict food intake to improve performance, achieve an ideal body image, or meet goals set by coaches, trainers, or parents are at risk for a syndrome of interrelated disorders referred to as the **female athlete triad**. This syndrome includes eating patterns that can lead to eating disorders, abnormalities in hormone levels that can lead to **amenorrhea**, and disturbances in bone formation and breakdown that can lead to osteoporosis (Figure 11.14). These occur when extreme energy restriction and excessive exercise create a physiological condition similar to starvation and contribute to hormonal abnormalities. Estrogen levels drop causing amenorrhea, and because estrogen is needed for calcium homeostasis in the bone and calcium absorption in the intestines, low levels lead to low peak bone mass, premature bone loss, and an increased risk of stress fractures. Neither adequate dietary calcium nor the increase in bone mass caused by weight-bearing exercise can compensate for bone loss due to low estrogen levels. Increasing energy intake and reducing activity so that menstrual cycles resume is essential for preventing long-term consequences to bone health.[15]

Low iron causes a decline in performance

For most individuals, exercise does not increase iron needs. However, in athletes, particularly female athletes, a reduction in the amount of stored iron is common. If this situation progresses to anemia, it can impair exercise performance as well as reduce immune function and affect other physiologic processes.[16]

Poor iron status may be caused by inadequate iron intake, increased iron needs, increased iron losses, or a redistribution of iron due to exercise training. Dietary iron intake may be limited in athletes who are attempting to keep body weight low, or in those who consume a vegetarian diet and therefore do not eat meat—an excellent source of readily absorbable heme iron. Iron needs may be increased in athletes because exercise stimulates the production of red blood cells, so more iron is needed for hemoglobin synthesis. Iron is also needed for the synthesis of muscle myoglobin and the iron-containing proteins needed for ATP production in the mitochondria. An increase in iron losses with prolonged training, possibly because of increased fecal, urinary, and sweat losses, also contributes to increased iron needs in athletes.[13] Iron balance may also be affected by the breaking of red blood cells from impact in events such as running (foot-strike hemolysis) or by the contraction of large muscles. However, this rarely causes anemia because the breaking of red blood cells stimulates the production of new ones.[17]

Some athletes experience a condition known as sports anemia, which is a temporary decrease in hemoglobin concentration that occurs during exercise training. This is an adaptation to training that does not seem to impair delivery of oxygen to tissues. It occurs when blood volume expands to increase oxygen delivery, but the synthesis of red blood cells lags behind the increase in plasma volume.

⚠ **Female athlete triad** The combination of disordered eating, amenorrhea, and osteoporosis that occurs in some female athletes, particularly those involved in sports in which low body weight and appearance are important.

⚠ **Amenorrhea** Delayed onset of menstruation or the absence of three or more consecutive menstrual cycles.

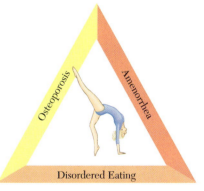

FIGURE 11.14

The female athlete triad includes disordered eating, amenorrhea, and osteoporosis. Women with these conditions typically have low body fat and may experience multiple or recurrent stress fractures. This syndrome is more common in women who are perfectionists, highly competitive, and have a low self-esteem.

Adequate Water Is Essential for Health and Performance

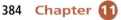

Remember

Does your face get red when you exercise? Chapter 9 discussed how water helps eliminate body heat by shunting blood to the body surface. This makes your skin appear red. Water also helps eliminate heat through the evaporation of sweat.

Heat-related illness Conditions, including heat cramps, heat exhaustion, and heat stroke, that can occur due to an unfavorable combination of exercise, hydration status, and climatic conditions.

Do you drink enough when you are exercising? Most people only drink enough to assuage their thirst. Therefore they end their exercise session in a state of dehydration and must restore fluid balance during the remainder of the day. Even when fluids are consumed at regular intervals throughout exercise, it may not be possible to drink enough to compensate for losses from sweat and evaporation through the lungs. Water is needed to eliminate heat during exercise; it is also needed to transport both oxygen and nutrients to your muscles, and to remove waste products from your muscles. Not consuming enough fluid to replace the water you lose can be hazardous to even the most casual exerciser.

Dehydration occurs when water losses exceed water intake

Dehydration occurs when water loss is great enough for blood volume to decrease, thereby reducing the ability to deliver oxygen and nutrients to exercising muscles. Dehydration hastens the onset of fatigue and makes a given exercise intensity seem more difficult. Even mild dehydration—a body water loss of 1 to 2% of body weight—can impair exercise performance. A 3% reduction in body weight can significantly reduce the amount of blood pumped with each heartbeat because of the lower volume of fluid. This reduces the ability of the circulatory system to deliver oxygen and nutrients to cells and remove waste products. The decrease in blood volume that occurs with dehydration reduces blood flow to the skin and sweat production, which limits the body's ability to sweat and cool itself. Core body temperature can then increase and with it the risk of various **heat-related illnesses** (Figure 11.15).

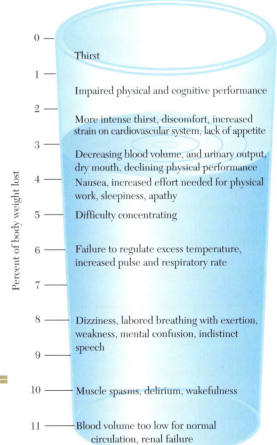

FIGURE 11.15

As the degree of dehydration increases, the adverse effects increase in severity. This can occur rapidly if water losses are excessive, as may occur with profuse sweating. (Robert Holmgren/Stone/Getty Images)

The risk of dehydration is greater in hot environments, but it may also occur when exercising in the cold. Cold air tends to be dry air so evaporative losses from the lungs are greater. Insulated clothing may increase sweat losses and fluid intake may be reduced because a chilled athlete may be reluctant to drink a cold beverage. Female athletes tend to limit fluid intake to avoid the inconvenience of removing clothing to urinate.[13]

Dehydration increases the risk of heat-related illness

Exercising in hot and humid weather increases the risk of heat-related illnesses. As environmental temperature rises it becomes more difficult to dissipate heat, and as humidity rises the ability to cool the body by evaporation decreases. When it is humid the same air temperature feels hotter than when the humidity is lower. For example, when the humidity is 100%, a temperature of 82°F feels the same as a temperature of 90°F and a humidity of only 40%. The risks associated with exercising in these conditions are similar. Acclimatizing with repeated exposure to hot environments combined with exercise can reduce the risk of heat-related illness but cannot compensate for a lack of water. If you are dehydrated it reduces your ability to cool your body and increases the risk of these disorders even when it is not extremely hot or humid.

Heat-related illnesses include heat cramps, heat exhaustion, and heat stroke. Heat cramps are involuntary muscle spasms that occur during or after intense exercise, usually in the muscles involved in exercise. They are caused by an imbalance of the electrolytes sodium and potassium at the muscle cell membranes and can occur when water and salt are lost during extended exercise. Heat exhaustion occurs when fluid loss causes blood volume to decrease so much that it is not possible to both cool the body and deliver oxygen to active muscles. It is characterized by a rapid weak pulse, low blood pressure, disorientation, profuse sweating, and fainting. Someone experiencing heat exhaustion symptoms should stop exercising and move to a cooler environment. If exercise continues, heat exhaustion may progress to heat stroke. Heat stroke, the most serious form of heat-related illness, occurs when the temperature regulatory center of the brain fails due to a very high core body temperature (greater than 105°F). Heat stroke is characterized by elevated body temperature, hot dry skin, extreme confusion, and unconsciousness. It requires immediate medical attention.

An imbalance of water and salt is as dangerous as too little water

Sweating helps us stay cool. Sweat is mostly water but also contains some minerals, primarily sodium and chloride with smaller amounts of potassium. For most activities sweat losses can be replaced with plain water, but when sweating continues for more than 4 hours enough sodium may be lost in sweat to affect electrolyte balance. A reduction in the level of sodium in the blood is referred to as **hyponatremia**. Hyponatremia can occur if an athlete loses large amounts of water and salt in sweat, and replaces the loss with water alone. This causes the sodium that remains in the blood to be diluted so the amount of water is too great for the amount of sodium. This is analogous to taking a full glass of salt water, dumping out half, and replacing what was poured out with plain water. The sodium in the glass is now more dilute. It is also possible to develop hyponatremia even when salt losses from sweating are not excessive. This can occur if an athlete drinks more water than is lost in sweat, which dilutes the sodium in the body; for example, if an athlete over-hydrates while exercising in a cooler climate where sweat losses are lower. It is the concentration of sodium that is important, not the absolute amount.

Hyponatremia causes a number of problems. Solutes in the blood help hold fluid in the blood vessels. As sodium concentration drops fluid will leave the bloodstream by osmosis and accumulate in the tissues causing swelling. Fluid accumulation in the lungs interferes with gas exchange and fluid accumulation in the brain causes disorientation, seizure, coma, and death. The early symptoms of hyponatremia may be similar

Hyponatremia Abnormally low concentration of sodium in the blood.

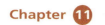
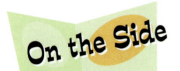

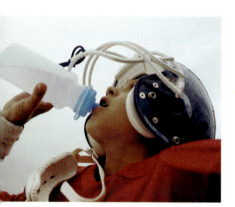

to dehydration: nausea, muscle cramps, disorientation, slurred speech, and confusion. Drinking water alone will make the problem worse.

Although imbalances of electrolytes can be life-threatening, the replacement of lost water during exercise is usually far more of a concern than replacement of lost electrolytes. For most types of exercise lost electrolytes can be replaced during the meals following exercise. Hyponatremia can be prevented by consuming a sodium-containing sports drink during long distance events, increasing sodium intake several days prior to competition, and avoiding Tylenol, aspirin, ibuprofen, and other nonsteroidal antiinflammatory agents. These medications interfere with kidney function and may contribute to the development of hyponatremia. Mild symptoms of hyponatremia can be treated by eating salty foods or drinking a sodium-containing beverage such as a sports drink. More severe symptoms require medical attention.

Fluid needs depend on the length of your workout

Anyone exercising should consume extra fluids. Since thirst is not a reliable indicator of fluid needs, it is important to schedule regular fluid breaks. Typically, however, exercising individuals ingest amounts of fluids that are equal to only about one- to two-thirds of the amount lost in sweat.[18] The amount and type of fluid that is best depends on how much water you lose and how long you exercise.

Drink enough fluid to minimize weight loss
To ensure hydration adequate fluids should be consumed before, during, and after exercise. Exercisers should drink generous amounts of fluid in the 24 hours before the exercise session and about 2 cups of fluid 2 hours before exercise. On warm days, athletes should consume an additional 1 to 2 cups about 30 to 60 minutes before exercising.[19] During exercise, whether casual or competitive, exercisers should try and drink enough water to prevent weight loss (Figure 11.16). Drinking 6 to 12 ounces of fluid every 15 to 20 minutes beginning at the start of exercise should maintain adequate hydration.[13] To restore lost water after exercise, each pound of weight lost should be replaced with 16 to 24 ounces (1 to 1.5 pounds) of fluid.

For exercise lasting less than an hour water is best
For exercise lasting less than an hour, water is the only fluid needed. For a 20-minute jog, 40 minutes at the gym, or a brisk walk through the park, sports drinks offer no advantage over a water bottle filled at the drinking fountain. And they may be counterproductive if the goal of exercise is losing weight. A typical sports drink contains about 50 Calories per cup, so drinking a 16-ounce bottle at the gym will replace about half of the 200 Calories expended during your 40-minute ride on the stationary bicycle.

For exercise lasting more than an hour add carbohydrate and salt to your water
For exercise lasting more than 60 minutes, beverages containing a small amount of carbohydrate and electrolytes are recommended. Exercise depletes body carbohydrate stores. Consuming carbohydrate in a beverage helps to maintain blood glucose levels, therefore providing a source of glucose for the muscle and delaying fatigue. Beverages containing 10 to 20 grams of carbohydrate per cup are best. This is the amount of carbohydrate found in popular sports beverages such as Gatorade and Powerade. A good sports drink should empty rapidly from the stomach, enhance intestinal absorption, and promote fluid retention. As the amount of carbohydrate in the beverage increases, the rate at which the solution leaves the stomach decreases. Therefore, beverages containing larger amounts of carbohydrate, such as fruit juices and soft drinks, are not recommended unless they are diluted with an equal volume of water. Water and carbohydrate trapped in the stomach do not benefit the athlete.

Small amounts of minerals, including sodium and chloride, are lost in sweat, but sweat consists mostly of water, so the amounts lost during exercise lasting less than 3 to 4 hours

FIGURE 11.16

It is important to stay well hydrated during any activity. (Yellow Dog Productions/The Image Bank/Getty Images)

TABLE 11.5

So, What Should You Drink?

Start exercise well hydrated
- Consume plenty of fluid in the 24 hours before exercise
- Consume about 2 cups of fluid in the 2 hours before exercise

Replace fluid losses during exercise
- Consume at least 3 to 6 ounces of fluid every 15 minutes
- Water is appropriate for exercise lasting less than 60 minutes
- For exercise lasting longer than 60 minutes, consuming a fluid containing about 14 grams of carbohydrate per cup may improve endurance
- For exercise lasting longer than 60 minutes, a fluid containing electrolytes can increase fluid intake by improving palatability

Restore fluid losses after exercise
- Begin fluid replacement immediately after exercise
- Consume 16 to 24 ounces of fluid for each pound of weight lost

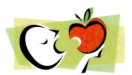

What to drink depends on how long you are exercising. For workouts over an hour, a sports drink is best. If your workout is less than an hour plain old water is fine, but there is nothing wrong with having a sports drink. Be aware however that adding a sports drink replaces some of the calories you just worked off.

are usually not enough to affect health or performance, particularly if sodium was present in the previous meal. Even though there may not be a physiological need to replace sodium, a beverage containing 500 to 700 mg of sodium per liter (around 150 mg in a cup) is recommended for exercise lasting 1 hour or more.[13] This is because the sodium enhances palatability and the drive to drink so it may cause an increase in fluid intake. The presence of small amounts of sodium and glucose also tend to slightly increase the rate of water absorption. A sodium-containing beverage will also help prevent hyponatremia in athletes who over hydrate and in those participating in endurance events, such as ultramarathons or iron man triathlons, when significant amounts of sodium may be lost in sweat.

Consuming salt alone in pill form is unnecessary and dangerous because the salt will draw water away from the tissues and may cause dehydration, nausea, and vomiting. Therefore, the common belief that salt pills are necessary to replace the sodium lost in sweat and prevent dehydration is a misconception (Table 11.5).

The Right Food and Drink Can Enhance Performance

Athletes need more calories and fluid than nonathletes. If nutrient-dense choices are made the extra calories will provide extra vitamins and minerals ensuring that all needs are met. The Food Guide Pyramid can be used to plan an athlete's diet. If their calorie needs exceed the highest recommended number of servings from each group, the number of servings from all groups can be increased; the resulting diet will still stack up to be a pyramid.

Athletes may also need to plan when they eat and what they eat before, during, and after competition. Food eaten at these times may give or take away the extra seconds that can mean victory or defeat.

Make sure you eat before you compete

You probably don't perform your best when you're hungry. The same is true for all athletes—they perform better after a small meal than when they haven't eaten. The size, composition, and timing of the pre-exercise meal is important. The wrong meal can hinder performance more than the right one can enhance it. The goal of meals eaten before exercise is to maximize glycogen stores and provide adequate hydration while minimizing any digestion, hunger, and gastric distress.

For more information on hydration and other sports nutrition and exercise science topics, go to the Gatorade Sports Science Institute at www.gssiweb.com/ and click on Sports Science Center.

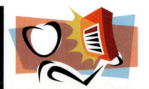

Off the Label: What Are You Getting from That Sports Bar?

Looking for a snack you can carry with you on your bike or stick in the pocket of your ski jacket? A sports bar may be the answer, but which should you choose? There are hundreds of varieties. Some are high in protein and low in carbohydrate; others are high in carbohydrate and low in fat; and some claim to have just the right balance of everything. They promise to optimize performance, build lean muscle, reduce body fat, increase strength, and speed recovery. But which will give you an energy boost during your bike ride or day of skiing?

To know what you are choosing, check out the label to see how much carbohydrate, fat, protein, and energy are in different bars. Carbohydrate is the fuel that becomes limiting during prolonged exercise, so if you want to have the energy to keep pedaling choose a high-carbohydrate bar. A bar that provides about 45 grams of carbohydrate will help to maintain your blood glucose level during exercise. Watch the fat and protein; in 300 Calories you want no more than about 8 grams of fat and 16 grams of protein. Bars higher in fat and protein or lower in carbohydrate will not give you the blood glucose boost that you need to continue exercising.

Are sports bars any better for you than a candy bar? With flavors like chocolate coconut, tropical crisp, and sesame raisin crunch they sound more like candy bars than high-performance snacks. A look at the label, however, shows that there is a difference. Typically sports bars are lower in fat, higher in fiber, and contain more vitamins and minerals than candy bars. Many contain vitamin C, vitamin E, calcium, iron, magnesium, copper, zinc, and a host of B vitamins. The % Daily Value of calcium, iron, and vitamins A and C must be listed. Many other vitamins and minerals may not be included in the Nutrition Facts portion of the label, but the nutrients added will appear in the ingredient list.

So, should you be packing a sports bar on your next outing? You don't need one, but if you can't fit a peanut butter sandwich and a banana in your pocket, they are a good alternative. Their biggest advantage is their convenience. They are pre-portioned, ready to eat, and transportable. They don't take the place of the whole grains, fresh vegetables and fruits, dairy products, and meats or meat substitutes that make up a healthy diet, but if having a compact, individually wrapped bar that can

travel with you means the difference between consuming this snack or no food at all, they can be beneficial. They may also provide a psychological edge if you believe they will enhance your performance.

If you choose to use these bars, wash them down with plenty of water. They provide carbohydrate, protein, fat, and many micronutrients, but they don't provide fluid—an essential during any activity. Also remember that sports bars provide Calories, generally about 200 to 300 per bar. Even though they are eaten to support activity they still add to your overall energy intake and can contribute to weight gain if consumed in excess.

Nutrition Facts	Amount/Serving	% DV*	Amount/Serving	% DV*
Serving Size 1 bar (65g)	**Total Fat** 2g	**3%**	**Potassium** 145mg	**4%**
Calories 230	Saturated Fat 0.5g	**3%**	**Total Carb** 45g	**15%**
Calories from Fat 20	Polyunsat Fat 1.0g		Dietary Fiber 3g	**12%**
Calories from Sat Fat 5	Monounsat Fat 0.5g		Sugars 14g	
*Percent Daily Values (DV) are based on a 2,000 calorie diet.	**Cholesterol** 0mg	**0%**	Other Carb 28g	
	Sodium 90mg	**4%**	**Protein** 10g	

Vitamin A 0% • Vitamin C 100% • Calcium 30% • Iron 35% • Vitamin E 100%
Thiamin 100% • Riboflavin 100% • Niacin 100% • Vitamin B$_6$ 100%
Folate 100% • Vitamin B$_{12}$ 100% • Biotin 100% • Pantothenic Acid 100%
Phosphorus 35% • Magnesium 35% • Zinc 35% • Copper 35% • Chromium 20%

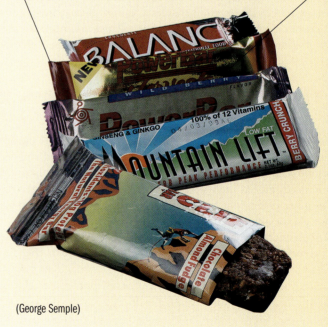

(George Semple)

Ideally a pre-exercise meal should provide enough fluid to maintain hydration and be high in carbohydrate (60 to 70% of Calories). This will help to maintain blood glucose and maximize glycogen stores. Muscle glycogen is depleted by exercise, but liver glycogen is used to supply blood glucose and is depleted even during rest if no food is ingested. So, first thing in the morning liver glycogen stores have been reduced by the overnight fast. A high-carbohydrate meal eaten 2 to 4 hours before the event will fill liver glycogen stores. In addition to being high in carbohydrate, the pre-exercise meal should contain about 300 Calories and be moderate in protein (10 to 20%) and low in fat (10 to 25%) and fiber to minimize GI distress and bloating during competition. A cup of pasta with tomato sauce and a slice of bread, or a turkey sandwich and a cup of juice are good choices. Spicy foods that could cause heartburn, and large amounts of simple sugars that could cause diarrhea, should also be avoided unless the athlete is accustomed to eating these foods.

In addition to providing nutritional clout, a meal that includes "lucky" foods may provide some athletes with an added psychological advantage. Meals should consist of foods familiar to the athlete. The effect of different meals and snacks should be tested during training, not during competition.

Keep eating and drinking even when you're on the move

Regardless of the type or duration of your exercise, maintaining adequate fluid intake is important while exercising (see Table 11.5). If your exercise lasts more than an hour, consuming some carbohydrate can also be beneficial. Consuming carbohydrate during exercise is particularly important for athletes who exercise in the morning when liver glycogen levels are low.

Carbohydrate intake should begin shortly after exercise commences and regular amounts should be consumed every 15 to 20 minutes during exercise. The carbohydrate should provide a combination of glucose and fructose. Fructose alone is not as effective and may cause diarrhea. Some athletes may prefer to obtain this carbohydrate from a sports drink but consuming a solid food snack or a carbohydrate gel with water is also appropriate.

During exercise, sodium and other minerals are lost in sweat. Although the amounts lost during exercise lasting less than 3 to 4 hours are usually not enough to affect health or performance, a snack or beverage containing sodium is recommended for exercise lasting 1 hour or more. The sodium enhances the palatability of beverages and increases the drive to drink so, even if sodium losses are small, consuming it during exercise may cause an increase in fluid intake.

Eat and drink to replenish and repair after exercise is done

When you stop exercising your body must shift from the task of breaking down glycogen, triglycerides, and muscle proteins for fuel to the job of restoring muscle and liver glycogen, depositing lipids, and synthesizing muscle proteins. The goal for meals after exercise is to replenish fluid, electrolyte, and glycogen losses and provide protein for building and repairing muscle tissue.

The first priority for all exercisers is to replace fluid losses. For serious athletes, appropriate postexercise intake can replenish muscle and liver glycogen within 24 hours of the athletic event. To maximize glycogen replacement, a high-carbohydrate meal or drink should be consumed as soon as possible after the competition and again every 2 hours for 6 hours after the event. Ideally the meals should provide about 0.7 to 1.5 grams of carbohydrate per kg of body weight, which is about 50 to 100 grams of carbohydrate for a 70-kg (150-pound) person—the equivalent of 1 1/2 to 2 cups of pasta. This type of regimen to restore glycogen is critical for athletes who must perform again the following day, but is not necessary if the athlete has one or more days to replace glycogen stores before the next intense exercise. If you aren't competing

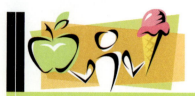

So, What Should I Eat?

Before you exercise drink and eat high-carbohydrate, low-fiber, low-fat foods
- Plan to have pasta but pass on the cream sauce
- Have a pancake breakfast
- Scarf down some cereal with low-fat milk
- Fill a water bottle 2 hours before exercise and finish it before you start
- Have a tall glass of juice

Pack lightly for a hike, bike, or ski
- Bring an apple and a bagel
- Fill your water bottle with a sports drink
- Bring a bar that's high in carbs
- Slip in a sack of raisins and granola
- Have a juicy fruit like orange sections
- Take a sip of water at every sign or intersection

If you are just going to the gym
- Bring your water bottle
- Wait for an hour after lunch, you need time to digest
- Refuel once you are done

again the next day, you can replace your glycogen more slowly by consuming high-carbohydrate foods for the next day or so. About 600 grams of carbohydrate, or about 8 to 10 grams per kilogram, is recommended for the 24 hours after exercise.[13] To provide amino acids for muscle protein synthesis and repair the postexercise meal should also provide protein. For example, a mixed meal such as pancakes and a glass of milk consumed soon after a strenuous competition or training session will help the athlete prepare for the next exercise session.

Most of us do not need a special glycogen replacement strategy to ensure our stores are full before our next gym visit. If your routine includes 30 to 60 minutes at the gym, a typical diet that provides about 55% carbohydrate will replace the glycogen used so you will be ready for a workout again tomorrow.

Do Supplements Enhance Athletic Performance?

Ergogenic aid Anything designed to increase work or improve performance.

"Citius, altius, fortius"—faster, higher, stronger—the Olympic motto. For as long as there have been competitions, athletes have yearned for something—anything—that would give them the competitive edge. Everything from bee pollen and brewer's yeast to high-dose vitamins, ancient herbs, and dangerous hormones have been used as **ergogenic aids** (Figure 11.17). Athletes are willing to go to great lengths to improve performance and are therefore susceptible to the lures of these products. Many of the vitamins, minerals, and other substances in these supplements are involved in producing energy for exercise or recovering from exercise. But others may carry more risks than benefits (see *Your Choice*: Ergogenic Hormones: Athletes Dying to Win).

When considering whether or not to use an ergogenic supplement, or any type of supplement, wise consumers weigh the health risks against potential benefits (Table 11.6). The following sections discuss some of the more popular products and others are reviewed in Table 11.7.

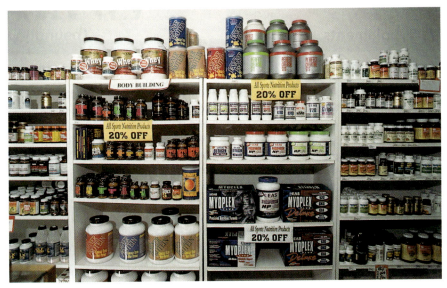

FIGURE 11.17

Many types of supplements are marketed to athletes as ergogenic aids. (George Semple)

Vitamin supplements are promoted to increase energy and antioxidant protection

More isn't always better. B vitamin supplements are promoted to enhance energy production. Although many of the B vitamins are important in producing energy in the body, having more of a vitamin around doesn't mean that you will produce more energy. For example, while it is true that vitamins B_6, B_{12}, and folic acid are needed to transport oxygen for aerobic metabolism, and that a deficiency of one or more of these would interfere with energy production and impair athletic performance, providing more than the recommended amount does not deliver more oxygen to the muscle, cause more ATP to be produced, or enhance athletic performance. Athletes who eat a balanced diet and meet their calorie needs usually get all the B vitamins they need without supplements.

TABLE 11.6
Is a Supplement Right for You?

Why do you want a supplement?
- What does the product contain?
- Has it been shown to provide the benefits you want?

Are the ingredients safe for you?
- Does it contain any ingredients that have been shown to be toxic to someone like you?
- Do you have a medical condition that would make it dangerous to take this product?
- Are you taking prescription medication that might interact with the supplement?

Is the dose safe?
- Does it contain potentially toxic levels of any nutrient? Check the % Daily Value for any nutrients that exceed 100%. If they do, do they exceed the UL?
- Follow the recommended dose on the package. More isn't always better and may cause side effects.

How much does it cost?
- More expensive is not always better.
- Compare costs and ingredients before you buy.

PIECE IT TOGETHER

Can Supplements Safely Give You a Boost?

Andrew is on the college track team. He would like to improve his performance and decides to try some ergogenic supplements. Based on the articles and advertisements he's read in sports magazines, he chooses creatine to improve his sprint times and chromium to increase his lean body mass. But before he begins taking these, he wants to explore their risks and benefits.

The ads and articles about these supplements make the following claims:

- Creatine will increase muscle creatine phosphate levels to provide quick energy and speed recovery after exercise.
- Chromium will increase lean body tissue and enhance fat loss.

DO THE CLAIMS MADE FOR THESE PRODUCTS MAKE SENSE?

Creatine is a precursor for creatine phosphate, which is a source of ATP for short-term exercise. Therefore, the claim that it will increase creatine phosphate levels and provide more energy for sprint activities seems logical.

Chromium is a mineral that is needed for insulin to perform its functions. Insulin has many essential roles, including getting glucose into cells, turning on protein synthesis, and stimulating the synthesis of fat. The claim that it will increase lean tissue makes some sense metabolically, but Andrew is not sure why taking chromium would enhance only the protein-building aspect of insulin's function.

IS THERE EVIDENCE THAT THESE SUPPLEMENTS WORK?

The advertisements show photographs of sprinters and bodybuilders and quote their testimonials on the effectiveness of these products. Andrew is not convinced by this type of anecdotal evidence, so he makes a trip to the library to explore the scientific literature.

WHERE SHOULD ANDREW LOOK FOR MORE INFORMATION?

In order to find sound scientific studies he should look for articles in well-respected, peer-reviewed journals in the field of nutrition and sports, such as the *International Journal of Sport Nutrition* and *Medicine and Science in Sports and Exercise.* He should then focus on studies that include athletes involved in the types of activities he performs. He can also look at the government nutrition site at www.nutrition.gov for links to information on dietary supplements.

DO THESE SUPPLEMENTS LIVE UP TO THEIR PROMOTERS' PROMISES?

Andrew finds several articles on creatine and chromium. The studies of creatine involve exercise that requires short bursts of activity such as sprinting and weight lifting and demonstrate enhanced performance when compared to a placebo. For chromium, the studies are contradictory. One shows an increase in the amount of weight gained and a decrease in body fat with weight training compared to a placebo, while another study finds no significant effects.

WHAT ARE THE RISKS OF TAKING CREATINE AND CHROMIUM?

No deleterious effects of creatine have been reported in healthy humans, but Andrew could not find any well-controlled studies on the long-term effects of this supplement. Because the doses of creatine are large (1 to 6 teaspoons), he has read that the purity of the product is a concern. He decides to select one that displays the USP verification mark on the label (see Chapter 10).

Chromium is an essential mineral, but the muscle-building effects of chromium are still questionable. The doses in supplements are about 200 μg per day. Although the evidence for chromium toxicity was not substantial enough to establish a UL, one study found that the picolinate form of chromium caused DNA damage in cells grown in the laboratory. Andrew decides that he will wait for more research to be done before he takes chromium picolinate as an ergogenic aid. Because he eats a balanced diet and takes a multivitamin and mineral supplement that contains chromium, he concludes that he is getting adequate chromium. He is still considering creatine but is unsure whether it will offer more benefits than risks.

WHAT WOULD YOU RECOMMEND ANDREW DO?

Your answer:

Creatine and bicarbonate can help for short-term intense exercise

Athletes in different events have different energy needs. For instance, a long-distance runner has to be concerned about running out of glycogen. Sprinters, however, are done with their event long before their glycogen tank is empty. They are looking for supplements that give them quick energy. For these athletes, creatine and bicarbonate may have some benefits.

Creatine supplements increase muscle creatine phosphate Creatine phosphate gives you instant energy. More of it should therefore increase the amount of short-term intense exercise that can be performed. Many athletes take creatine supplements for this reason (Figure 11.18). Creatine is a nitrogen-containing compound found in the body, primarily in muscle, where it is used to make creatine phosphate. It is synthesized by the kidney, liver, pancreas, and other tissues and is consumed in the diet in meat and milk. The more creatine in the diet, the greater the muscle creatine stores. Creatine supplements have been shown to increase levels of both creatine and creatine phosphate in muscle.[29] Higher levels of these provide muscles with more quick energy for activity, delay fatigue, prevent the accumulation of lactic acid, and allow creatine phosphate to be regenerated more quickly after exercise.[30] These effects make creatine supplementation beneficial for exercise that requires explosive bursts of energy, such as sprinting and weight lifting, but not for long-term endurance activities such as marathons. Creatine supplements have also been found to increase lean body mass. This increase is believed to be due to water retention related to creatine uptake in the muscle. An increase in muscle mass and strength may also occur in response to the greater amount and intensity of training that may be achieved.[29]

A number of studies have suggested that creatine supplements are safe, but controlled toxicology studies have not been done and the safety and efficacy of the long-term use of high-dose supplements is unknown.[31] Product purity is also a concern. Because large doses of 5 to 30 grams (1 to 6 teaspoons) are needed to be effective, even a minor contaminant might be consumed in significant amounts. Ingestion of creatine before or during exercise is not recommended, and the FDA has advised consumers to consult a physician before using the supplement.

Bicarbonate boosts buffering capacity Intense anaerobic exercise produces lactic acid. If too much accumulates in the muscles it impairs muscle function and causes pain and fatigue. Bicarbonate acts as a buffer in the body, so supplements have been hypothesized to neutralize lactic acid and thus delay fatigue and improve performance. Taking sodium bicarbonate, which is just baking soda from the kitchen cupboard, before exercise has been found to improve performance and delay exhaustion in sports such as sprint cycling, which involve intense exercise lasting only 1 to 7 minutes, but it is of no benefit for lower-intensity aerobic exercise.[22] However, just because baking soda is an ingredient in your cookies doesn't make it risk-free. Many people experience abdominal cramps and diarrhea after taking bicarbonate and other possible side effects have not been carefully researched.

Healthy eating helps performance more than herbs or hoaxes

Supplements may get most of the press when it comes to performance, but they are only the very tip of the iceberg when it comes to the things you can do to enhance your performance. The foundation of good athletic performance is a healthy diet, talent, and hard work. A healthy diet is one that provides the right number of calories to keep your weight in the desirable range; the proper balance of carbohydrate, protein, and fat to fuel your activity and maintain your tissues; plenty of water; and sufficient but not excessive amounts of essential vitamins and minerals. It is rich in whole grains, fruits, and vegeta-

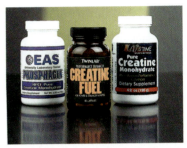

FIGURE 11.18

Creatine supplements are promoted to delay fatigue and increase muscle mass. (George Semple)

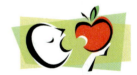

Most dietary supplements do little to enhance athletic performance, but there are a few with proven benefits for specific types of activities. Even the safest are not risk-free and the benefits they provide are very small compared to the benefits of a healthy overall diet and training routine.

FIGURE 11.19

This pyramid illustrates the relative value of various nutrition strategies for exercise performance. The most significant benefit is achieved by eating a healthy overall diet. Foods and beverages used to supply energy and ensure hydration during an event can provide additional benefits but ergogenic aids provide little or no performance boost. (Adapted from Burke, L. Supplements in sport-nutritional ergogenic aids. 2001 Available online at www.ausport.gov.au/fultext/2001/ascpub/FactSupp2.asp Accessed February 26, 2004)

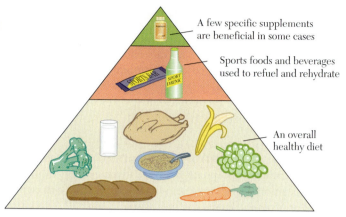

A few specific supplements are beneficial in some cases

Sports foods and beverages used to refuel and rehydrate

An overall healthy diet

The Impact of Nutritional Strategies on Excercise Performance

bles, high in fiber, moderate in fat and sodium, and low in saturated fat, cholesterol, *trans* fat, and added sugars. Whether you are a couch potato or an Olympic hopeful the recommendations from the Food Guide Pyramid and the Dietary Guidelines can help you choose such a diet. This diet provides the foundation from which to optimize performance. Your performance can be further improved by using appropriate foods and fluids to help you refuel and rehydrate during workouts and events. Where do supplements fit in? Most of them don't but a few specific types of athletes in specific events will receive an additional small benefit from a few select supplements (Figure 11.19).

THINKING FOR YOURSELF

1. How much exercise do you get?
   a. Keep a log of your activity for one day.
   b. Refer to Table 7.5 to help you determine how many hours you spend engaged in:
      1. activities of daily living?
      2. moderate intensity activity?
      3. vigorous activity?
   c. Use Table 7.6 to determine your physical activity level and PA value.
   d. Use Table 7.7 to calculate your estimated energy expenditure (EER).
   e. If you increased your exercise enough to move to the "active" physical activity level, what would your new EER be? (If you are already active, what would your EER be in the "very active" level?)
   f. Make a list of foods that you could add to your diet to balance the added expenditure of this increase in activity.

2. What types and amounts of exercise work for you?
   a. Taking into consideration your typical weekly schedule of activities and events, design a reasonable exercise program for yourself using the Activity Pyramid. Include the types of activities, the times during the week you will be involved in each activity, and the length of time you will engage in each activity. Choose activities you enjoy and schedule them for reasonable lengths of time and at reasonable frequencies.
   b. What everyday changes have you made that will increase the energy expended in day-to-day activities?
   c. Of the activities you have included, which are aerobic, which improve flexibility, and which are for strength training?
   d. Can each of these activities be performed year-round? Suggest alternative activities and locations for inclement weather.

3. Are ergogenic aids safe and beneficial?
   a. Choose an ergogenic aid and use information from the Internet to determine its promised benefits, its actual benefits, its potential risks.
   b. Write a conclusion as to why you would or would not take this substance.

SUMMARY

1. Regular exercise improves fitness in individuals of all ages and can reduce the risk of chronic diseases such as obesity, heart disease, diabetes, and osteoporosis. Exercise can also delay some of the changes in body composition and metabolism that occur with age.

2. A well-designed fitness program involves aerobic exercise, stretching, and strength training. To maintain a healthy body weight and maximize health, 60 minutes per day of moderate exercise should be performed in addition to the activities of daily living. One way to create a more active lifestyle is to choose enjoyable activities and follow the recommendations of the Activity Pyramid.

3. Activity is fueled by ATP. The source of ATP depends on how long you have been exercising. During the first 10 to 15 seconds of exercise stored ATP and creatine phosphate fuel activity. During the next 2 to 3 minutes the amount of oxygen at the muscle remains limited so ATP is generated by the anaerobic metabolism of glucose. After a few minutes the delivery of oxygen at the muscle increases and ATP can be generated by aerobic metabolism. Aerobic metabolism is more efficient than anaerobic metabolism and can utilize glucose, fatty acids, and amino acids as energy sources.

4. For lower-intensity exercise of longer duration, aerobic metabolism predominates, and both glucose and fatty acids are important fuel sources. Protein becomes an important source of energy only when exercise continues for many hours. Training improves oxygen delivery and utilization, allowing aerobic exercise to be sustained for longer periods at higher intensity.

5. For short-term, high-intensity activity, ATP is generated primarily from the anaerobic metabolism of glucose from muscle glycogen stores. Anaerobic metabolism uses glucose more rapidly and produces lactic acid. Both of these factors hasten the onset of fatigue.

6. The diet of an active individual should provide sufficient energy to fuel activity. In general, it should contain about 45 to 65% of total energy as carbohydrate from whole grains, fruits, vegetables, and milk to ensure that glycogen stores are replenished after daily exercise; 20 to 35% of energy as fat; and about 10 to 35% of energy as protein.

7. Sufficient micronutrients are needed to generate ATP from macronutrients, to maintain and repair tissues, and to transport oxygen and wastes to and from the cells. Most athletes who consume a varied diet that meets their calorie needs also consume enough vitamins and minerals. Those who restrict their intake, may be at risk for deficiencies.

8. The pressure to compete and maintain a body weight that is optimal for their sport puts some athletes at risk for eating disorders. A combination of excessive exercise and energy restriction puts female athletes at risk for the female athlete triad, a combination of menstrual irregularities and disordered eating that leads to bone loss and increases osteoporosis risk.

9. Adequate fluid intake before exercise ensures that athletes begin exercise well hydrated. Fluid intake during and after exercise must replace water lost in sweat and from evaporation through the lungs. Water is needed to ensure that the body can be cooled and that nutrients and oxygen can be delivered to body tissues. If water intake is inadequate, dehydration can lead to a decline in exercise performance and thermal distress may occur.

10. Plain water is an appropriate fluid to consume for most exercise. Beverages containing carbohydrate are also appropriate and are recommended for exercise lasting more than an hour because they provide carbohydrate that helps spare glycogen. Electrolyte replacement is not necessary during exercise lasting less than 3 to 4 hours but is recommended for exercise lasting more than an hour because it enhances the palatability of the drink and may increase fluid intake.

11. Meals eaten before competition should provide about 300 Calories; should be high in carbohydrate, low in fat, moderate in protein, and low in fiber; and should satisfy the psychological needs of the athlete. Postcompetition meals should replace lost fluids and electrolytes, provide carbohydrate to restore muscle and liver glycogen, and provide protein for muscle protein synthesis and repair.

12. Many types of ergogenic aids are marketed to improve athletic performance. Some are beneficial for certain types of activity, but many offer little or no benefit. An individual risk-benefit analysis should be used to determine if a supplement is appropriate for you.

REVIEW QUESTIONS

1. List 5 of the health benefits of exercise.
2. What is aerobic exercise?
3. What is strength training?
4. How does aerobic exercise affect resting heart rate?
5. Suggest an exercise plan for someone who is just starting to exercise. What types of exercise should they include? How long and how frequently should they perform each type?
6. From where does the ATP to fuel the first few minutes of exercise come?
7. What fuels are used to produce ATP in anaerobic metabolism?
8. Which is more efficient, aerobic or anaerobic metabolism?
9. What fuels are used in exercise of long duration such as marathon running?
10. What are the recommendations for fluid intake before, during, and after exercise?
11. How does exercise affect protein needs?
12. List the steps you might take to evaluate the safety and effectiveness of an ergogenic acid.

REFERENCES

1. Gallagher, D., Heymsfield, S. Heo, M., et al. Healthy percentage body fat ranges: An approach for developing guidelines based on body mass index *Am. J. Clin. Nutr.* 72:694–701, 2000.
2. Institute of Medicine, Food and Nutrition Board. *Dietary Reference Intakes for Energy, Carbohydrates, Fiber, Fat, Protein and Amino Acids.* Washington, DC: National Academy Press, 2002.
3. Albright, A., Franz, M., Hornsby, G. et al. American College of Sports Medicine Position Stand. Exercise and type 2 diabetes. *Med. Sci. Sports Exerc.* 32:1345–1360, 2000.
4. Stein, C. J., and Colditz, G. A. Modifiable risk factors for cancer. *Br. J. Cancer* 90:299–303, 2004.
5. Lee, I. M. Physical activity and cancer prevention—data from epidemiologic studies. *Med. Sci. Sports Exerc.* 35:1823–1827, 2003.
6. Fontaine, K. R. Physical activity improves mental health. The Physician and Sportsmedicine. Available online at www.physsportsmed.com/issues/2000/10_00/fontaine.htm/ Accessed August 24, 2004.
7. Centers for Disease Control and Prevention Physical Activity and Health: A Report of the Surgeon General. Available online at www.cdc.gov/nccdphp/sgr/adults.htm/Accessed August 24, 2004.
8. U.S. Department of Agriculture, U.S. Department of Health and Human Services. *Nutrition and Your Health: Dietary Guidelines for Americans*, 5th ed. Home and Garden Bulletin No. 232. Hyattsville, MD: U.S. Government Printing Office, 2000.
9. Healthy People 2010. Available online at www.healthypeople.gov/ Accessed August 24, 2002.
10. Exploring the Activity Pyramid. Institute for Research and Education. Healthsystem Minnesota. Available online at www.hsmnet.com/HSM/BHC/IRE/HEC/EXPLORE.HTM/ Accessed January 10, 2000.
11. Andersen, R. E., Crespo, C. J., Bartlett, S. J., et al. Relationship of physical activity and television watching with body weight and level of fatness among children: Results from the Third National Health and Nutrition Examination Survey. *JAMA* 279:938–942, 1998.
12. Manore, M., and Thompson, J. *Sport Nutrition for Health and Performance.* Champaign, IL: Human Kinetics, 2000.
13. American Dietetic Association. Nutrition and Athletic Performance—Position of the American Dietetic Association, Dietitians of Canada, and American College of Sports Medicine. *J. Am. Diet. Assoc.* 100:1543–1556, 2000.
14. Tipton, K. D., and Wolfe, R. R. Protein and amino acids for athletes. *J. Sports Sci.* 22:65–79, 2004.
15. Kazis, K., Iglesias, E. The female athlete triad. *Adolesc. Med.* 14:87–95, 2003.
16. Beard, J., and Tobin, B. Iron status and exercise. *Am. J. Clin. Nutr.* 72(Suppl.):594S–597S, 2000.
17. Food and Nutrition Board, Institute of Medicine. *Dietary Reference Intakes: Vitamin A, Vitamin K, Arsenic, Boron, Chromium, Copper, Iodine, Iron, Manganese, Molybdenum, Nickel, Silicon, Vanadium, and Zinc.* Washington, DC: National Academy Press, 2001.
18. Senay, L. C. Water and electrolytes during physical activity. In *Nutrition in Exercise and Sport*, 3rd ed. Wolinski, I., ed. Boca Raton, FL: CRC Press, 1998:257–276.
19. American College of Sports Medicine. Position stand on exercise and fluid replacement. *Med. Sci. Sports Exerc.* 28:i–vii, 1996.
20. Dekkers, J. C., van Doornen, L. J. P., and Kemper, H. C. G. The role of antioxidant vitamins and enzymes in the prevention of exercise-induced muscle damage. *Sports Med.* 21:213–238, 1996.
21. Vincent, J. B. The potential value and toxicity of chromium picolinate as a nutritional supplement, weight loss agent and muscle development agent. *Sports Med.* 33:213–230, 2003.
22. Williams, M. H. Facts and fallacies of purported ergogenic amino acid supplements. *Clin. Sports Med.* 18:633–649, 1999.
23. van Hall, G., Saris, W. H., van de Schoor, P. A., and Wagenmakers, A. J. The effect of free glutamine and peptide ingestion on the rate of muscle glycogen resynthesis in man. *Int. J. Sports Med.* 21:25–30, 2000.
24. Davis, J. M., Welsh, R. S., De Volve, K. L., and Alderson, N. A. Effects of branched-chain amino acids and carbohydrate on fatigue during intermittent, high-intensity running. *Int. J. Sports Med.* 20:309–314, 1999.
25. Brass, E. P. Supplemental carnitine and exercise. *Am. J. Clin. Nutr.* 72(Suppl.):618S–623S, 2000.
26. Misell, L. M., Lagomarcino, N. D., Schuster, V., and Kern M. Chronic medium-chain triacylglycerol consumption and

endurance performance in trained runners. *J. Sports Med. Phys. Fitness* 41:210–215, 2001.

27. Horowitz, J. F., Mora-Rodriguez, R., Byerley, L. O., and Coyle, E. F. Preexercise medium-chain triglyceride ingestion does not alter muscle glycogen use during exercise. *J. Appl. Physiol.* 88:219–225, 2000.

28. Spriet, L. L. Caffeine and performance. *Int. J. Sport Nutr.* 5(Suppl.):84S–99S, 1995.

29. Terjung, R. L., Clarkson, P., Eichner, E. R., et al. American College of Sports Medicine Roundtable: The physiological and health effects of oral creatine supplementation. *Med. Sci. Sports Exerc.* 32:706–717, 2000.

30. Feldman, E. B. Creatine: A dietary supplement and ergogenic aid. *Nutr. Rev.* 57:45–50, 1999.

31. Poortmans, J. R., and Francaux, M. Adverse effects of creatine supplementation: Fact or fiction? *Sports Med.* 30:155–170, 2000.

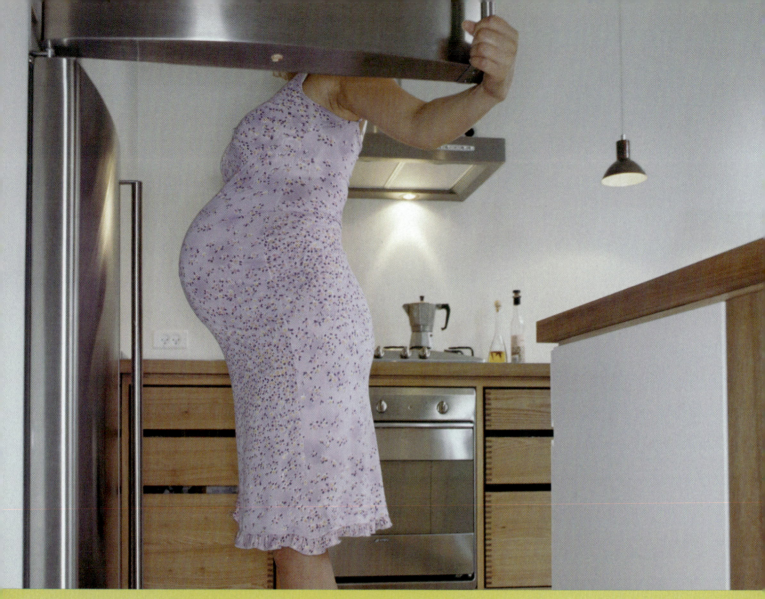

(Henrik Sorensen/Photonica)

CHAPTER 12 CONCEPTS

- Over the 40 weeks of pregnancy, a single cell develops into a fully formed child and the pregnant woman's body undergoes many changes to provide for the growing fetus.
- Energy, protein, water, vitamins, and minerals needs increase during pregnancy.
- The developing child is vulnerable to nutrient imbalances and toxins.
- High blood glucose or high blood pressure during pregnancy put mother and child at risk.
- Nutritional status, income, and age affect the risks to mother and child during pregnancy.
- Nutrient needs are even greater during lactation than pregnancy.
- A newborn infant's energy and protein needs are higher per unit of body weight than at any other time of life.
- Breast-feeding is the ideal way to nourish most infants.
- Infants' growth rates are the best measure of the adequacy of their diets.
- After 4 to 6 months of age, solid foods can gradually be introduced into the infant's diet.

Just A Taste

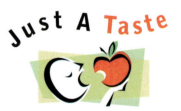

Should overweight women gain weight during pregnancy?

Is a pregnant woman really eating for two?

Do pregnant women need vitamin and mineral supplements?

Is breast-feeding the best option for all newborn infants and their mothers?

Nutrition, Pregnancy, and Infants

12

INTRODUCTION

USA Today

Study: Pregnant Women Eating Too Much Fish

By *Elizabeth Weise*

Apr. 7, 2004—Of the 4 million babies born in the USA in 2000, more than 300,000 of them—and as many as 600,000—may have been exposed to "unacceptable" levels of methyl mercury because their mothers ate a diet rich in fish, a study finds.

The new study, by researchers at the Office of Prevention, Pesticides and Toxic Substances at the Environmental Protection Agency, repeats a warning by numerous studies that the neurotoxin is particularly dangerous for growing fetuses.

Exposure to even low levels of mercury *in utero* can cause developmental problems and difficulties with visual and motor integration.

_____
To read the entire article, go to www.usatoday.com/news/health/2004-04-07-mercury-usat_x.htm.

Human development is an extremely complex process, but miraculously most babies are born healthy. In 9 months, a single cell grows and develops into a complete human being. During this time all nutrients are delivered to the developing child through the mother's body. Her diet must provide everything needed to grow a healthy baby. Too much or too little of a nutrient can affect the development of the child and the outcome of the pregnancy. Toxins, like mercury, are also transferred from mother to child and can interfere with normal development of the baby.

Babies Begin as a Single Cell

⚠ **Implantation** The process by which the cells derived from the fertilized egg embed in the uterine lining.

⚠ **Embryo** The developing human from 2 to 8 weeks after fertilization. All organ systems are formed during this time.

⚠ **Placenta** An organ produced from both maternal and embryonic tissues. It secretes hormones, transfers nutrients and oxygen from the mother's blood to the fetus, and removes wastes.

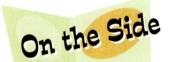

When an egg from the mother is fertilized by a sperm from the father, the genetic material from each parent combines to form a genetically unique individual. Only identical twins have the same genetic makeup. They develop from a single fertilized egg.

⚠ **Fetus** The developing human from the 9th week to birth. Growth and refinement of structures occur during this time.

⚠ **Gestation** The time between conception and birth, which lasts about 9 months (or about 40 weeks) in humans.

Whether you are 6 foot 4 or 5 foot 3, you started out as a single fertilized egg. The fertilized egg, which is called a zygote, divides rapidly to form a ball of smaller cells. The cells begin to differentiate and to move to form structures. After about 2 weeks, it is still not any bigger than the zygote, but consists of many cells and has begun burrowing its way into the lining of the mother's uterus. After this **implantation** process is complete, the ball of cells is called an **embryo**. At first the embryo gets its nourishment by breaking down the lining of the uterus, but soon this is inadequate to meet needs and the **placenta** begins to take over the role of nourishing it. The placenta is formed when branchlike projections grow from the implanted ball of cells into the lining of the uterus. These projections contain blood vessels that end up in close proximity to maternal blood. The fully developed placenta contains a network of blood vessels that allows nutrients and oxygen to be transferred from the mother's blood to the baby and waste products to be transferred from the baby to the mother's blood for elimination (Figure 12.1). The placenta also secretes hormones necessary to maintain pregnancy.

In the first 8 weeks all organs begin to form

The embryonic stage of development lasts until the 8th week after fertilization. During this time, the cells rapidly differentiate to form the multitude of specialized cell types that make up the human body. They arrange themselves in the proper shapes and locations to form organs and structures. At the end of this stage the embryo is approximately 3 cm long (a little more than an inch) and has a beating heart. All major external and internal structures have been formed (Figure 12.2a).

Between the 9th and the 40th week, the fetus grows and organs mature

Beginning at the 9th week of development and continuing until birth, the developing offspring is known as a **fetus** (Figure 12.2b). During the fetal period of development, structures that appeared during the embryonic period continue to grow and mature. The size of the fetus increases from about 3 cm to around 50 cm at birth. The fetal period usually ends after 40 weeks of **gestation** with the birth of an infant weighing about 3 to 4 kg (6.6 to 8.8 pounds).[1]

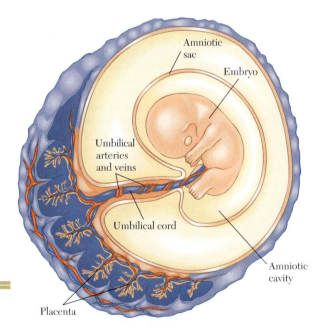

FIGURE 12.1

During pregnancy, the amniotic sac and the fluid it contains protect the fetus, and the placenta allows nutrients and wastes to be transferred between mother and baby.

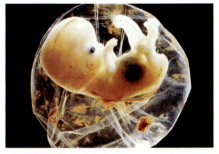 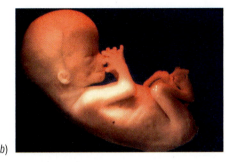

(a)   (b)

FIGURE 12.2

(a) At 5 to 6 weeks the embryo is less than 3 cm long but has a beating heart and the rudiments of all the major organ systems. (b) At 16 weeks, the fetus is about 16 cm (6.4 inches) long and organ systems continue to mature. (a: Biophoto Associates/Photo Researchers; b: Meitchik/Custom Medical Stock Photo, Inc.)

Infants who are born on time but have failed to grow well in the uterus are said to be **small-for-gestational-age**. Those born before 37 weeks of gestation are said to be **preterm** or **premature**. Whether born too soon or just too small, **low-birth-weight** infants and **very-low-birth-weight** infants are at increased risk for illness and early death.[2] They often require special care and a special diet in order to successfully continue to grow and develop. Survival improves with increasing gestational age and birth weight. Today, with advances in medical and nutritional care, infants born as early as 25 weeks of gestation and those weighing as little as 1 kg (2.2 pounds) can survive.

Small-for-gestational-age An infant born at term weighing less than 2.5 kg (5.5 lb).

Preterm or **premature** An infant born before 37 weeks of gestation.

Low-birth-weight A birth weight of less than 2.5 kg (5.5 lb).

Very-low-birth-weight A birth weight of less than 1.5 kg (3.3 lb).

A Woman's Body Undergoes Many Changes During Pregnancy

During pregnancy, a woman's body must undergo many changes to support the development of her child. Her blood volume increases by 50%, and her heart, lungs, and kidneys work harder to deliver nutrients and oxygen and remove wastes. The placenta develops to allow nutrients to be delivered to the growing fetus and the hormones it produces orchestrate other changes. Body fat increases to provide the energy needed late in pregnancy, the uterus enlarges, muscles and ligaments relax to accommodate the growing fetus and allow for childbirth, and the breasts develop to prepare for **lactation**. These changes all result in weight gain and can affect the type and level of physical activity that is safe. In some cases they can also cause uncomfortable side effects.

Lactation Milk production and secretion.

Trimester A term used to describe each third, or 3-month period, of a pregnancy.

Adequate weight gain during pregnancy is essential for mother and child

A healthy, normal-weight woman should gain 25 to 35 pounds (11.4 to 15.9 kg) during her pregnancy. An average healthy baby weighs about 7 pounds at birth. The rest of the weight gained during pregnancy is due to changes in the mother's body (Figure 12.3).

The rate of weight gain during pregnancy is as important as the total amount of weight. Little gain is expected in the first 3 months, or **trimester**, of pregnancy—usually about 2 to 4 pounds (0.9 to 1.8 kg). In the second and third trimesters, when the fetus grows from less than a pound to 6 to 8 pounds, the recommended weight gain for the mother is about 1 pound (0.45 kg) per week. Women who are underweight or overweight at conception should also gain weight at a slow, steady rate (Figure 12.4). Weight gains of up to 40 pounds (18 kg) are recommended for women who begin pregnancy underweight. Overweight women should gain less, only about 15 to 25 pounds (6.8 to 11.4 kg) over the course of pregnancy.

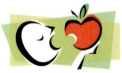

Even women who are overweight at the start of pregnancy need to gain weight during pregnancy to allow for the growth of the child and expansion of the mother's blood volume and growth of other maternal tissues.

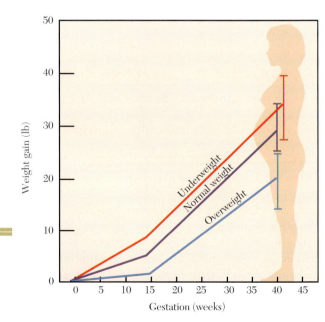

Total	25-35 lb
Fetus	7-8 lb
Amniotic fluid	2 lb
Placenta	1-2 lb
Uterus	2 lb
Maternal blood	3-4 lb
Breast tissue	2 lb
Extracellular fluids	4 lb
Maternal fat	4-11 lb

FIGURE 12.3

The weight gained by the mother during pregnancy includes increases in the weight of her tissues as well as the weight of the fetus, placenta, and amniotic fluid.

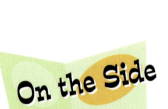

On the Side

Most women lose all but about 2 pounds of the weight gained during pregnancy within a year of delivery. Typically, a woman loses about 10 pounds at delivery and another 5 pounds during the first week after delivery. Further weight loss requires a balanced low-calorie diet combined with moderate exercise.

✳ **Cesarean section** The surgical removal of the fetus from the uterus.

✳ **Large-for-gestational-age** An infant weighing greater than 4 kg (8.8 pounds) at birth.

Gaining too much or too little weight as well as being underweight or overweight can affect the health of both mother and child.[1] Being underweight by 10% or more at the onset of pregnancy or gaining too little weight during pregnancy increases the risk of producing a low-birth-weight baby. Excess weight, whether present before conception or gained during pregnancy, can also compromise the outcome of the pregnancy. The mother's risks for high blood pressure, diabetes, a difficult delivery, and a **cesarean section** are increased by excess weight, as is the risk of having a **large-for-gestational-age** baby. However, dieting during pregnancy is not advised even for obese women. If possible, excess weight should be lost before the pregnancy begins or, alternatively, after the child is born and weaned.

FIGURE 12.4

The same pattern of weight gain is recommended for women who are normal weight, underweight, or overweight at the start of pregnancy, but the recommendations for total weight gain are different. (Adapted from Committee on Nutritional Status During Pregnancy and Lactation. *Nutrition During Pregnancy.* Washington, D.C.: National Academy Press, 1990.)

TABLE 12.1

Moderate Exercise Is Recommended for Most Healthy Pregnant Women

- Check with your physician before beginning an exercise program during pregnancy
- Drink plenty of liquids before, during, and after exercise
- Increase your activity gradually and limit strenuous exercise
- Exercise regularly, at least three times per week, rather than intermittently
- Stop exercising when you are tired
- Avoid exercising in hot or humid environments
- Choose activities that have a minimal risk of falls or abdominal injury
- Avoid exercises that require lying on your back
- After recovering from delivery, gradually resume prepregnancy exercise routines

Adapted from American Dietetic Association. Nutrition and lifestyle for a healthy pregnancy outcome. *J. Am. Diet. Assoc.* 102:1470–1490, 2002.

Most pregnant women don't need to give up their regular routines

Pregnant women may need more rest, but they usually don't need to give up their regular exercise routines. Physical activity during pregnancy improves overall fitness, mood, and body image; reduces stress; improves digestion; prevents excess weight gain, low back pain, and constipation; reduces the risk of diabetes; and speeds recovery from childbirth. Therefore, for healthy, well-nourished women, carefully chosen moderate exercise is recommended during pregnancy. Women who were physically active before their pregnancy can continue their exercise programs, but women who begin an exercise program after becoming pregnant should start slowly, with low-intensity, low-impact activities such as walking.[3] During pregnancy, the risk of injury is greater because women weigh more and carry that weight in the front of their bodies where it can interfere with balance and place stress on the bones, joints, and muscles. Activities that have a risk of abdominal trauma, falls, or joint stress, such as contact and racquet sports, should be avoided (Figure 12.5).[4] To ensure adequate delivery of oxygen and nutrients to the fetus, intense exercise should be limited. Guidelines have been developed to minimize the risks and maximize the benefits of exercise during pregnancy (Table 12.1).

Some physiological changes of pregnancy have uncomfortable side effects

During pregnancy, a woman experiences changes in the amount and distribution of body fluids and the types and levels of certain hormones. These physiological changes can cause uncomfortable side effects. Most of these problems are minor, but in some cases they may endanger the mother and the fetus.

Blood volume increases during pregnancy During pregnancy, blood volume expands to nourish the fetus, but this expansion may also cause the accumulation of extracellular fluid in the tissues, known as **edema**. Edema is characterized by swelling, particularly in the feet and ankles (Figure 12.6). It can be uncomfortable but does not increase medical risks unless it is accompanied by a rise in blood pressure. Reducing water or salt intake is not beneficial in preventing edema.

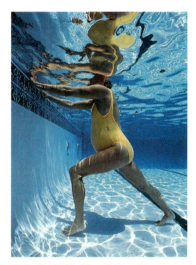

FIGURE 12.5

During pregnancy, exercising in the water can reduce stress on joints and help keep the body cool. (Tracy Frankel/The Image Bank/ Getty Images)

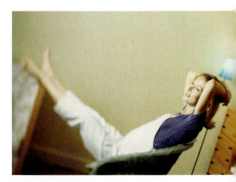

FIGURE 12.6

Edema in the feet and ankles is a common problem during pregnancy. Elevating the feet will help reduce swelling. (Elie Bernager/ Stone/Getty Images)

⚠ **Edema** Swelling due to the buildup of extracellular fluid in the tissues.

Morning sickness Nausea and vomiting that affects many women during the first few months of pregnancy and in some women can continue throughout the pregnancy.

Hormonal changes cause morning sickness Morning sickness is a syndrome of nausea and vomiting that occurs during pregnancy. The term is somewhat of a misnomer because symptoms can occur anytime during the day or night. It is thought to be related to the hormonal changes of pregnancy and may be alleviated to some extent by eating small, frequent snacks of dry starchy foods, such as plain crackers or bread. In most women symptoms decrease significantly after the first trimester, but in some cases the symptoms last for the entire pregnancy and, in severe cases, may require intravenous nutrition to assure that needs are met.

Digestive complaints are common as muscles in the GI tract relax The hormones produced to relax the muscles of the uterus also relax the muscles of the gastrointestinal tract. This relaxation along with the crowding of the organs by the growing baby can cause digestive complaints such as heartburn and constipation. Heartburn is common because the relaxation of the sphincter between the stomach and the esophagus allows the acidic stomach contents to back up into the esophagus, causing irritation. The problem gets more severe as pregnancy progresses because as the growing baby crowds the stomach, its contents are more likely to back up into the esophagus. Heartburn can be reduced by avoiding substances such as caffeine and chocolate that are known to cause heartburn, and eating many small meals throughout the day rather than a few large ones. Limiting intake of high-fat foods, such as fried foods, rich sauces, and desserts, which leave the stomach slowly, can also help reduce heartburn. Because a reclining position makes it easier for acidic juices to flow into the esophagus, remaining upright after eating can also help.

Constipation is also common during pregnancy because the relaxed muscles of the colon are less efficient. Maintaining a moderate level of physical activity and consuming plenty of fluid, as well as high-fiber foods such as whole grains, vegetables, and fruits, are recommended to prevent constipation. Hemorrhoids are more common during pregnancy, as a result of both constipation and physiological changes in blood flow.

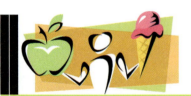

So, What Should I Eat?

To ease the nausea of morning sickness
- Try some crackers or dry toast in the morning—before you even get out of bed
- Have half your lunch now and half later
- Sip water throughout the day

To reduce constipation
- Focus on fiber by eating whole grains and lots of fruits and vegetables
- Keep all of you moving by getting regular exercise
- Drink an extra glass of water after each meal

To prevent heartburn
- Relax and enjoy your meal—you won't have time once the baby is born
- Save your fluids for between meals so your stomach doesn't get too full
- Skip the spicy, fatty foods
- Eat sitting up and stay upright to let gravity keep food in your stomach

Diet During Pregnancy Affects Mother and Child

During pregnancy the mother's intake must provide all the nutrients needed for the growth and development of the baby while continuing to meet the mother's needs. Because the increase in calorie requirement is proportionately smaller than the increased need for protein, vitamins, and minerals, a nutrient-dense diet is essential. Because the developing child is vulnerable, deficiencies and excess of nutrients as well as other damaging substances must be avoided during pregnancy.

Pregnant women have increased calorie needs

It is often said of a pregnant woman that she is eating for two. Although she doesn't need to eat twice as much, during most of the pregnancy she does need to eat more than a nonpregnant woman. This extra energy is needed to provide for the baby and new maternal tissues. During the first trimester, total energy expenditure changes little, so the EER is not increased above nonpregnant levels. During the second and third trimesters, an additional 340 and 452 Calories per day, respectively, are recommended (Figure 12.7). This is the number of calories contained in a snack such as a sandwich, an apple, and a glass of milk.

Pregnant women need more protein

During pregnancy blood volume increases, the placenta develops and grows, the uterus and breasts enlarge, and the baby grows from a single cell to a fully formed infant. Protein is needed for the structure of new cells so this growth increases the need for dietary protein. An additional 25 grams of protein per day above the RDA for nonpregnant women or 1.1 grams per kilogram per day is recommended for the second and third trimesters of pregnancy. For a woman weighing 136 pounds (62 kg), this increases protein needs to about 75 grams per day (see Figure 12.7). This is the

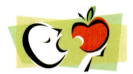

A pregnant woman is eating for two because she must provide for all her nutrient needs as well as for those of the fetus. But eating for two doesn't mean eating twice as much. The equivalent of having 2 lunches every day toward the end of pregnancy will provide the extra energy and nutrients needed.

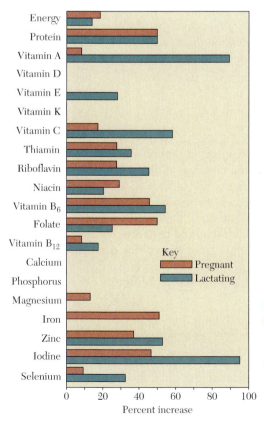

FIGURE 12.7

This graph illustrates the increase in recommended nutrient intakes for a 25-year-old woman during the third trimester of pregnancy and during lactation. The RDA for iron during lactation is equal to half the RDA for nonpregnant, nonlactating women.

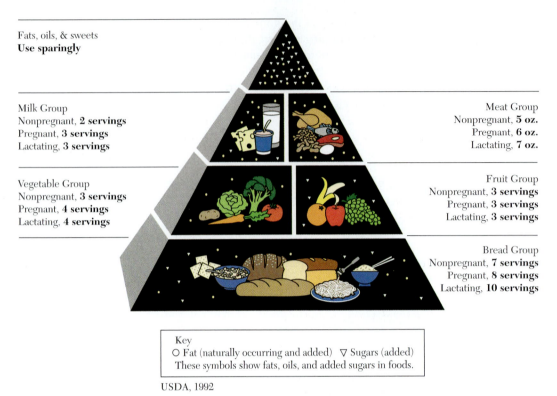

Food Guide Pyramid
A Guide to Daily Food Choices

Fats, oils, & sweets
Use sparingly

Milk Group
Nonpregnant, **2 servings**
Pregnant, **3 servings**
Lactating, **3 servings**

Meat Group
Nonpregnant, **5 oz.**
Pregnant, **6 oz.**
Lactating, **7 oz.**

Vegetable Group
Nonpregnant, **3 servings**
Pregnant, **4 servings**
Lactating, **4 servings**

Fruit Group
Nonpregnant, **3 servings**
Pregnant, **3 servings**
Lactating, **3 servings**

Bread Group
Nonpregnant, **7 servings**
Pregnant, **8 servings**
Lactating, **10 servings**

Key
○ Fat (naturally occurring and added) ▽ Sugars (added)
These symbols show fats, oils, and added sugars in foods.

USDA, 1992

FIGURE 12.8

The Food Guide Pyramid can be used for diet planning during pregnancy and lactation. Shown here are the recommended servings for a 25-year-old woman before pregnancy and during pregnancy and lactation. (U.S. Department of Agriculture, Home and Garden Bulletin No. 252, 1992)

amount of protein in three servings of milk or yogurt and two servings of meat. Following the Food Guide Pyramid recommendations for pregnant women can ensure that these needs are met (Figure 12.8).

Fluid needs are increased slightly during pregnancy

The need for water is increased during pregnancy because of the increase in blood volume, the production of amniotic fluid, and the needs of the fetus. During a pregnancy a woman will accumulate about 6 to 9 liters of water. Some is intracellular, but most is due to increases in the volume of blood and interstitial fluid between cells. The need for water is therefore increased from 2.7 liters per day in nonpregnant women to 3 liters per day of total water—that from both food and beverages.[5] Adequate fluid consumption throughout pregnancy is also important in preventing constipation. Despite changes in the amount and distribution of body water there is no evidence that the requirement for potassium, sodium, or chloride is different from that of nonpregnant women.

The need for many vitamins and minerals is increased during pregnancy

In order to grow new tissues in the mother and the child, the requirements for many vitamins and minerals increase during pregnancy. The need for B vitamins, such as thiamin, niacin, and riboflavin, increases as energy needs increase. The requirements for vitamin B_6 and zinc rise to meet the needs for increased protein synthesis. The requirements for calcium, vitamin D, and vitamin C increase to provide for the growth and development of bone and connective tissue. The needs for folate, vitamin B_{12}, zinc, and iron are increased to support the formation of new maternal and fetal cells. For many of these nutrients, intake is easily increased when energy intake is increased to meet needs, but for others there is a risk that inadequate amounts will be consumed.

Increased calcium absorption helps meet needs

Over the course of gestation the fetus accumulates about 30 grams of calcium. Most of this is deposited during the last trimester when the fetal bones are growing most rapidly and the teeth are forming. Many women have trouble consuming enough calcium to meet their own needs, let alone enough to provide this amount for the fetus. Fortunately they don't need to eat any more than is recommended for nonpregnant women because calcium absorption increases during pregnancy. At one time there was concern that the calcium needed by the fetus would come from maternal bones if intake was not adequate. It is now known that the increased need for calcium does not increase maternal bone resorption, and studies have found no correlation between the number of pregnancies a woman has had and the density of her bones. The AI for calcium for pregnant women age 19 and older—1000 mg per day—is therefore not increased above nonpregnant needs.[6] The AI for calcium can be met by consuming three to four servings of milk or other dairy products daily. Women who are lactose intolerant can meet their calcium needs with yogurt, cheese, reduced-lactose milk, calcium-rich vegetables, calcium-fortified foods, and calcium supplements.

Vitamin D is needed to ensure adequate calcium absorption

Adequate vitamin D is essential to ensure efficient calcium absorption, but the recommended intake for vitamin D is not increased above nonpregnant levels. Pregnant women who receive regular exposure to sunlight can make sufficient vitamin D in their bodies. If exposure to sunlight is limited, dietary sources such as milk must supply the needed amounts. Inadequate vitamin D may be a particular problem in African American women because their consumption of milk, which is a good source of vitamin D, is often low due to lactose intolerance and their darker pigmentation reduces the synthesis of vitamin D in the skin. It is also a concern in women who remain covered when outdoors. If sufficient vitamin D is not consumed in the diet, careful supplementation should be considered. Most prenatal supplements provide 10 μg of vitamin D, which is twice the AI but well below the UL for pregnancy of 50 μg.[6]

Vitamin C is needed for healthy connective tissue

Vitamin C is important for bone and connective tissue formation because it is needed for the synthesis of collagen, which gives structure to skin, tendons, and the protein matrix of bones. Vitamin C deficiency during pregnancy increases the risk for premature birth and other complications. The RDA is increased by 10 mg per day during pregnancy.[7] The requirement for vitamin C can easily be met with foods such as strawberries and citrus fruit; supplements are generally not necessary.

Low folate increases the risk of neural tube defects

Folate is needed for the synthesis of DNA, and thus, for cell division. During pregnancy, cells multiply to form the placenta, expand maternal blood, and allow for fetal growth. Adequate folate intake is crucial even before conception because rapid cell division occurs in the first days and weeks of pregnancy.

Folate deficiency can cause megaloblastic anemia in the mother. In the baby, low folate levels increase the risk of abnormalities in the formation of the **neural tube**. The neural tube is the portion of the embryo that develops into the brain and spinal cord. During development, neural tissue forms a groove; the groove closes when the sides fold together to form a tube (Figure 12.9). This neural tube closure occurs between 21 and 28 days of development. If it does not occur normally, the infant will be born with a neural tube defect, such as spina bifida, a defect in which the neural tube does not close completely (see Chapter 8). Folate continues to be important even after the

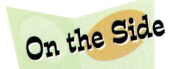

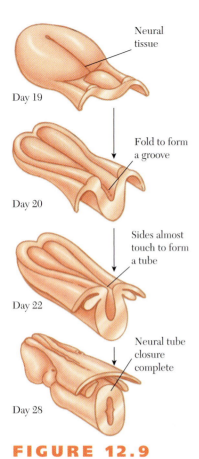

Neural tissue

Day 19

Fold to form a groove

Day 20

Sides almost touch to form a tube

Day 22

Neural tube closure complete

Day 28

FIGURE 12.9

During embryonic development, a flat plate of neural tissue forms a groove and then the edges fold up and join to form the neural tube, which will become the brain and spinal cord.

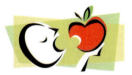

Pregnant women don't necessarily need vitamin and mineral supplements, but they are typically recommended during the last two trimesters. The supplement can help ensure that a pregnant woman and her baby are getting all the micronutrients they need.

neural tube closes. Inadequate folate intake is associated with premature and low-birth-weight births and fetal growth retardation.[8]

Because the neural tube closes so early in development, often before a woman even knows she is pregnant, the DRIs recommend that women capable of becoming pregnant consume 400 μg daily of synthetic folic acid from fortified foods, supplements, or a combination of the two, in addition to consuming a varied diet rich in natural sources of folate (see Chapter 8, Piece it Together: Is it Hard to Meet Folate Recommendations?). During pregnancy, the RDA is 600 μg of dietary folate equivalents per day.[9] Natural sources of folate include orange juice, legumes, leafy green vegetables, and organ meats. Fortified sources include breads, cereals, and other enriched grain products. Folic acid supplements can also be used to meet this goal. Most prenatal supplements contain 400 μg of folic acid.

Vitamin B_{12} is needed to activate folate Vitamin B_{12} is essential for the regeneration of active forms of folate, so a deficiency of vitamin B_{12} can also result in megaloblastic anemia. Based on the amount of vitamin B_{12} transferred from the mother to the fetus during pregnancy, and the increased efficiency of vitamin B_{12} absorption that occurs during pregnancy, the RDA for pregnancy is set at 2.6 μg per day.[9] This recommendation is easily met by a diet containing even small amounts of animal products. Vegetarian diets are generally safe for pregnant women but vegans must consume foods fortified with vitamin B_{12} or take vitamin B_{12} supplements to meet the needs of mother and fetus.

Zinc is important for growth and development Zinc is involved in the synthesis and function of DNA and RNA and the synthesis of proteins. It is therefore extremely important for growth and development. Zinc deficiency during pregnancy is associated with an increased risk of fetal malformations, premature birth, and low birth weight.[10] Because zinc absorption is inhibited by high iron intakes, iron supplements may compromise zinc status if the diet is low in zinc. The RDA is 11 mg per day for pregnant women 19 years of age and older.[11]

Iron needs increase by 50% during pregnancy Iron needs are high during pregnancy to provide for the synthesis of hemoglobin and other iron-containing proteins in both maternal and fetal tissues. The RDA for pregnant women is 27 mg per day, which is 50% higher than the 18 mg per day recommended for non-pregnant women.[11] Many women fail to meet their iron needs even when not pregnant. Because low iron stores are so common among women of childbearing age, women often start pregnancy with diminished iron stores and quickly become deficient. This occurs despite the fact that iron absorption is increased during pregnancy and iron losses are decreased due to the cessation of menstruation. Iron deficiency anemia during pregnancy has been associated with an increased risk of low birth weight and preterm delivery.[12] Babies born at term usually have adequate iron stores even if the mother is deficient. But, because most of the transfer of iron from mother to child occurs during the last trimester, babies born prematurely may not have had time to accumulate sufficient iron.

It takes an exceptionally well-planned diet to meet iron needs during pregnancy. Red meats, leafy green vegetables, and fortified cereals are good sources of iron. Foods that enhance iron absorption, such as citrus fruit and meat, should also be included in the diet. Iron supplements are typically recommended during the second and third trimesters.

Prenatal supplements are typically recommended Even when a healthy diet is consumed it is difficult to meet all the vitamin and mineral needs of pregnancy. Generally supplements of folic acid are recommended before and during pregnancy, and iron supplements are recommended during the second and third trimesters.[1] A multivitamin and mineral supplement may also be necessary for those whose food choices are limited, such as vegetarians, and for those whose needs are very high, such as pregnant teenagers. A prenatal supplement, however, must be taken in conjunction with, not in place of, a carefully planned diet.

PIECE IT TOGETHER

Nutrient Needs for a Successful Pregnancy

Tina is 4 months pregnant. From the start—before she tried to conceive—she has been careful about her diet. She has paid attention to her folate intake by eating plenty of leafy greens, which are naturally high in folate, and enriched grain products, which are fortified with folic acid. Now that she is entering her second trimester, her doctor is concerned that her diet may be deficient in iron and has prescribed a prenatal supplement. Tina follows his advice and takes the supplement, but she is curious about whether her diet meets the nutrient needs of pregnancy without supplements. She records her intake for a typical day:

Food	Food Guide Pyramid Group/Serving
Breakfast	
1 cup corn flakes	1 grain
with 1 cup reduced-fat milk	1 milk
3/4 cup orange juice	1 fruit
1 cup decaffeinated coffee with sugar and cream	fats, oils, and sweets
Lunch	
Tuna sandwich	
3 oz tuna	1 meat
2 tsp mayonnaise	fats, oils, and sweets
2 slices white bread	2 grain
20 french fries	2 vegetable
1 can orange soda	fats, oils, and sweets
3 chocolate chip cookies	1 grain
1 apple	1 fruit
Dinner	
3 oz chicken leg	1 meat
1/2 cup peas	1 vegetable
1 piece corn bread	2 grain
1 tsp margarine	fats, oils, and sweets
1 cup lettuce and tomato salad	1 vegetable
1 Tbsp dressing	fats, oils, and sweets
1 cup reduced-fat milk	1 milk

Tina's current diet meets the recommendations of the Food Guide Pyramid for a nonpregnant woman, but during her second and third trimesters, she will need an extra 340 to 450 Calories per day. To obtain this extra energy she should add a serving of vegetables, a serving of milk, an ounce of meat, and a serving of grain products.

WHAT NUTRIENTS ARE PROVIDED BY THESE ADDITIONS?

An added serving of whole grains will add iron, zinc, fiber, and B vitamins. The extra serving of vegetables will add folate, fiber, and vitamin C or A. The extra serving of dairy products will add protein, riboflavin, vitamin D, and calcium. Even though the recommendation for calcium intake is not increased during pregnancy, most young women do not meet calcium needs, and three servings from this group provide about 1000 mg, which is the AI for young adults. The extra meat adds protein, and if it is from red meat, it provides an excellent source of absorbable iron and zinc as well as vitamins B_{12} and B_6.

TINA IS OVERWEIGHT. SHOULD SHE STILL ADD THESE FOODS TO HER DIET? WHY OR WHY NOT?

Your answer:

DOES TINA'S DIET MEET THE IRON NEEDS OF PREGNANCY WITHOUT SUPPLEMENTS?

Her current diet provides 10.5 mg of iron—significantly less than the RDA of 27 mg for pregnant women.

COULD TINA MODIFY HER DIET TO MEET THE IRON RECOMMENDATIONS WITHOUT INCREASING HER CALORIE INTAKE? SUGGEST SOME CHANGES.

Your answer:

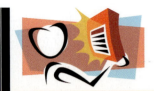

Off the Label: What's in Your Prenatal Supplement?

Most pregnant women leave their first prenatal doctor's visit with a prescription for a prenatal vitamin and mineral supplement. What's in these supplements? Do they meet all the needs of pregnancy?

A look at the supplement label shows you that a typical prenatal supplement contains more than 15 vitamins and minerals. It contains enough folate and iron to meet recommendations and the same can be said for many of the other nutrients, but taking a prenatal supplement does not mean you can ignore your diet. Even though they supply many vitamins and minerals at levels that meet or slightly exceed the recommended intake for pregnancy, some are present in amounts that do not meet the needs of pregnancy, and others are missing altogether. For example, the tablet shown in the table contains only 200 mg of calcium, which is only 20% of the recommended intake for a pregnant woman age 19 or older. The reason it does not contain more is that the tablet would have to be very large to provide the recommendation of 1000 mg. To meet her needs, a pregnant woman would need to consume this tablet plus the amount of calcium in about three glasses of milk. For similar reasons, the tablet doesn't meet the recommendation for magnesium.

Even if all the calcium and magnesium needed for pregnancy could be packed into a little pill, it still would not provide everything needed in an adequate diet. Prenatal supplements do not contain the protein needed for tissue synthesis or the complex carbohydrates needed for energy. They lack fiber, which helps prevent constipation, and they do not contain fluid for expanding blood volume and maintaining normal bowel function. They also don't contain other food components such as the phytochemicals that are supplied by a diet rich in whole grains, fruits, and vegetables. Taking a multivitamin and mineral supplement during pregnancy can be beneficial as long as the recommended dosage is not exceeded and they do not take the place of a carefully planned diet.

Nutrient	Amount per Tablet	Recommendations for Pregnancy*
Vitamin A (μg)	800	770
Vitamin D (μg)	10	5
Vitamin E (mg α-tocopherol)	11–15	15
Vitamin C (mg)	80–120	85
Folate (μg DFE)	680–1700	600
Thiamin (mg)	1.5	1.4
Riboflavin (mg)	1.6–3.0	1.4
Niacin (mg)	17–20	18
Vitamin B$_6$ (mg)	2.6–10	1.9
Vitamin B$_{12}$ (μg)	2.5–12	2.6
Biotin (μg)	30	30
Pantothenic acid (mg)	7	6
Calcium (mg)	200	1000
Iron (mg)	60–65	27
Magnesium (mg)	100	350
Copper (mg)	2–3	1.0
Zinc (mg)	25	11

*Values represent recommendations for a pregnant woman 19 to 30 years of age during her third trimester.

The developing child is vulnerable to poor nutrition and damaging substances

Cells that are rapidly dividing, differentiating, and moving to form organs and other structures are particularly vulnerable. Anything that interferes with development can cause a baby to be born too soon or too small or can result in birth defects. Any chemical, biological, or physical agent that causes birth defects is called a **teratogen**. The placenta prevents some teratogens from passing from the mother's blood to the embryonic or fetal blood, but it cannot prevent the passage of all hazardous substances. Because the majority of cell differentiation occurs during the embryonic period, this is the time when exposure to teratogens can do the most damage, but vital body organs can still be affected during the fetal period (Figure 12.10). Each organ system develops at a different rate and time, so each has a critical period when exposure to a teratogen or other insult can disrupt development causing irreversible damage. If the damage is severe, it may result in a **spontaneous abortion** or **miscarriage**.

Teratogen A substance that can cause birth defects.

Spontaneous abortion or **miscarriage** Interruption of pregnancy prior to the 7th month.

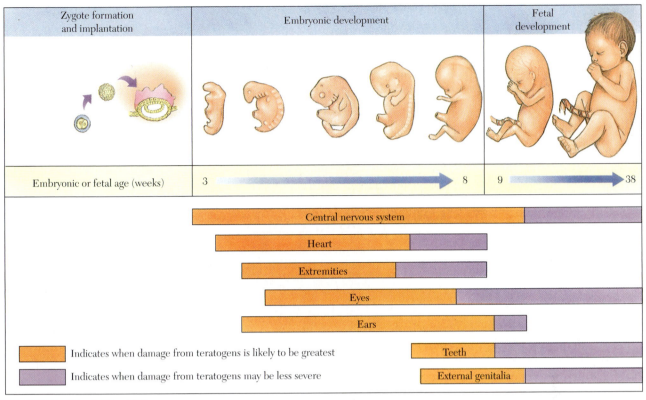

| | Zygote formation and implantation | Embryonic development | Fetal development |

Embryonic or fetal age (weeks)   3 ———————————→ 8   9 ——————————→ 38

Central nervous system
Heart
Extremities
Eyes
Ears
Teeth
External genitalia

■ Indicates when damage from teratogens is likely to be greatest

■ Indicates when damage from teratogens may be less severe

FIGURE 12.10

The critical periods of development vary for different body systems, but for most, exposure to teratogens is most damaging during the embryonic period. (Adapted from Moore, K., and Persaud, T. *The Developing Human*, 5th ed. Philadelphia: W. B. Saunders Company, 1993.)

Deficiencies or excesses of nutrients can cause birth defects

Consuming a diet that is low in energy or nutrients can affect the development of the fetus. Maternal malnutrition can cause fetal growth retardation, low infant birth weight, birth defects, premature birth, spontaneous abortion, and stillbirth. The effect of malnutrition depends on what is missing from the diet and when during the pregnancy it occurs. In general, poor nutrition early in pregnancy affects embryonic development and the potential of the embryo to survive and poor nutrition in the latter part of pregnancy affects fetal growth. Vitamin and mineral intake is crucial early in pregnancy when cell division and differentiation are taking place; malformations or death can result if the embryo does not receive adequate nutrients. After the first trimester, low intakes of micronutrients are less likely to cause birth defects because most organs and structures have already formed, but a low-calorie intake will interfere with fetal growth. Even a mild energy restriction during the last trimester, when the fetus is growing rapidly, can affect birth weight.

Excesses of some nutrients can cause birth defects. For example, excess vitamin D can cause mental retardation in the newborn. Too much preformed vitamin A is of particular concern because the risk of abnormalities in the offspring increases even when maternal intake is not extremely high. Too much vitamin A early in pregnancy is the most damaging. A UL of 3000 µg per day has been established for pregnant women, ages 19 to 50 years.[11] Supplements consumed during pregnancy should therefore contain β-carotene, which is not teratogenic.

Food cravings and aversions during pregnancy are usually harmless

When you think of food and pregnancy, pickles and ice cream may come to mind, but most women just crave the ice cream. The foods most commonly craved during pregnancy are ice cream, sweets, candy (especially chocolate), fruit, and fish. Common aversions include coffee and other caffeinated drinks, highly seasoned foods, or fried foods.[13] Why women have these cravings and aversions is still a matter for debate. It has been suggested that hormonal or physiological changes during pregnancy—in particular, changes in taste and smell—may be the physiological basis. But there are also psychological and behavioral factors involved.

Usually the things women crave during pregnancy are foods, and generally they have no harmful effects and can be consumed within reason. After all, a healthy diet not only meets your nutritional needs, but also your emotional needs and individual preferences. But when the things craved, and consumed, are not food, the health consequences can be serious. The abnormal craving for and ingestion of nonfood substances having little or no nutritional value is called **pica**. Women with pica commonly consume clay, laundry starch, ice and freezer frost, baking soda, cornstarch, and ashes. Consuming large amounts of these can reduce the intake of nutrient-dense foods, reduce nutrient absorption from food, increase the risk of consuming toxins, and even cause intestinal obstructions. Complications of pica include iron-deficiency anemia, lead poisoning, and parasitic infestations.[14] Anemia and high blood pressure are more common in mothers who practice pica, but it is not clear if pica is a result of these conditions or a cause. In newborns, anemia and low birth weight are often related to pica in the mother.

Pica has been described since antiquity but its cause is still a mystery. It was once thought that pica was an attempt to meet micronutrient needs. It is now believed that pica may be more related to cultural factors than the need for micronutrients. It is more common in areas of low socioeconomic status and among women (especially pregnant women) and children.[14]

Exposure to environmental toxins can be dangerous
In a pregnant woman, exposure to toxic substances—such as cleaning solvents, lead, mercury, insecticides, and paint—can affect her developing child. Therefore, pregnant women need to be aware of the potential toxins in their food, water, and environment. In the case of mercury, exposure can be controlled by avoiding excess consumption of fish such as shark, swordfish, king mackerel, or tilefish and by limiting tuna intake to no more than 6 ounces of albacore per week. Up to 12 ounces (about 2 meals) a week of varieties of fish and shellfish that are lower in mercury, such as shrimp, canned light tuna, salmon, pollock, and catfish, can be safely consumed.[15]

Cigarette smoke affects the baby before birth and throughout life
If a woman smokes cigarettes during pregnancy, her baby will be affected before birth and throughout life. Compounds in tobacco smoke bind to hemoglobin and reduce oxygen delivery to fetal tissues. The nicotine absorbed from cigarette smoke constricts arteries and limits blood flow, reducing both oxygen and nutrient delivery to the fetus. Low birth weight is about 58% more common in offspring of smokers than nonsmokers.[16] Even exposure to cigarette smoke from the environment has been found to increase the risk of low birth weight.[17] The risks of miscarriage, stillbirth, and premature birth are also increased in mothers who smoke. The risk of **sudden infant death syndrome (SIDS, or crib death)** and respiratory problems are increased in children exposed to cigarette smoke both in the uterus and after birth. The effects of maternal smoking follow children throughout life; they are more likely to have frequent colds and develop lung problems later in life.[18]

Alcohol consumption is a major cause of birth defects
You wouldn't serve your baby a glass of wine, yet about 13% of women report drinking alcohol during pregnancy.[19] Alcohol consumption during pregnancy is one of the leading causes of preventable birth defects. Alcohol is a teratogen that is particularly damaging to the developing central nervous system.[20] It also indirectly affects fetal growth and development because it is a toxin that reduces blood flow to the placenta, thereby decreasing the delivery of oxygen and nutrients to the fetus. The consumption of alcohol can also impair maternal nutritional status, further increasing the risk to the embryo or fetus.

Pica An abnormal craving for and ingestion of unusual food and nonfood substances.

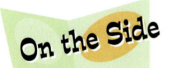

On the Side

The word *pica* is Latin for magpie—a bird notorious for eating almost anything.

Sudden infant death syndrome (SIDS) or **crib death** The unexplained death of an infant, usually during sleep.

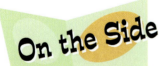

On the Side

Coffee is part of our culture, but many pregnant women limit coffee intake because they are afraid the caffeine in coffee will harm their baby. Research, however, has found little consistent evidence that caffeine consumption increases the risk of any reproductive problem.

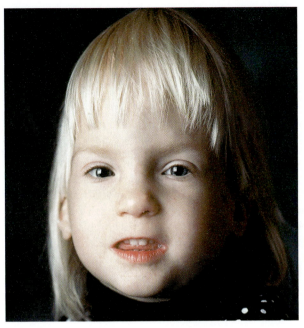

FIGURE 12.11

Children with fetal alcohol syndrome have common facial characteristics. The head circumference is small, the cheekbones are poorly developed, the nose is short with a low nasal bridge between the eyes, the area under the nose is flat, and the upper lip is thin. (George Steinmetz)

Prenatal exposure to alcohol can cause a spectrum of disorders depending on the dose, timing, and duration of the exposure. One of the most severe effects of drinking during pregnancy is **fetal alcohol syndrome (FAS)**, which causes facial deformities, growth retardation, and permanent brain damage (Figure 12.11). Newborns with the syndrome may be shaky and irritable, with poor muscle tone and alcohol withdrawal symptoms. Other problems include heart and urinary tract defects, impaired vision and hearing, and delayed language development. Mental retardation is the most common and most serious effect. Not all babies exposed to alcohol have FAS, but many have some alcohol-related problems. Alcohol-related neurodevelopmental disorders (ARND) are functional or mental impairments linked to prenatal alcohol exposure, and alcohol-related birth defects (ARBD) are malformations in the skeleton or major organ systems. These conditions are less severe than FAS, but occur about three times more often.

Because alcohol consumption in each trimester has been associated with abnormalities, and because there is no level of alcohol consumption that is known to be safe, complete abstinence from alcohol is recommended during pregnancy. Warning labels that appear on containers of beer, wine, and hard liquor state that "According to the Surgeon General, women should not drink alcoholic beverages during pregnancy because of the risk of birth defects."

Illegal drugs can affect pregnancy outcome
Substance abuse during pregnancy is a national health issue. Prenatal exposure to cocaine, opiates, or amphetamines has been shown to affect infant behavior and impact learning and attention span during childhood.[21] It is estimated that from 1 to 11% of babies born each year have been exposed to drugs during the prenatal period. These numbers include only the use of illicit drugs and would be much larger if alcohol and nicotine were included.[22]

Marijuana and cocaine are drugs that are commonly used during pregnancy. Both cross the placenta and enter the fetal blood. There is little evidence that marijuana affects fetal outcome, but cocaine use increases the risk of complications to the mother and creates problems for the infant before, during, and after delivery.[23] Cocaine is a central nervous system stimulant, but many of its effects during pregnancy occur because it constricts blood vessels, thereby reducing the flow of oxygen and nutrients to the rapidly dividing fetal cells. Cocaine use during pregnancy is associated with a high rate of miscarriages, intrauterine growth retardation, spontaneous abortion, premature labor and delivery, low-birth-weight infants, and birth

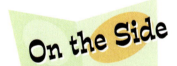

Fetal alcohol syndrome A characteristic group of physical and mental abnormalities in an infant resulting from maternal alcohol consumption during pregnancy.

On the Side

Fetal alcohol syndrome is 100% preventable if a woman does not drink while she is pregnant. It occurs in 0.2 to 1.5 per 1000 live births from the general population and 43 of every 1000 babies born to heavy drinkers.

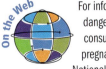

For information on the dangers of alcohol consumption during pregnancy go to the National Organization on Fetal Alcohol Syndrome at **www.nofas.org/**

defects.[24] Babies exposed to cocaine show signs of withdrawal and abnormalities in arousal, attention, and neurological function, but there is little evidence that these problems continue beyond early infancy and childhood.[23,24]

Complications During Pregnancy Put Mother and Baby at Risk

Most of the 4 million women who give birth every year in the United States are healthy during pregnancy and produce healthy babies. However, childbearing is not without risks. In the United States, 300 to 500 women die yearly as a result of childbirth. Eleven percent of babies are born too soon, 7.4% are low birth weight, and 7.2 out of each 1000 born alive die within the first year of life.[25] If complications such as diabetes and hypertension that occur during pregnancy are caught early they can often be managed, allowing for a healthy delivery (Figure 12.12).

Gestational diabetes makes delivery difficult for mother and child

Gestational diabetes A consistently elevated blood glucose level that develops during pregnancy and returns to normal after delivery.

Diabetes that develops during pregnancy is known as **gestational diabetes**. It occurs in 2 to 6% of all pregnancies and is most common in obese women.[26] It usually disappears when the pregnancy is completed, but the mother remains at higher risk for developing type 2 diabetes later on in life (see Chapter 4). In addition to its effects on the mother's health, gestational diabetes increases risks for the baby. Because glucose in the mother's blood passes freely across the placenta, when the mother's blood levels are high, the growing fetus receives extra calories. This extra energy promotes growth, resulting in babies who are large for gestational age and consequently at increased risk of complications. As with other types of diabetes, the treatment of gestational diabetes involves consuming a carefully planned diet, moderate daily exercise, and in some cases, insulin.

Pregnancy-induced hypertension can be life-threatening

Pregnancy-induced hypertension A spectrum of conditions involving elevated blood pressure during pregnancy.

Pregnancy-induced hypertension is a spectrum of conditions involving elevated blood pressure that occurs in about 6 to 8% of pregnancies. It is a major risk factor for maternal and fetal illness and death; it accounts for nearly 15% of pregnancy-related maternal deaths in the United States.[27] It is more common in mothers under 20 or over 35 years of age, those in low-income groups, and women with chronic hypertension or kidney disease.

Gestational hypertension High blood pressure that develops after the 20th week of pregnancy and returns to normal after delivery. It may be an early sign of preeclampsia.

The mildest form of pregnancy-induced hypertension is **gestational hypertension**, which is an abnormal rise in blood pressure that occurs after the 20th week of pregnancy. If the rise in blood pressure is accompanied by excretion of protein in the urine

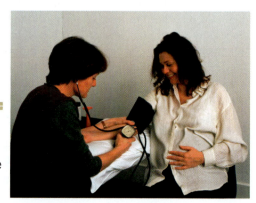

FIGURE 12.12

Prenatal care helps prevent complications during pregnancy. By monitoring the mother's blood pressure as shown here, as well as her blood sugar and the baby's size and heartbeat, problems can be identified and treated early. (Faye Norman/Science Photo Library/Photo Researchers)

and edema the condition is called **preeclampsia**. Its onset is often signaled by a weight gain of several pounds within a few days. It can progress to a more severe form of pregnancy-induced hypertension called **eclampsia**, in which life-threatening seizures occur.

The cause of pregnancy-induced hypertension is not known. At one time low-sodium diets were prescribed to prevent preeclampsia but more recent studies have found reducing sodium intake to be of no benefit.[5] Calcium may play a role in preventing pregnancy-induced hypertension but the evidence of a connection is not strong enough to support routine supplementation. Pregnant teens, individuals with inadequate calcium intake, and women known to be at risk of developing pregnancy-induced hypertension may benefit from additional dietary calcium during pregnancy.[28] Treatment includes bed rest and careful medical attention. The condition usually resolves after delivery.

Preeclampsia A condition characterized by an increase in body weight, elevated blood pressure, protein in the urine, and edema. It can progress to eclampsia which can be life-threatening to mother and fetus.

Eclampsia A life-threatening condition that can occur during pregnancy. It is characterized by high blood pressure, protein in the urine, convulsions, and coma.

Nutrition, Income, and Age Can Affect Pregnancy Outcome

Some women and their babies are at increased risk for complications because they start their pregnancy poorly nourished. Others may be at risk because they have limited access to nutritious foods and prenatal care. The mother's age can also affect the chances of a healthy pregnancy.

Nutritional health is important for conception and pregnancy outcome

Being well nourished before pregnancy is important to support conception and maximize the likelihood of a healthy pregnancy. If a woman is consuming a diet that meets her needs for energy and all essential nutrients and that is plentiful in whole grains, fruits, and vegetables, it will help ensure that her body is prepared for a pregnancy. Deficiencies or excesses can reduce fertility and affect pregnancy outcome. Starvation diets, eating disorders, and excessive athletic activity, such as marathon running, can interfere with ovulation and therefore make conception less likely. Obesity can alter hormone levels and decrease fertility. Excess vitamin A early in pregnancy can cause birth defects and poor folate status can increase the likelihood of birth defects.

The use of certain birth control methods can affect nutritional status, and these can therefore have an impact on a subsequent pregnancy. Oral contraceptives may cause a rise in fasting blood sugar and a tendency toward abnormal glucose tolerance in those with a family history of diabetes. They may also cause changes in body composition, including weight gain due to water retention and an increase in lean body mass. Oral contraceptives may reduce the need for iron by reducing menstrual flow and increasing iron absorption. Therefore, a special RDA for iron of 11.4 mg per day has been established for those taking oral contraceptives (the RDA for menstruating women not using oral contraceptives is 18 mg per day). Blood levels of some B vitamins have been found to be low in oral contraceptive users, although it is not known whether these changes in blood levels reflect an increased need for these nutrients.[9] For example, oral contraceptive use is associated with reduced blood levels of vitamins B_6 and B_{12}. If conception occurs soon after oral contraceptive use stops, these levels will not have had time to return to normal before pregnancy begins.

A woman's pregnancy history also affects her chances of having a healthy pregnancy. Frequent pregnancies, with little time between, increase the risk for malnutrition because the mother may not have replenished nutrient stores depleted in the first pregnancy when she becomes pregnant again. A short interval between pregnancies also increases the risk of preterm and low-birth-weight infants. Women with a history of poor pregnancy outcome are generally at increased risk. For example, a woman who has had a number of miscarriages is more likely to have another, and a woman who has had one child with a birth defect has an increased risk for defects in subsequent children.

On the Web

For information about prenatal care, risks and problems during pregnancy, and postnatal care, go to the New York Online Access to Health (NOAH) at **www.noah-health.org/** and click on "Pregnancy" under Health Topics.

Poverty increases the risks of pregnancy

One of the greatest risk factors for poor pregnancy outcome is low-income level. Poverty limits access to food, education, and health care.[29] Low-income women have a higher incidence of low-birth-weight and preterm infants. Low-income women are unlikely to receive any prenatal care until late in pregnancy. One federally funded program that addresses the nutritional needs of pregnant women is the Special Supplemental Nutrition Program for Women, Infants, and Children (WIC). WIC has been shown to reduce health-care costs by providing preventive care to low-income pregnant women through nutrition education and food vouchers. This program provides services to pregnant women, to nonlactating women for 6 months after birth, to lactating women for 12 months after birth, and to infants and children up to 5 years of age, but it does not address the need for good nutrition for women planning a pregnancy.

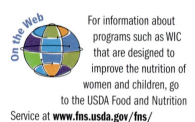

For information about programs such as WIC that are designed to improve the nutrition of women and children, go to the USDA Food and Nutrition Service at **www.fns.usda.gov/fns/**

Pregnant teenagers face economic, social, medical, and nutritional problems

Pregnancy places a stress on the body at any age, but this is compounded when the mother herself is still growing. Although the rate of teen pregnancy has been decreasing over the past decade, from 62.1 babies per 1000 teens in 1991, to 48.5 per 1000 in 2001, it remains a major public health problem.[30] Pregnant teens are at greater risk of pregnancy-induced hypertension and are more likely to deliver preterm and low-birth-weight babies. To produce a healthy baby, a pregnant teenager needs early medical intervention and nutritional counseling.

Adolescent girls continue to grow and mature physically for about 4 to 7 years after menstruation begins. Therefore the diet of a pregnant teen must provide both for her growth and that of her baby. Because the nutrient needs of a pregnant teen may be higher than those of a pregnant adult, the DRIs include a special set of nutrient recommendations for pregnant teens (Figure 12.13). Consuming a diet that meets these needs can be challenging. Even nonpregnant teens often fall short of meeting their nutrient needs. Nutrients that are commonly low in the diets of pregnant teens are calcium, iron, zinc, magnesium, vitamin D, folate, and vitamin B$_6$.[6,9,11]

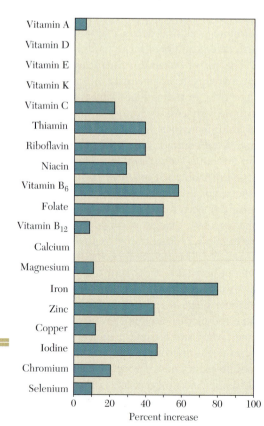

FIGURE 12.13

The need for many micronutrients increases during pregnancy. The percentage increases in micronutrient needs above nonpregnant levels are shown here for a 14- to 18-year-old teen during pregnancy.

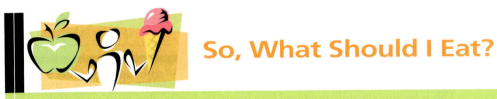

So, What Should I Eat?

Make nutrient-dense choices to meet the extra nutrient needs of pregnancy
- Have yogurt for a mid-morning snack
- Put some peanut butter on your banana to add some protein to your snack
- Have a plate of pasta—it's fortified with folic acid

Drink plenty of fluids
- Have a glass of milk and get calcium with your fluids
- Keep a bottle of water at your desk or in your car
- Relax with a cup of tea

Indulge your cravings, within reason
- That bowl of ice cream does add calcium and protein
- Enjoy your cookies, with a glass of milk

Older mothers are more likely to begin pregnancy with health problems

The nutritional requirements for older women during pregnancy are no different than for women in their 20's, but pregnancy after the age of 35 does carry additional risks because older women are more likely to start pregnancy with health problems such as cardiovascular disease, kidney disorders, obesity, and diabetes.[31] During pregnancy, older women are more likely to develop gestational diabetes, pregnancy-induced hypertension, and other complications. They also have a higher incidence of low-birth-weight deliveries and of chromosomal abnormalities, especially **Down syndrome**. Today, careful medical monitoring throughout pregnancy is reducing the risks to older mothers and their babies (Figure 12.14).

Medications used to treat existing illness can also affect nutritional status and consequently both fertility and pregnancy outcome. A woman who is considering pregnancy should discuss her plans with her physician in order to determine the risks associated with any medication she is taking.

Down syndrome A disorder caused by extra genetic material that results in distinctive facial characteristics, mental retardation, and other abnormalities.

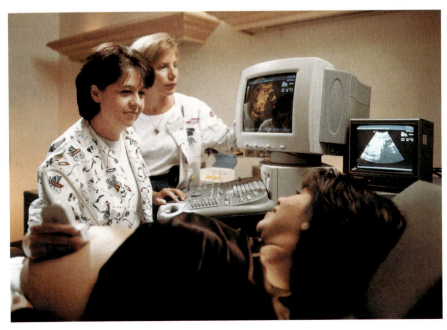

FIGURE 12.14

Prenatal care with careful medical monitoring can help older women have uncomplicated pregnancies and produce healthy babies. (Steward Cohen/Stone/Getty Images)

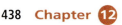

5. The hormones that direct changes in maternal physiology and the growth and development of the fetus sometimes cause unwanted side effects. Changes in fluid volume may cause edema. Digestive system discomforts that are common in pregnancy include morning sickness, heartburn, constipation, and hemorrhoids.

6. During pregnancy the requirements for energy, protein, water, vitamins, and minerals increase. The B vitamins are needed to support increased energy and protein metabolism; calcium, vitamin D, and vitamin C are needed for bone and connective tissue growth; protein, folate, vitamin B_{12}, and zinc are needed for cell replication; and iron is needed for red blood cell synthesis. Supplements containing iron and folic acid are recommended.

7. Because the embryo and fetus are rapidly developing and growing, they are susceptible to damage from poor nutrition and physical, chemical, or other environmental teratogens. Severe defects in development often result in miscarriage. Foods consumed due to food cravings are generally safe unless nonfood items are craved. Environmental toxins such as mercury in fish cause birth defects. Exposure to cigarette smoke causes low birth weight. Alcohol consumption during pregnancy is a leading cause of mental retardation and other birth defects. The use of illegal drugs such as cocaine also increases the risk of low birth weight and birth defects.

8. Complications during pregnancy increase risk for mother and child. Gestational diabetes involves a high blood sugar in the mother that provides extra calories to the growing baby. Pregnancy-induced hypertension may involve high blood pressure (gestational hypertension), edema, weight gain, and protein in the urine (preeclampsia), and in severe cases can be life-threatening (eclampsia).

9. Nutritional status, income, and age affect pregnancy outcome. Risks of pregnancy are increased by poor nutritional status before pregnancy; poverty, which limits access to food and health care; age that is under 20 years because the mother is still growing, or over 35 years because the mother is more likely to have preexisting health conditions.

10. During lactation the need for protein, fluid, and many vitamins and minerals is even greater than during pregnancy.

11. Newborns grow more rapidly and require more energy and protein per kilogram of body weight than at any other time in life. Fat and fluid needs are also proportionately higher than in adults. A diet that meets energy, protein, and fat needs may not necessarily meet the need for iron, fluoride, and vitamins D and K. Growth is the best indicator of adequate nutrition in the infant.

12. Breast milk is the ideal food for new babies. It is designed specifically for the human newborn; it is always available; it requires no special equipment, mixing, or sterilization; and it provides immune protection. If breast-feeding is not chosen, there are many infant formulas on the market that are patterned after human milk and provide adequate nutrition to the baby. Formula is the best option when the mother is ill or is taking prescription or illicit drugs, or when the infant has special nutritional needs.

13. Introducing solid foods between 4 and 6 months of age adds iron and other nutrients to the diet and aids in muscle development. Newly introduced foods should be appropriate to the child's stage of development and offered one at a time to monitor for food allergies. Food allergies occur when the immune system reacts to a food. They can be confirmed by an elimination diet and a food challenge. Food intolerances cause GI symptoms but are not caused by antibody production by the immune system.

REVIEW QUESTIONS

1. Why is the adequacy of the mother's diet so important early in pregnancy?
2. List three physiological changes that occur in the mother's body during pregnancy.
3. How much weight should a woman gain during pregnancy?
4. How do the recommendations for weight gain differ for overweight and underweight women?
5. What kind of exercise is safe during pregnancy?
6. How do the requirements for energy and protein change during pregnancy?
7. Why does the mother's recommended intake for iron increase during pregnancy?
8. How do a woman's energy and protein requirements change during lactation?

9. How does alcohol consumed by a woman during pregnancy affect the child?
10. Why does gestational diabetes cause babies to be born too big?
11. How does maternal age affect nutrient requirements during pregnancy?
12. Why do babies need a higher fat diet than adults?
13. What are the advantages of breast-feeding?
14. When is bottle-feeding a better choice?
15. When should solid and semisolid foods be introduced into an infant's diet?
16. Why is it important to introduce new foods one at a time?
17. What steps can caregivers take to reduce the risk of a child developing food allergies?

REFERENCES

1. Committee on Nutritional Status during Pregnancy and Lactation, National Academy of Sciences. *Nutrition During Pregnancy.* Washington, DC: National Academy Press, 1990.

2. Bryson, S. R., Theriot, L., Ryan, N. J., et al. Primary follow-up care in a multidisciplinary setting enhances catch-up growth of very-low-birth-weight infants. *J. Am. Diet. Assoc.* 97:386–390, 1997.

3. American College of Sports Medicine. *ACSM's Guidelines for Exercise Testing and Prescription,* 6th ed. Baltimore: Lippincott Williams & Wilkins, 2000.

4. Food and Nutrition Board, Institute of Medicine. *Dietary Reference Intakes for Energy, Carbohydrates, Fiber, Fat, Protein and Amino Acids.* Washington, DC: National Academy Press, 2002.

5. Food and Nutrition Board, Institute of Medicine. *Dietary Reference Intakes for Water, Potassium, Sodium, Chloride, and Sulfate.* Washington, DC: National Academy Press, 2004.

6. Food and Nutrition Board, Institute of Medicine. *Dietary Reference Intakes for Calcium, Phosphorus, Magnesium, Vitamin D, and Fluoride.* Washington, DC: National Academy Press, 1997.

7. Food and Nutrition Board, Institute of Medicine. *Dietary Reference Intakes for Vitamin C, Vitamin E, Selenium, and Carotenoids.* Washington, DC: National Academy Press, 2000.

8. Scholl, T. O., and Johnson, W. G. Folic acid: Influence on the outcome of pregnancy. *Am. J. Clin. Nutr.* 71(Suppl.):1295S–1303S, 2000.

9. Food and Nutrition Board, Institute of Medicine. *Dietary Reference Intakes for Thiamin, Riboflavin, Niacin, Vitamin B-6, Folate, Vitamin B-12, Pantothenic Acid, Biotin, and Choline.* Washington, DC: National Academy Press, 1998.

10. King, J. C. Determinants of maternal zinc status during pregnancy. *Am. J. Clin. Nutr.* 71(Suppl.):1334S–1343S, 2000.

11. Food and Nutrition Board, Institute of Medicine. *Dietary Reference Intakes for Vitamin A, Vitamin K, Arsenic, Boron, Chromium, Copper, Iodine, Iron, Manganese, Molybdenum, Nickel, Silicon, Vanadium, and Zinc.* Washington, DC: National Academy Press, 2001.

12. Allen, L. H. Anemia and iron deficiency: Effects on pregnancy outcome. *Am. J. Clin. Nutr.* 71(Suppl.):1280S–1284S, 2000.

13. Mitchell, M. K. *Nutrition Across the Life Span.* Philadelphia: W. B. Saunders, 1997.

14. Rose, E. A., Porcerelli, J. H., and Neale, A. V. Pica: Common but commonly missed. *J. Am. Board Fam. Pract.* 13:353–358, 2000.

15. U.S. DHHS and U.S. EPA. FDA and EPA announce the revised consumer advisory on methylmercury in fish. Available online at www.fda.gov/bbs/topics/news/2004/NEW01038.html/Accessed August 25, 2004.

16. Magee, B. D., Hattis, D., and Kivel, N. M. Role of smoking in low birth weight. *J. Reprod. Med.* 49:23–27, 2004.

17. Goel, P., Radotra, A., Singh, I., et al. Effects of passive smoking on outcome in pregnancy. *J Postgrad. Med.* 50:12–16, 2004.

18. National Center for Chronic Disease Prevention and Health Promotion. Women and Smoking: A Report from the Surgeon General 2001. Available online at www.cdc.gov/tobacco/sgv/index.htm/Accessed August 25, 2004.

19. CDC. Alcohol Use Among Women of Childbearing Age—United States, 1991–1999. *MMWR* 51:273–276, 2002. Available online at www.cdc.gov/mmwr/preview/mmwrhtml/mm5113a2.htm/Accessed August 25, 2004.

20. Goodlett, C. R., and Horn, K. H. Mechanisms of alcohol-induced damage to the developing nervous system. *Alcohol Res. Health* 25:175–184, 2001. Available online at www.niaaa.nih.gov/publications/arh25-3/175-184.htm/Accessed August 25, 2004.

21. Wagner, C. L., Katikaneni, L. D., Cox, T. H., and Ryan, R. M. The impact of prenatal drug exposure on the neonate. *Obstet. Gynecol. Clin. North Am.* 25:169–194, 1998.

22. The National Council on Alcoholism and Drug Dependence. Alcohol- and other drug-related birth defects. Facts and information. Available online at www.ncadd.org/facts/defects.html/Accessed August 25, 2004.

23. Chiriboga, C. A. Fetal alcohol and drug effects. *Neurologist* 9:267–279, 2003.

24. Fajemirokun-Odudeyi, O., and Lindow, S. W. Obstetric implications of cocaine use in pregnancy: A literature review. *Eur. J. Obst. Gyncol. Reprod. Biol.* 112:2–8, 2004.

25. Centers for Disease Control and Prevention. Available online at www.cdc.gov/Accessed August 25, 2004.

26. Centers for Disease Control and Prevention. National Agenda for Public Health Action: A National Public Health Initiative on Diabetes and Women's Health. Available online at www.cdc.gov/diabetes/pubs/action/facts.htm/Accessed August 25, 2004.

27. Report of the National High Blood Pressure Education Program Working Group on High Blood Pressure in Pregnancy. *Am. J. Obstet. Gynecol.* 183:S1–S22, 2000.

28. Hofmeyr, G. J., Roodt, A., Atallah, A. N., and Duley, L. Calcium supplementation to prevent pre-eclampsia—a systematic review. *Afr. Med. J.* 93:224–228, 2003.

29. Kramer, M. S., Seguin, L., Lydon, J., and Goulet, L. Socio-economic disparities in pregnancy outcome: Why do the poor fare so poorly? *Paediatr. Perinat. Epidemiol.* 14:194–210, 2000.

30. Women are having more children: New report shows teen births continue to decline. US Department of Health and Human Services. www.hhs.gov/news/press/2002pres/20020212.html/Accessed September 13, 2004.

31. Prysak, M., and Kisly, A. Age greater than thirty-four years is an independent pregnancy risk factor in nulliparous women. *J. Perinatol.* 17:296–300, 1997.

32. Prentice, A. Calcium requirements of breast-feeding mothers. *Nutr. Rev.* 56:124–130, 1998.

33. U.S. Department of Health and Human Services, Centers for Disease Control and Prevention, National Center for Health Statistics. CDC growth charts: United States, advance data. pub. No. 314, June 8, 2000 (revised). Available online at www.cdc.gov/growthcharts/Accessed August 25, 2004.

34. Kelsey, J. J. Hormonal contraception and lactation. *J. Hum. Lact.* 12:315–318, 1996.

35. American Dietetic Association. Breaking the barriers to breastfeeding. *J. Am. Diet. Assoc.* 101:1213–1219, 2001.

36. WHO Fact Sheet No. 180. Reducing mortality from major childhood killer diseases, September 1997. Available online at www.who.int/child-adolescent-health/New_Publications/IMCI/fs_180.html/Accessed September 13, 2004.

37. Golding, J. Unnatural constituents of breast milk—medication, lifestyle, pollutants, viruses. *Early Hum. Dev.* 29 (Suppl.):S29–S43, 1997.

38. Formanek, R. Food allergies: When food becomes the enemy. U.S. Food and Drug Administration. *FDA Consumer,* July/Aug, 2001. Available online at www.fda.gov/fdac/features/2001/401_food.html/Accessed August 25, 2004.

39. Chandra, R. K. Food hypersensitivities and allergic disease: A selective review. *Am. J. Clin. Nutr.* 66(Suppl):526S–529S, 1997.

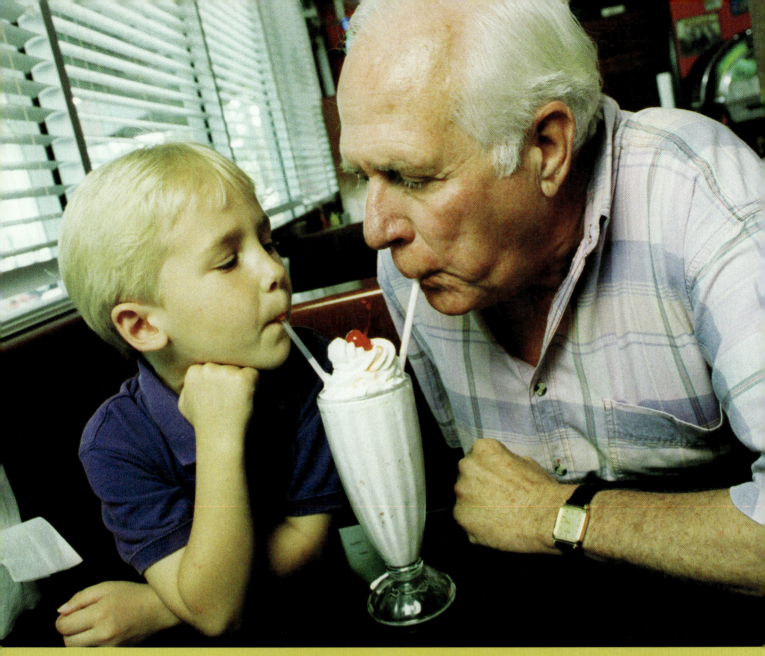

(Jeff Cadge/The Image Bank/Getty Images)

CHAPTER 13 CONCEPTS

- Eating patterns can affect health and nutrition throughout life.
- Children's nutrient intakes must meet their needs for growth and development as well as for maintenance and activity.
- Normal growth is the best indicator of adequate intake.
- Sexual maturation affects nutrient needs.
- Eating disorders and the use of fad diets, sports supplements, and alcohol use all increase during adolescence.
- Americans are living longer than ever before; good nutrition can help to increase the number of healthy years.
- The physiological, social, and economic changes that occur with aging increase the risk of malnutrition.
- Older adults need to consume nutrient-dense diets to meet nutrient needs without exceeding their calorie needs.
- Alcohol consumption can affect nutritional status, judgment, and health.

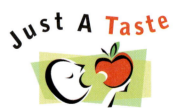

Just A Taste

Does a child's diet affect their risk of heart disease as an adult?

Can fast food and sweetened cereals be part of a healthy diet?

Can a healthy diet keep you young?

Does getting older increase your risk of malnutrition?

Nutrition from 2 to 102

13

INTRODUCTION

The Orlando Sentinel

See How They Run Ocoee Elementary. . . .

By *Kate Santich*

April 12, 2004 . . . At a time when childhood obesity is a national crisis, when kids are casualties in an epidemic of type 2 diabetes and high blood pressure, tiny Ocoee Elementary School has become a microcosm of hope. Professionals from the Health Central Foundation have teamed with teachers and administrators to spread the gospel of healthy living—regular exercise, good eating habits, taking care of yourself. . . .

In January, the entire elementary school—nearly 600 students, kindergarten through fifth grade—launched a "wellness challenge." They walk or run at least once a week, in addition to other exercise. In the classroom, they learn about the food pyramid and the importance of eating fruits and vegetables. On the school's morning announcements, guest speakers talk about drinking water instead of soda and sum up the latest health findings on children.

No one is chastised for being out of shape. The word "diet" is never uttered. The idea is to inspire, not ridicule. And parents are encouraged to join in as well.

To read the entire article, go to www.orlandosentinel.com/.

Why does it matter if you eat doughnuts for breakfast and french fries for lunch when you're 8 years old? It doesn't, if you do it occasionally, but a diet based on foods like these that are high in calories and low in nutrients can affect your growth and increase your risk of developing obesity, heart disease, or diabetes as a child and later on in life. Unfortunately most 8-year-olds, and other children and adolescents in the United States today, are eating doughnuts for breakfast, french fries for lunch, burgers and shakes for dinner, and sodas and chips for snacks a lot more often than is healthy.

441

Good Nutrition Early On Is Key to Health Throughout Life

A healthy diet is important throughout life. As an infant, the nutrients in formula or breast milk allow for optimal brain development. As a young child, consuming the right balance of nutrients is key to optimal growth and development. In the teen years, good nutrition allows for continued growth, maturation, and sexual development. As an adult, a diet that provides enough of the right mix of nutrients can help postpone or avoid the chronic diseases that are common in the developed world. And in older adults, a nutritious diet can help maintain health despite diminishing function in organ systems.

A poor diet at any time in life can affect your immediate and future health. We all know that undernourished children do not grow well and get sick more often and that malnutrition during childhood has long-term effects on growth and development. But, we don't always think about the fact that dietary excesses during childhood and adolescence can also affect health throughout life. Therefore, learning to eat a healthy diet early in life can be one of the most significant factors affecting lifelong health.

Healthy eating habits keep children healthy

We used to think of diabetes, high blood pressure, high cholesterol, and obesity as adult problems. Not any more. These conditions are occurring more and more often in children and teens. The reason is believed to be due to changes in the dietary and exercise patterns of America's youth. The high-calorie, high-salt, high-saturated fat diet and low-activity lifestyle that contributes to chronic disease in adults is having the same effect in children. Fortunately, as with adults, a healthy diet and active lifestyle can prevent or delay the onset of many of these conditions.

Overweight and obesity are major problems for U.S. children It is estimated that more than 15% of U.S. children and adolescents ages 6 through 19 are at risk for becoming overweight.[1] As with adults, children who carry excess body fat are at increased risk of developing chronic diseases. Obese children may have high blood cholesterol and glucose levels and elevated blood pressure, all of which increase their chances of developing heart disease, diabetes, and hypertension. In addition to the health issues, obese children in the United States have social and psychological challenges. They are less well accepted by their peers than normal-weight children and are frequently ridiculed and teased. They often have a poor self-image and low self-esteem, particularly during the teenage years. Obese adolescents may be discriminated against by adults as well as by their peers. This can lead to feelings of rejection, social isolation, and low self-esteem. The isolation of obese adolescents from teen society results in boredom, depression, inactivity, and withdrawal—all of which can cause an increase in eating and a decrease in energy output, worsening the problem (Figure 13.1).

Type 2 diabetes is no longer just an adult disease Until recently, type 2 diabetes was considered a disease that primarily affected adults over 40 years of age, but it is now on the rise among America's youth.[2] Little is known about this disease in children, but based on experience with adults, it is thought to be a progressive disease that increases in severity with time from diagnosis. It occurs most often in overweight children with a family history of the disease. The longer an individual has diabetes, the greater the risk of complications that involve the circulatory system or nervous system and that can lead to blindness, kidney failure, heart disease, or amputations (see Chapter 4).[3]

Many children and teens have elevated blood cholesterol The recommended level for blood cholesterol in children 2 through 18 years is less than 170 mg per 100 ml. In the United States, many children have blood

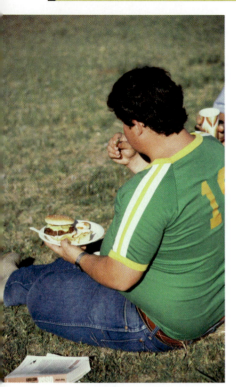

FIGURE 13.1

Overweight teens may become socially isolated, which reduces physical activity. (Robert E. Daemmrich/Stone/Getty Images)

✳ Remember

Obesity is due to a combination of genetic and environmental factors. Obese parents are more likely to have obese offspring not only because they pass on their genetic tendencies but also because their children may learn eating and exercise habits that lead to weight gain. If sound nutrition and exercise habits are developed early and are followed throughout life, obesity can be avoided despite a genetic predisposition. See Chapter 7.

cholesterol levels higher than this. Elevated blood cholesterol levels during child-hood and adolescence are associated with higher blood cholesterol and higher mor-tality rates from cardiovascular disease in adulthood. The American Academy of Pediatrics recommends blood cholesterol monitoring for high-risk children and teenagers. This includes those with parents or grandparents who developed heart disease before age 55, and those whose parents have cholesterol levels over 240 mg per 100 ml.

Higher blood pressure in childhood leads to hyperten-sion later Children who have blood pressure at the high end of normal are more likely to develop high blood pressure as adults. High blood pressure increases the risk of stroke, heart disease, and kidney disease. As with adults, blood pressure can be affected by the amount of body fat, activity level, and sodium intake, as well as by the total pattern of dietary intake. So, even in childhood, a diet that meets but doesn't exceed nutrient recommendations and includes plenty of exercise can help prevent hypertension. This is particularly important if there is a family history of hypertension.

Healthy eating habits are learned

Much of what we eat depends on what we have learned to eat. This is not to say that personal preferences don't affect intake, but the foods that we learn to eat from our parents and caregivers as well as our culture have a significant impact on the foods we choose to eat. If a child's role models eat a diet high in fat and low in fruits and veg-etables, the child will likely follow suit. Offering children a variety of healthy, nutri-tious foods allows them to meet their nutrient needs for growth and development and to prevent or delay the onset of the chronic diseases that plague American adults. Unfortunately most children and adolescents in the United States today consume a dietary pattern that is low in fruits and vegetables and high in sweet and salty processed foods. They eat more than the recommended amount of fat and not enough calcium. As children get older, the quality of their diet gets worse; they drink less milk and eat less fruit (Figure 13.2). These eating habits developed during child-hood and adolescence may last a lifetime and affect how healthy and how long your later years are.

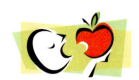

A child who eats a poor diet has an increased risk of developing elevated blood cholesterol, blood sugar, and blood pressure levels, all of which increase the risk of developing heart disease in adulthood. On the other hand, a healthy diet in childhood can delay or prevent the onset of heart disease.

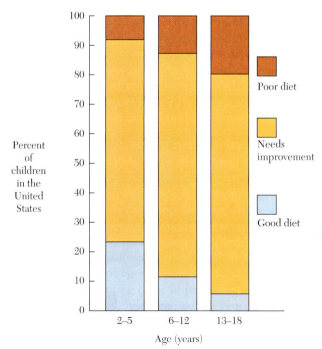

FIGURE 13.2

This graph shows us the percentage of U.S. children between the ages of 2 and 18 who have a good diet, a diet that needs improvement, and a poor diet. The classification is based on the Healthy Eating Index. A Healthy Eating Index score of 80 out of 100 is considered a good diet, a score between 51 and 80 is classified as a diet that needs improvement, and a score less than 51 indicates a poor diet. As children grow older, the percentage that eats a good diet decreases. (U.S. Department of Agriculture, Center of Nutrition Policy and Promotion. Continuing Survey of Food Intakes by Individuals, 1996)

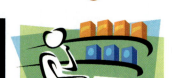

Your Choice: Breakfast Is Brain Food

Do you eat breakfast? If not, you probably should. It feeds your body and fuels your brain. When you haven't eaten since the night before, your brain and other tissues have to rely on nutrients released from your body stores. But after you've eaten breakfast, you have a ready supply of glucose and other nutrients to get you going. Research studies have found that those who eat breakfast perform better on achievement tests and have fewer behavior problems in school.[1] Breakfast eaters are also more likely to meet their nutritional needs than breakfast skippers.[2] Many children and teens are not particularly hungry first thing in the morning and will gladly go off with an empty stomach. Whether the child is in preschool or high school, this may be detrimental to both school performance and total nutrient intake.[3]

So, what should you have for breakfast? A good breakfast should provide a quarter to a third of the day's nutrient needs. For example, a bowl of oatmeal with milk and raisins, and a glass of orange juice provides about 300 Calories as well as B vitamins; vitamins C, A, and D; and calcium and iron. Though not every child will eat this good breakfast, even children who do not like breakfast may be willing to consume a slice of toast with peanut butter or a bowl of interestingly shaped colored cereal. Although a bowl of oatmeal is preferable to a breakfast of Cookie Crisp, even the most sugary cereal has some redeeming features. For example, while 40% of the energy in Cap'n Crunch is from simple sugars, it provides 20% or more of the Daily Value for thiamin, riboflavin, niacin, vitamin B$_6$, folate,

vitamin B$_{12}$, pantothenic acid, and iron. When 1/2 cup of reduced-fat milk is added to the cereal, it also provides 15% of the Daily Value for calcium. Children who eat ready-to-eat cereals, sugared or not, have a higher overall intake of vitamins and minerals than children who do not eat cereal.[3]

Children who cannot or will not eat breakfast before they leave the house can take a snack to be eaten on the way to school or during recess. Fruit, yogurt, a bag of dry cereal, or half a sandwich is certainly a better alternative than no breakfast at all. Having breakfast at school is also an option. The National School Breakfast Program is available in about half the nation's schools and serves more than 7 million children. For families who meet income guidelines the meals are free or offered at a reduced cost. Children participating in the National School Breakfast Program have higher achievement test scores than eligible nonparticipants.[1] The breakfasts served must provide at least 25% of the 1989 RDA for certain nutrients and furnish at least 1 serving of milk; 1 serving of fruit, juice, or vegetables; and either 2 servings of bread, 2 servings of meat, or 1 serving of each. This is probably a good guideline for the breakfast you serve at home as well.

References
1. Kennedy, E., and David, C. USDA School Breakfast Program. *Am. J. Clin. Nutr.* 67:798S–803S, 1998.
2. Nahikian-Nelms, M. Influential factors of caregivers' behaviors at mealtime: A study of 24 child care providers. *J. Am. Diet. Assoc.* 97:505–509, 1997.
3. Nicklas, T. A., O'Neil, C. E., and Berenson, G. S. Nutrient contribution of breakfast, secular trends, and the role of ready-to-eat cereals: A review of the data from the Bogalusa Heart Study. *Am. J. Clin. Nutr.* 67:757S–763S, 1998.

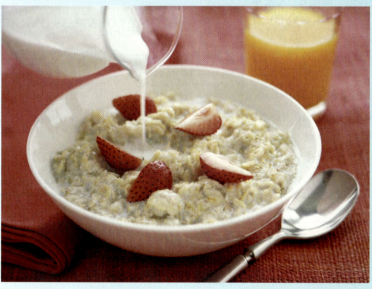

(Leigh Beisch/Foodpix/PictureArts Corp.)

to soups and casseroles; fruit can be served on cereals or in milkshakes; cheese can be included in recipes such as macaroni and cheese and pizza; milk can be added to hot cereal, cream soups, and puddings; powdered milk can be used in baking; and meats can be added to spaghetti sauce, stews, casseroles, burritos, and pizza.

Children often have periods known as food jags, when they will eat only certain foods and nothing else. For example, a child may refuse to eat anything other than peanut butter and jelly sandwiches for breakfast, lunch, and dinner. The general guideline is to continue to offer other foods along with those the child is focused on. What children will not touch at one meal, they may eat the next day or the next week.

Vitamin and mineral supplements are not necessary As with adults, children who consume a varied diet based on healthy choices can meet all their vitamin and mineral requirements with food. Occasional skipped meals and unfinished dinners are a normal part of most children's eating behavior and do not necessarily indicate that a supplement is needed. On the other hand, supplements that provide no more than 100% of the Daily Values are not harmful and may be beneficial for children with particularly erratic eating habits, those on regimens to manage obesity, those with limited food availability, and those who consume a vegan diet. If a children's supplement is offered, it should be monitored by caregivers and stored safely.

Nutritious meals at day care or school are important All meals need to contribute to a child's nutrient intake, but parents may have little input into what children eat while at day care or school. Ensuring that meals eaten away from home are nutritious is not easy because there is no guarantee that what is served or brought from home will be eaten. A packed lunch should contain foods the child likes and that do not require refrigeration (even if a refrigerator is available, the child is likely to forget to put the lunch in it). Even the most carefully planned lunch doesn't provide nutrients if it is not eaten.

For children who buy their lunch at school, the National School Lunch Program provides low-cost meals designed to meet nutrient needs and promote healthy diets. The goals of this program are to improve the dietary intake and nutritional health of America's children, and to promote nutrition education by teaching children to make appropriate food choices.[11] Each lunch meal must provide one-third of the 1989 RDA for protein, vitamin A, vitamin C, iron, calcium, and energy and meet the Dietary Guidelines recommendations of no more than 30% of energy from fat and 10% from saturated fat. Within these guidelines, each school or school district can decide which foods to serve and how they are prepared. In addition to lunches, federal guidelines regulate foods sold in snack bars and vending machines that compete with school lunch programs. These must provide at least 5% of the RDA for one or more of the following: protein, vitamin A, vitamin C, niacin, riboflavin, calcium, and iron. An analysis of the foods students choose to eat from the meal offered found that students who participated in the school lunch program consumed one-third of the RDA for energy, protein, vitamin A, vitamin C, vitamin B_6, calcium, iron, and zinc and drank twice as much milk as students not participating in school lunch programs.

Normal growth is the best indicator of adequate intake

Children don't always eat what and when they should, so how can you tell if they are meeting their needs? The best indicator of adequate nourishment is a pattern of growth that follows normal growth curves. Growth is most rapid in the first year of life, when an infant's length increases by 50%, or about 10 inches. In the second year of life, children generally grow about 5 inches; in the third year, 4 inches; and thereafter, about 2 to 3 inches per year. During adolescence, there is a period of growth that is almost as rapid as that of infancy.

On the Side

Supplements containing iron include the following on the label: "Warning: close tightly and keep out of reach of children. Contains iron, which can be harmful or fatal to children in large doses. In case of accidental overdose, seek professional assistance or contact a poison control center immediately."

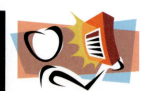

Off the Label: Labeling Food for Young Children

Children have different nutrient needs than adults. Therefore, the labels on foods designed for young children must follow different rules. The most obvious difference relates to how fat is listed in the Nutrition Facts section. Labels for foods intended for children under 2 years of age are not permitted to list the amount of saturated fat, polyunsaturated fat, monounsaturated fat, cholesterol, Calories from fat, and Calories from saturated fat on the label.[1] These labels are also not allowed to carry most of the claims about a food's nutrient content or health effects. This is because dietary fat is needed for brain development and as an energy source during the rapid growth and development that occurs in infancy and early childhood. Eliminating this information from the label may prevent caregivers from restricting fats in the diets of young children.

As children develop, the amount of fat in the diet can safely be reduced. Therefore, labels on foods designed for 2- to 4-year-olds must include information on the amount of cholesterol and saturated fat per serving and can voluntarily provide information on the number of Calories from fat and saturated fat and the amount of polyunsaturated and monounsaturated fat per serving. The serving sizes listed are based on servings appropriate for small children.

Another difference between standard food labels and those for foods designed for children under age 4 is the absence of percent Daily Values for total fat, saturated fat, cholesterol, total carbohydrate, fiber, and sodium.[1] Daily Values for these nutrients have not been established for children under 4; for this age group, the FDA has set Daily Values only for vitamins, minerals, and protein. Labels include the percent Daily Values for these nutrients when they are present in significant amounts.

A few nutrient and health claims are allowed on young children's foods. These include claims that describe the percentage of vitamins or minerals in a food as they apply to the Daily Values for children under age 2, such as "provides 50% of the Daily Value for vitamin C." Also, for children under 2, the terms "unsweetened" and "unsalted" are allowed. "No sugar added" and "sugar free" are approved only for use on dietary supplements for children.

The labels of foods intended for young children provide information needed to make wise food selections, but many of the foods consumed by young children do not have special labels because they are also adult foods. When selecting these foods, keep in mind that the needs of young children, especially for fat, are different than the needs of adults.

Reference
1. Kurtzweil, P. Labeling rules for young children's foods. *FDA Consumer* 29:14–18, March 1995.

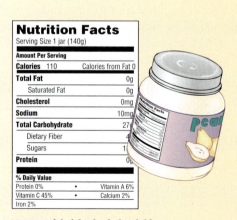

Nutrition label for foods for children under age two

Nutrition Facts

Serving Size 1/4 cup (15g)
Servings Per Container About 30

Amount Per Serving

Calories 60

Total Fat		1g
Sodium		0mg
Potassium		50mg
Total Carbohydrate		10g
Fiber		1g
Sugars		0g
Protein		2g

	Infants **0-1**	Children **1-4**
Daily Value		
Protein	7%	6%
Vitamin A	0%	0%
Vitamin C	0%	0%
Calcium	15%	10%
Iron	45%	60%
Vitamin E	15%	8%
Thiamin	45%	30%
Riboflavin	45%	30%
Niacin	25%	20%
Phosphorus	15%	10%

Nutrition Facts

Serving Size 1 jar (140g)

Amount Per Serving

Calories 110	Calories from Fat 0	
Total Fat		0g
Saturated Fat		0g
Cholesterol		0mg
Sodium		10mg
Total Carbohydrate		27g
Dietary Fiber		4
Sugars		1
Protein		0

% Daily Value		
Protein 0%	•	Vitamin A 6%
Vitamin C 45%	•	Calcium 2%
Iron 2%		

Nutrition label for foods for children ages two to four

Child and adolescent growth can be monitored by comparing growth to standard patterns using growth charts (see Appendix B).[12] For children and teens ages 2 through 20, weight-for-age, height-for-age, and BMI-for-age charts are available. The BMI-for-age growth chart is the recommended method for identifying children and adolescents who are over- and underweight (Figure 13.6).

Growth occurs in spurts and plateaus, but overall growth patterns are predictable. The ultimate size (height and weight) that a child will attain is affected by genetic, environmental, and lifestyle factors. A child whose parents are 5 feet tall may not have the genetic potential to grow to 6 feet, but when adequately nourished, most children follow standard patterns of growth. If a child's overall pattern of growth changes, his or her dietary intake should be evaluated to determine the reason for the sudden change. There are critical periods in childhood when malnutrition can cause lasting damage to physical, emotional, and cognitive development for which adequate nutrition later on may not be able to compensate.[5]

Too little growth may mean undernutrition When a child's calorie intake is too low to meet needs, weight will decrease. If the deficiency continues, growth in height will slow or stop. A child who falls below the fifth percentile of the BMI-for-age distribution is considered underweight and should be evaluated to

CDC Growth Charts: United States

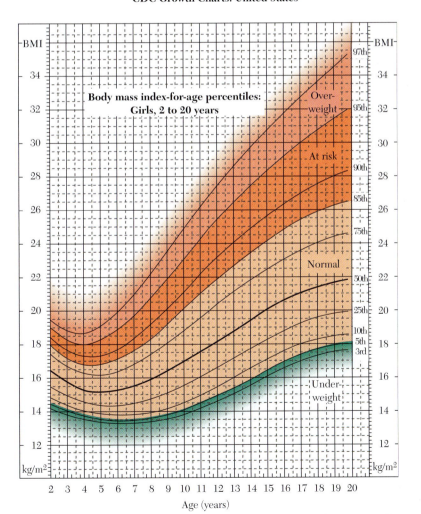

FIGURE 13.6

Growth charts are helpful for monitoring a child's pattern of growth. This example illustrates BMI-for-age percentiles for girls ages 2 through 20. BMI can be used beginning at 2 years of age, when height can be measured accurately. BMI is predictive of body fat and has been recommended to screen for underweight and overweight children, ages 2 years and older. The colored areas represent BMI values that are associated with underweight, normal weight, at-risk of overweight, and overweight.

SOURCE: Developed by the National Center for Health Statistics in collaboration with the Nation Center for Chronic Disease Prevention and Health Promotion (2000).

determine the cause of his or her low body weight (see Figure 13.6). Nutritional interventions such as offering children small, frequent, nutritious meals and snacks can increase energy intake and help increase body weight. Underweight adolescents can increase their weight by combining muscle-building exercises with increases in energy intake.

A high BMI may indicate a risk of becoming overweight

A drastic increase in BMI may be due to an energy intake that exceeds output. Research has found that overweight children and adolescents are more likely than their normal-weight counterparts to be overweight as adults.[13] As with adults, excess body weight in childhood and adolescence increases the risk of chronic disease. A child is considered overweight when BMI falls at or above the 95th percentile and is at risk of being overweight when BMI is greater than or equal to the 85th percentile and less than the 95th percentile (see Figure 13.6).

Excessive weight gain in children is related to both eating and exercise habits. Reducing weight into the healthy range involves a permanent change in lifestyle. Because children, like adults, may overeat for comfort, self-reward, or out of boredom, parent involvement in helping the child find other sources of gratification can be vital.

Mild calorie restriction can allow for growth with little weight gain

The goal of weight management for children and teens is to slow their rate of weight gain and allow them to grow into their current weight. As long as the rate of weight gain is slowed, a child at the 95th percentile for weight at age 7 can be at the 90th percentile by age 9 and at the 75th percentile by age 11. The diet should be moderate in calories and include whole grains, fruits and vegetables, lean meats, and reduced-fat dairy products. Both meals and snacks are important. Breakfast and lunch are important because skipping meals may actually increase energy intake by increasing the amount of food consumed later in the day. Denying food may promote further overeating by making the child feel that there will not be enough to satisfy hunger. Planning ahead can help manage eating at social events. For example, a teenage boy with a weight problem could plan how much he will eat at a pizza party and then increase his exercise to burn off the excess calories.

Increasing physical activity increases energy expenditure

Although energy intake among American children overall is not increasing, they are getting heavier, suggesting that a major contributor to the increase in body weight is lack of physical activity.[14] Watching television, playing video games, and surfing the Web have replaced neighborhood games of tag and soccer for many children (Figure 13.7).

Overweight children are less likely to be physically active than lean children. They may be embarrassed by their bodies and shy away from participating in group activities. Increases in physical activity need to be gradual in order to make exercise a positive experience. A good way to start is to encourage activities such as games, walks after dinner, bike rides, hikes, swimming, and volleyball that can be enjoyed by the whole family. This sends a positive message to "be more active" rather than a negative message of "do not eat so much." Again, involvement of the whole family is key. Parents who are active, play with their children, watch their children compete or play, or take children to physical activities or sports events have more active children.

Whether or not a child is overweight, he or she should be active. The Dietary Guidelines and the DRIs recommend that children be physically active for at least an hour per day.[15] Children have short attention spans, so their activities should be intermittent. Periods of moderate to vigorous activity lasting 10 to 15 minutes or more each day should be interspersed with periods of rest and recovery. Preadolescent children should be exposed to a variety of different types of activities that are of various levels of intensity (Figure 13.8). Learning to enjoy sports and exercise in childhood will set the stage for an active lifestyle in adulthood.

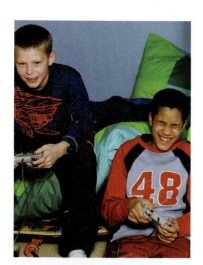

FIGURE 13.7

Video games provide children with an inactive way to spend their spare hours. (Mel Yates/Taxi/Getty Images)

Fitness Pyramid for Kids

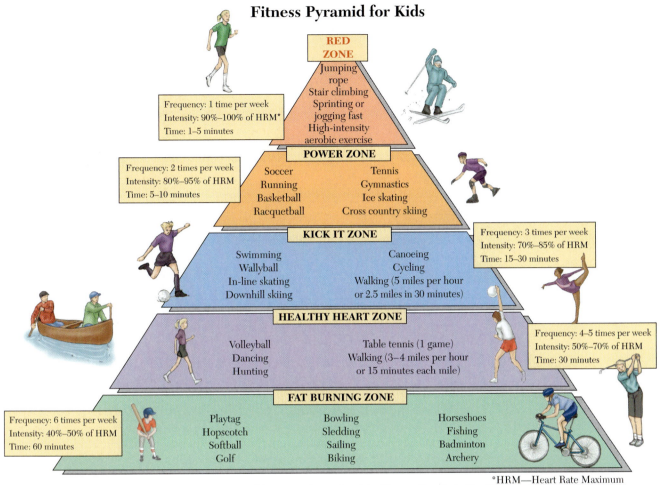

Frequency: 1 time per week
Intensity: 90%–100% of HRM*
Time: 1–5 minutes

RED ZONE
Jumping rope
Stair climbing
Sprinting or jogging fast
High-intensity aerobic exercise

Frequency: 2 times per week
Intensity: 80%–95% of HRM
Time: 5–10 minutes

POWER ZONE
Soccer   Tennis
Running   Gymnastics
Basketball   Ice skating
Racquetball   Cross country skiing

Frequency: 3 times per week
Intensity: 70%–85% of HRM
Time: 15–30 minutes

KICK IT ZONE
Swimming   Canoeing
Wallyball   Cycling
In-line skating Walking (5 miles per hour
Downhill skiing or 2.5 miles in 30 minutes)

Frequency: 4–5 times per week
Intensity: 50%–70% of HRM
Time: 30 minutes

HEALTHY HEART ZONE
Volleyball   Table tennis (1 game)
Dancing   Walking (3–4 miles per hour
Hunting   or 15 minutes each mile)

Frequency: 6 times per week
Intensity: 40%–50% of HRM
Time: 60 minutes

FAT BURNING ZONE
Playtag   Bowling   Horseshoes
Hopscotch   Sledding   Fishing
Softball   Sailing   Badminton
Golf   Biking   Archery

°HRM—Heart Rate Maximum

(Adapted from: American Dietetic Association. Position of the American Dietetic Association: Dietary guidance for healthy children ages 2 to 11 years. *J. Am. Diet. Assoc.* 99:93–101, 1999)

FIGURE 13.8

Children should enjoy participating in a variety of activities of varying intensity.

Diet and lifestyle affect nutritional risks in children

A number of diet and lifestyle factors can put children at risk for illness and malnutrition. Some of these are a greater risk in young children because of their size and stage of development and others may continue to be problems into adolescence.

A high sugar intake reduces nutrient density and promotes tooth decay Children often eat more sugar than is recommended. Added sugars reduce the nutrient density of foods and too many foods high in added sugars make it difficult to meet nutrient needs. In addition, a diet high in sugary foods promotes tooth decay. Decay occurs when there is prolonged contact between sugar and bacteria on the surface of the teeth.

Much of the added sugars in children's diets come from soft drinks and other sweetened beverages; when these are sipped slowly between meals the contact time between sugar and teeth increases and hence, increases the risk of tooth decay. Although sugary foods are the most cavity-promoting, any carbohydrate-containing food can cause tooth decay, especially if the food sticks to the teeth (see Chapter 4).

Preventing tooth decay involves limiting carbohydrate snacks, especially those that stick to teeth; brushing teeth frequently to remove sticky sweets; and consuming adequate fluoride (Figure 13.9). Because the primary teeth guide the growth of the permanent teeth, maintaining healthy primary teeth is just as important as preserving

On the Web

For more information on weight control in children, go to the National Institute of Diabetes and Digestive and Kidney Disorders at **www.niddk.nih.gov** and click on "weight loss & control" under Health Information.

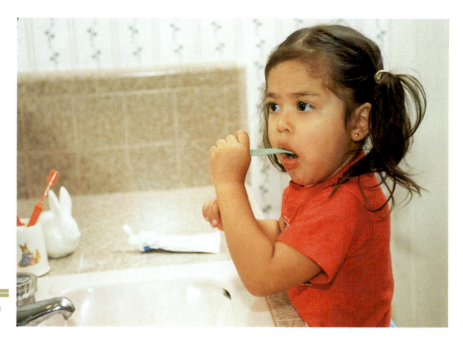

FIGURE 13.9

Frequent tooth brushing can help prevent cavities in children. (David Young-Wolff/PhotoEdit)

 Attention deficit hyperactivity disorder A condition that is characterized by a short attention span and a high level of activity, excitability, and distractibility.

permanent ones. Children's teeth should be brushed as soon as they erupt, and those 3 years of age and over should be examined by a dentist regularly.

Hyperactivity has not been found to be related to sugar intake

Diet, in particular sugar intake, has been blamed for hyperactivity in children. Hyperactivity is a problem in 5 to 10% of school-age children, occurring more frequently in boys than in girls. It involves extreme physical activity, excitability, impulsiveness, distractibility, short attention span, and a low tolerance for frustration. Hyperactive children have more difficulty learning but usually are of normal or above-average intelligence. Hyperactivity is now considered part of a larger syndrome known as **attention deficit hyperactivity disorder**.

Although sugar is often blamed for hyperactivity, research on sugar intake and behavior has failed to support this hypothesis.[16] The hyperactive behavior that follows sugar intake is more likely due to other factors. For example, at a birthday party the excitement rather than the sugary cake that is served is a more likely reason for over activity. Other situations that might cause hyperactivity include lack of sleep, overstimulation, the desire for more attention, or lack of physical activity.

Specific foods and food additives have also been implicated as a cause of hyperactivity. Numerous studies have been done to test the hypothesis that food sensitivities cause hyperactivity, but the results have been inconsistent.[17] Some children with this disorder seem to improve when particular foods or additives are eliminated, while others do not.

Another possible cause of hyperactive behavior in children is caffeine. Caffeine is a stimulant that can cause sleeplessness, restlessness, and irregular heartbeats. Beverages, food, and medicines containing caffeine are often a part of children's diets. For example, children's fast-food meals are typically accompanied by caffeinated beverages such as Coke and Mountain Dew.

Lead from the environment harms the developing nervous system

Lead is an environmental contaminant that can be toxic, especially in children under 6 years of age. Children are particularly susceptible because they absorb lead much more efficiently than do adults. It is estimated that children may absorb as much as 30 to 75% of ingested lead, whereas adults absorb only about 11%.[18]

Once absorbed from the gastrointestinal tract, lead circulates in the bloodstream and then accumulates in the bones and, to a lesser extent, the brain, teeth, and kidneys. Lead disrupts the functioning of neurotransmitters and thus interferes with the

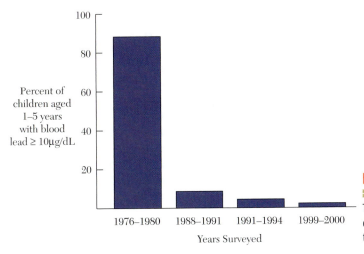

FIGURE 13.10

The prevalence of children ages 1 to 5 with elevated blood lead levels has decreased dramatically over the last 25 years due to interventions such as the elimination of lead from paint, gasoline, and solder. *Source:* NHANES.

functioning of the nervous system. Higher levels of lead can contribute to iron deficiency anemia, changes in kidney function, nervous system damage, and even seizures, coma, and death. In young children, lead poisoning can cause learning disabilities and behavior problems.[19] In adults, lead poisoning can damage the reproductive organs and cause high blood pressure.[20] During pregnancy, lead toxicity can damage the fetal nervous system.

Lead is found naturally in the earth's crust, but over the years industrial activities have redistributed it in the environment. Lead is now found in soil contaminated with lead paint dust; it also enters drinking water from old corroded lead plumbing, lead solder on copper pipes, or brass faucets. It is found in polluted air, in leaded glass, and in glazes used on imported and antique pottery. These can contaminate food and beverages. Because of the risks of lead toxicity from environmental contamination, lead is no longer used in house paint, gasoline, or solder. As a result, the number of children with elevated blood lead levels has decreased dramatically (Figure 13.10).[21] The U.S. Department of Health and Human Services has established a national goal of eliminating blood lead levels greater than 10 μg per dL in children younger than 6 years of age by 2010.[19] Despite these gains, there are still nearly a million children under 6 years of age who have blood lead levels that are high enough to cause damage. For a number of reasons, the problem is greatest among children living in poverty. Their exposure is likely to be greater because they tend to live in older buildings where chipped paint and old plumbing may be contaminated with lead. In addition, children living in poverty are more likely to be malnourished, and malnutrition increases lead absorption because lead is better absorbed from an empty stomach and when other minerals such as calcium, zinc, and iron are deficient.

Children should have their blood lead levels tested.[19] The effects of lead poisoning are permanent, but if high levels are detected early, the lead can be removed with medical treatment, preventing damage (Table 13.2).

Too much television reduces activity and influences food choices Many children today spend more time watching television than they do in any activity other than sleep. Television affects nutritional status in a number of ways: it introduces children to foods they might otherwise not be exposed to, it promotes snacking, and it reduces physical activity (Figure 13.11).

Through advertising, television has a strong influence on the foods selected by young children. A review of commercials broadcast during children's programming found that over 60% were for food products—primarily sweetened breakfast cereals; sweets such as candy, cookies, doughnuts, and other desserts; snacks; and beverages—that are high in sugar, fat, or salt.[22] Television also promotes snacking behavior. Although snacks are an important part of a growing child's diet, while watching TV many children snack on sweet and salty foods that are low in nutrient density.

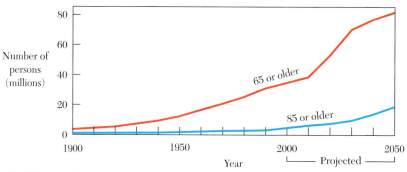

FIGURE 13.17

This graph illustrates the increase in the total number of persons age 65 and older and 85 and older from 1900 to 2050. Data through 2050 are based on projections of the population and indicate that in the next few decades there will be almost 80 million people in the United States who are 65 or older. (U.S. Census Bureau. *Decennial Census Data and Population Projections.* Available online at www.agingstats.gov)

Even though average life expectancy in the United States is over 77 years, the average healthy life span is only about 69 years.[33] This means that on average the last 8 years of life are restricted by disease and disability. The goal of successful aging is to increase not only life expectancy but the number of years of healthy life that an individual can expect. Achieving this goal is important because we live in an aging population. Currently about 12.4% of the U.S. population is 65 years of age or over and this is expected to increase to about 19.6% by the year 2030 (Figure 13.17).[34] The fastest-growing segment of the population in industrialized nations is individuals over the age of 85, called the oldest old.[35] Individuals in this age group tend to have more activity limitations, experience more chronic conditions, and require more services than younger adults. This oldest old population accounts for a large part of the public health budget. Keeping older adults healthy will benefit not only the aging individuals themselves but also the family members who must find the time and resources to care for them and the public health programs that attempt to meet their needs.

Good nutrition can prolong our healthy years Although nutrition is not the key to immortality, a healthy diet can prevent malnutrition and delay the onset of chronic disease. The diseases that are the major causes of disability in older adults—cardiovascular disease, hypertension, diabetes, cancer, and osteoporosis—are all nutrition-related. Exercise and a lifetime of healthy eating will not necessarily prevent these diseases, but they may slow the changes that accumulate over time, postponing the onset of disease symptoms. For example, the risk of developing cardiovascular disease can be decreased by exercise and a diet low in cholesterol, *trans* fat, and saturated fat and high in whole grains, fruits, and vegetables. The risk of osteoporosis may be reduced by adequate calcium intake and an active lifestyle. And the likelihood of developing certain types of cancer can be reduced by consuming a diet low in fat and high in whole grains, vegetables, and fruits.

Aging affects recommendations for some nutrients

The physiological and health changes that accompany aging affect the requirements for some nutrients, how nutrient requirements must be met, and the risk of malnutrition (Figure 13.18). In order to best recommend nutrient intakes for adults, the DRIs include four adult age categories: young adulthood, ages 19 through 30; middle age, 31 through 50 years; adulthood, ages 51 through 70; and older adults, those over 70 years of age. Recommendations are developed to meet the needs of the majority of healthy individuals in each age group. Although the incidence of chronic diseases and disabilities increases with advancing age, these are not considered when making general nutrient intake recommendations.

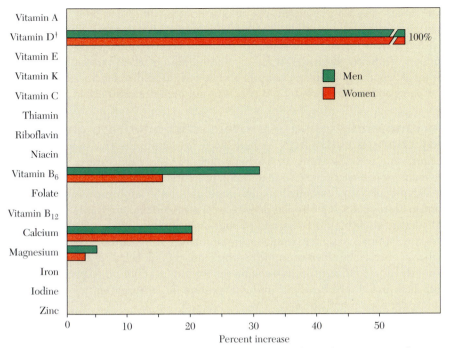

†This represents the AI for individuals 51 to 70 years old. For those over age 70 the AI is increased by 200%

FIGURE 13.18

The nutrient needs of older adults are not drastically different from those of young adults. This graph illustrates the percentage increase in micronutrient recommendations for adults age 51 and older compared to those of young adults ages 19 through 30. The RDA for vitamin B_{12} is not increased, but it is recommended that vitamin B_{12} be obtained from fortified foods or supplements. The RDA for iron for women over 50 years of age is reduced by 50%.

Energy needs are reduced in the elderly

Energy needs generally decrease with age in adults. Some of this decline is related to a decrease in lean body mass, which reduces basal metabolism and therefore total energy requirements (Figure 13.19). For example, the EER for an 80-year-old man is almost 600 Calories per day less than that for a 20-year-old man of the same height, weight, and physical activity level. For women, the difference in EER between an 80-year-old and a 20-year-old of the same height, weight, and physical activity level is about 400 Calories per day.[4] The decrease in energy needs with age is even greater if activity level declines. Some of this decrease can therefore be prevented by maintaining an active lifestyle.

Even though energy needs decline with age, some older adults don't consume enough to maintain a healthy body weight. People tend to gain weight in their 20's, 30's, and 40's, but after age 65, it is more common for people to lose weight. Even in

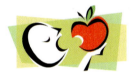

A healthy diet won't actually keep you young but it can help keep you fit and healthy for more of your years.

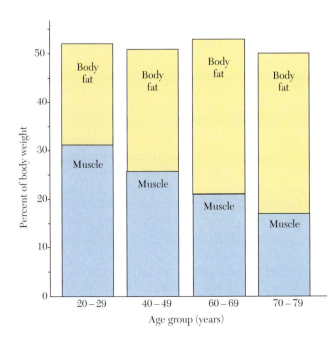

FIGURE 13.19

In most individuals, the proportion of muscle mass decreases and body fat increases with age. (Adapted from Cohen, S. H., et al. Compartmental body composition based on the body nitrogen, potassium, and calcium. *Am. J. Physiol.* 239:192–200, 1980)

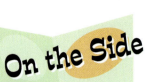

older adults who are overweight, the risks associated with excess body fat are lower than they are for younger adults.[36] Stable body weight is a sign of good health. Weight loss may reduce the ability to ward off disease or be a symptom of disease. Extreme thinness or unintentional weight loss is a health risk, especially among older adults. Although laboratory studies in animals have found that a diet deficient in energy can slow aging and extend life span, this effect has not been demonstrated in humans.[37]

Recommendations for protein, carbohydrate and fat do not change with age

Unlike calorie needs, the need for protein does not decline with age. Therefore, an adequate diet for older adults must be somewhat higher in protein relative to calorie intake in order to meet needs.

The proportion of carbohydrate recommended in the adult diet also remains the same in older adults, but nutrient density becomes more important. Most dietary carbohydrates should be from less refined sources in order to ensure adequate vitamin and mineral intake despite a reduction in calorie needs. In addition, whole grains are higher in fiber. Fiber, when consumed with adequate fluid, helps prevent constipation, hemorrhoids, and diverticulosis—conditions that are common in older adults. High-fiber diets may also be beneficial in the prevention and management of diabetes, cardiovascular disease, and obesity.

The digestion and absorption of fat does not change as adults age; therefore the recommendations regarding dietary fat apply to older as well as younger adults. A diet with 20 to 35% of energy from fat that contains adequate amounts of the essential fatty acids and limits saturated fat, *trans* fat, and cholesterol is recommended. Following these recommendations will allow older adults to meet their nutrient needs without exceeding their energy requirements and may delay the onset of chronic disease. However, there are certain situations, such as being underweight, where greater fat intake may be warranted.

Fluid intake is a concern in older adults

The recommended water intake for older adults is the same as that for younger adults; but meeting these needs may be more challenging. With age there is a reduction in the sense of thirst, which can decrease fluid intake.[7] Changes in mobility may limit access to water even in the presence of thirst. In addition, the kidneys are no longer as efficient at conserving water, so water loss increases. Depression, which decreases water intake, and medications that increase water loss, such as laxatives and diuretics, also increase the risk of dehydration in the elderly. Inadequate fluid intake along with low-fiber intake and lack of activity increase problems with constipation.

Older adults should consume supplemental sources of vitamin B₁₂

The RDA for vitamin B_{12} is not increased for older adults, but it is recommended that individuals over the age of 50 meet their RDA for vitamin B_{12} by consuming foods fortified with the vitamin, such as breakfast cereals or soy-based products, or by taking a supplement containing vitamin B_{12}. This is because food-bound vitamin B_{12} is not absorbed efficiently in many older adults due to **atrophic gastritis**, an inflammation of the stomach lining accompanied by a decrease in the secretion of stomach acid.[38,39] It is estimated that 10 to 30% of American adults over age 50 and 40% of those in their 80's have atrophic gastritis. The vitamin B_{12} in fortified foods and supplements is not bound to proteins, so it is absorbed even when stomach acid is low. Atrophic gastritis may also reduce the absorption of iron, folate, calcium, and vitamin K. Reduced stomach acid secretion also allows microbial overgrowth in the stomach and small intestine. This increased population of microbes in the gut further reduces vitamin B_{12} absorption by competing for available vitamin B_{12}.

Reduced absorption and low intakes of calcium affect bone health

Calcium status is a problem in the elderly because intakes are low and intestinal absorption decreases with age. Without sufficient calcium, bone mass

⚠ **Atrophic gastritis** An inflammation of the stomach lining that causes a reduction in stomach acid and allows bacterial overgrowth.

✱ **Remember**
Vitamin B₁₂ that is found naturally in foods is bound to food proteins. Chapter 8 discussed how acid and protein digesting enzymes in the stomach release it from food proteins so it can bind to intrinsic factor, which is essential for adequate for absorption.

decreases and the risk of bone fractures increases. The loss of calcium from bone is accelerated in women due to the normal hormonal changes of **menopause**. During menopause, which normally occurs around the age of 50, the cyclical release of the female hormones estrogen and progesterone slows and eventually stops, causing ovulation and menstruation to cease. The decrease in estrogen is accompanied by changes in mood, skin, and body composition, with body fat increasing and lean tissue decreasing. Reduced estrogen also increases the risk of osteoporosis by increasing the rate of bone breakdown and decreasing calcium absorption from the intestine. As a result of age-related bone loss the AI for adults over age 51 is 1200 mg, 200 mg greater than the AI set for younger adults. Although the decrease in estrogen that occurs at menopause causes bone loss, it cannot be prevented by increasing calcium intake alone, so the recommended intakes for men and women are not different.

Vitamin D is a concern because intake is low and skin synthesis is decreased

Vitamin D is necessary for adequate calcium absorption, so a deficiency may contribute to bone loss. Vitamin D status is a concern in the elderly for a number of reasons. First, intakes are often low, usually due to limited consumption of dairy products. In addition, vitamin D synthesis in the skin is reduced due to limited exposure to sunlight, which is necessary for the formation of provitamin D, and because the capacity to synthesize provitamin D in the skin and to form active vitamin D in the kidneys decrease with age (Figure 13.20). Using bone loss as an indicator of adequacy, the AI for men and women 51 to 70 years has been set at 10 μg per day—twice as much as that of younger age groups. For individuals over age 70, this is further increased to 15 μg per day.

A diet high in antioxidant nutrients helps prevent chronic disease

Antioxidant nutrients will not keep you young, but adequate intakes may reduce the incidence of disease. Antioxidants, including vitamin E, vitamin C, and β-carotene, have been found to improve immune function and may therefore help protect the body from infectious disease. Diets high in antioxidants have also been associated with a reduced risk of heart disease and certain types of cancer. Oxidative damage is believed to cause two of the most common causes of visual disorders in older adults, **macular degeneration** and **cataracts**. Macular degeneration is the most common cause of blindness in older Americans. The macula is a small area of the retina of the eye that distinguishes fine detail. If the number of viable cells in the macula is reduced, visual acuity declines, ultimately resulting in blindness. Cataracts are cloudy spots on the lens and sometimes the cornea, which obscure vision (Figure 13.21). Of people who live to age 85, half will have cataracts that impair vision. A diet high in foods containing antioxidant nutrients might slow or prevent these eye disorders.[40]

But, don't run to the supplement counter just yet. The evidence that antioxidants in supplement form will prevent many of these chronic diseases is not as strong as the evidence supporting a diet plentiful in foods high in these nutrients. When these nutrients are obtained from foods, they bring with them phytochemicals, some of which offer additional antioxidant protection and some of which protect us from chronic disease in other ways.

Menopause Physiological changes that mark the end of a woman's capacity to bear children.

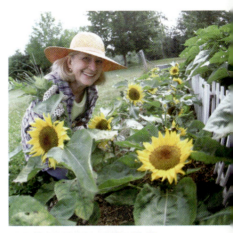

FIGURE 13.20

Sun exposure is often limited in the elderly because they spend less time outdoors or tend to wear clothing that covers or shades their skin when they go out. (Tom Stewart/ Corbis Images)

Macular degeneration Degeneration of a portion of the retina that results in a loss of visual detail and blindness.

Cataracts A disease of the eye that results in cloudy spots on the lens (and sometimes the cornea), which obscure vision.

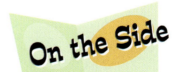

On the Side

Supplements of lutein, an antioxidant phytochemical found in dark green leafy vegetables, have been found to delay the onset of macular degeneration and possibly reverse some of the symptoms. You can get your lutein in a pill or eat 3 to 4 ounces of spinach, which provides the amount found in most supplements.

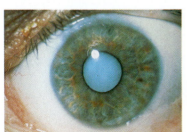

FIGURE 13.21

Cataracts cause the lens of the eye to become cloudy and impair vision. (© Science VU/Visuals Unlimited)

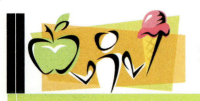

So, What Should I Eat?

Consume plenty of fluids and fiber
- Drink a beverage with every meal
- Keep a bottle of water handy to sip on
- Use whole wheat bread
- Bake bran muffins

Pay attention to B₁₂, calcium, and vitamin D
- Make sure your cereal is fortified with vitamin B₁₂
- Drink milk; it gives you both calcium and vitamin D
- Sit in the sun to get some vitamin D with no calories at all
- Add some canned salmon to a salad for lunch
- Have yogurt for dessert

Antioxidize
- Have a bowl of strawberries
- Choose colorful vegetables to boost carotenoids
- Use vegetable oils in cooking to supply vitamin E
- Eat some nuts but not too many—they are high in calories

Work on your meals for one
- Ask the grocer to break up larger packages of eggs and meats
- Buy in bulk and share with a friend
- Make a whole pot but freeze it in meal-size portions
- Top a baked potato with leftover vegetables or sauces

The physical, mental, and social changes of aging increase nutritional risks

The aging process itself is usually not a cause of malnutrition in healthy active adults, but nutritional health can be compromised by the physical changes that occur with age, the presence of disease, and economic, psychological, and social circumstances[41] (Table 13.3). These can increase the risk of malnutrition by altering nutrient needs and decreasing the motivation to eat and the ability to acquire and enjoy food.

A decline in muscle strength leads to frailty With age there is a decline in muscle size and strength. It affects both the skeletal muscles needed to move the body and the heart and respiratory muscles needed to deliver oxygen to the tissues (Figure 13.22). Therefore, both strength and endurance are decreased, making the

FIGURE 13.22

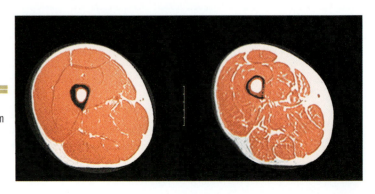

With age total muscle mass declines, leading to a loss of strength. These magnetic resonance images of thigh cross-sections from a 25-year-old man (*left*) and a 65-year-old man (*right*) illustrate that the older man has a greater amount of fat (shown in white) around and through the muscle, indicating significant muscle loss. (Courtesy S. A. Jubias and K. E. Conley, University of Washington Medical Center)

TABLE 13.3
Aging Can Affect Nutrition

Organ or Process	How It Changes	How It Affects Nutrition and Health
Sensory Organs	Ability to taste and smell declines.	Reduces food intake by decreasing the appeal and enjoyment of food.
	Vision typically declines, often due to macular degeneration or cataracts.	Reduces food choices by making shopping for and preparation of food difficult.
Mouth	Secretion of saliva decreases.	Decreases the appeal of food by causing dryness, which decreases the taste of food and makes swallowing difficult. Increases the likelihood of tooth decay and gum disease because saliva is needed to wash material away from the teeth and kill bacteria.
Stomach	Stomach emptying is slower and gastric secretions are reduced.	Reduces hunger and, therefore, nutrient intake. Reduced gastric secretions can affect the absorption of some nutrients.
Colon	Motility and elasticity are reduced, abdominal and pelvic muscles are weakened, and sensory perception is decreased.	Increases the likelihood of constipation.
Liver	Liver size and blood flow are decreased and fat accumulation increases.	Decreases the liver's ability to metabolize nutrients and break down drugs and alcohol.
Pancreas	Responsiveness to blood glucose levels decreases and the body cells may become more resistant to insulin, resulting in diabetes.	Increases blood glucose.
Kidneys	Kidneys shrink and their ability to filter blood and to excrete the products of protein breakdown declines. The ability to concentrate urine decreases.	Increases blood urea levels when protein intake is high. Increases the risk of dehydration, which is made worse by a decline in the sensation of thirst with age.
Body Composition	Body fat increases, especially in the abdomen. Lean tissue, including muscle and bone mass, decreases.	Decreases in strength and endurance. An increased risk of falls and fractures due to weakness and a loss of bone mass.
Hormones	Levels of growth hormone, DHEA (dehydroepiandosterone), melatonin, estrogen, and testosterone all decline.	Decreases in muscle and bone mass, changes in body rhythms, and immune function.
Immune System	Ability to fight disease declines.	Increases the incidence of infections, cancers, and autoimmune diseases, and decreases the effectiveness of immunizations.

tasks of day-to-day life more difficult. The changes in muscle strength contribute not only to physical frailty, which is characterized by general weakness, impaired mobility and balance, and poor endurance, but also to the risk of falls and fractures. In the oldest old, loss of muscle strength becomes the limiting factor determining whether they can continue to live independently.

Some of the reduction in muscle strength and mass is due to changes in hormone levels and in muscle protein synthesis, but a lack of exercise is also an important contributor.[42] Regular exercise can help maintain muscle mass, bone strength, and cardiorespiratory function and can increase energy needs. Exercise can reduce the loss of lean body mass, maintain fitness and independence, and allow an increase in food

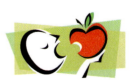

The changes that occur with aging including an increase in the prevalence of disease and the likelihood of social and economic changes, increase the risk of malnutrition.

intake without weight gain so micronutrient needs are more easily met. Therefore, maintaining regular physical activity remains important throughout life.

Medical conditions can limit the ability to meet nutrient needs
More than half of the older population suffers from some form of physical illness or disability, and the incidence increases with advancing age. These limitations affect the ability to maintain good nutritional health by changing nutrient requirements, decreasing the appeal of food, and impairing the ability to obtain and prepare an adequate diet.

Some illnesses change nutrient recommendations. For instance, kidney failure reduces the ability to excrete protein waste products. Therefore, the diet has to be limited in protein. Blood pressure is affected by sodium intake so a low sodium diet is recommended for those with high blood pressure. Dietary restrictions such as these limit food choices and can affect the palatability of the diet. These dietary restrictions may contribute to malnutrition if the elderly individuals and their families are not provided with enough information about how to substitute foods that will provide adequate energy, nutrients, and eating pleasure.

Physical disabilities can limit the ability to obtain and prepare food and therefore reduce food intake and increase the risk of malnutrition. The most common cause of physical disability among older adults is **arthritis**, a condition that causes pain upon movement. Osteoarthritis is a type of arthritis that affects over 33 million Americans.[43] It occurs when the cartilage that prevents the bones in joints from rubbing together degenerates over time, causing pain. Arthritis is treated with drugs that reduce inflammation, such as aspirin and ibuprofen, and with pain relievers such as acetaminophen. Supplements containing glucosamine and chondroitin sulfate are also used by arthritis sufferers. Glucosamine and chondroitin sulfate are not essential nutrients. But in the body, they are needed for the synthesis of large molecules that bind water to form a porous, gel-like material that allows cartilage to resist crushing forces and cushion the joints. It has been suggested that when consumed in the diet, glucosamine and chondroitin sulfate provide the raw materials needed to synthesize these large cushioning molecules. Glucosamine may also inhibit inflammation and increase the production of a compound that contributes to the lubricating and shock-absorbing properties of cartilage. Supplements of both glucosamine and chondroitin sulfate are said to reduce arthritis pain, stop cartilage degeneration, and possibly stimulate the repair of damaged joint cartilage. Results of studies of the effectiveness of these supplements have been mixed but the National Institutes of Health (NIH) is currently conducting a large trial in centers across the country to evaluate the effects of glucosamine and chondroitin sulfate, given separately and in combination, for reducing pain and improving function in patients with osteoarthritis of the knee.[44]

Mental changes can affect nutritional status
Mental changes in the elderly may be due to depression or to **dementia**. Regardless of the cause, these mental problems can affect the ability to consume a healthy diet.

Depression in the elderly may be caused by social, psychological, and physical factors. For example, retirement and the death or relocation of friends and family can cause social isolation, which contributes to depression. The inability to engage in normal daily activities, visit with friends and family easily, and provide for personal needs also contributes to depression as does the loneliness of living, cooking, and eating by oneself. Depression can make meals less appetizing and decrease the quantity and quality of foods consumed, thereby increasing the risk of malnutrition.

Many individuals maintain adequate nervous system function into old age, but the incidence of dementia does increase with age. Dementia involves an impairment in memory, thinking, or judgment that is severe enough to cause personality changes and affect daily activities and relationships with others. It may be caused by multiple strokes, alcoholism, vitamin B_{12} deficiency, or **Alzheimer's disease**. Alzheimer's disease is the cause of over half of the cases of dementia in the elderly. It involves a progressive, incurable loss of mental function. The brains of patients with Alzheimer's disease

---

Arthritis A disease characterized by inflammation of the joints, pain, and sometimes changes in structure.

Dementia A deterioration of mental state resulting in impaired memory, thinking, and/or judgment.

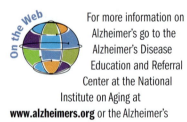

For more information on Alzheimer's go to the Alzheimer's Disease Education and Referral Center at the National Institute on Aging at **www.alzheimers.org** or the Alzheimer's Association at **www.alz.org**

Alzheimer's disease A disease that results in the relentless and irreversible loss of mental function.

are characterized by the accumulation of an abnormal protein in the spaces between nerve cells and tangled protein fibers inside the nerve cells. Together these block the normal passage of electrical signals between nerve cells that allow us to think, talk, remember, and move. As the disease progresses nerve cells die, the brain shrinks, and function deteriorates. Its cause is unknown, but there does appear to be a genetic component in some cases. Drugs can treat some of the symptoms, but there is no cure and it is eventually fatal. Many ineffective nutritional cures have been marketed for Alzheimer's disease. Supplements of choline and lecithin have been promoted to increase levels of the neurotransmitter acetylcholine, which is deficient in Alzheimer's patients, and antioxidant supplements have been suggested to prevent free radical damage. To date, there is little evidence that nutritional supplements are helpful in treating or preventing Alzheimer's disease.

Increased use of medications can affect nutritional status

The medications required to treat the diseases that become more common with age can also affect nutritional status. Almost half of older Americans take multiple medications daily (Figure 13.23).[45] The more medications taken, the greater the chance of side effects that affect nutritional status such as increased or decreased appetite, changes in taste, constipation, weakness, drowsiness, diarrhea, and nausea. Complications related to incorrect doses or inappropriate combinations of medications are also a significant problem in the elderly. Medications can affect nutritional status and nutritional status can alter the effectiveness of drugs. This is true whether the medication is a prescription drug, an over-the-counter medication, or a dietary supplement.

Medications can alter nutrient intake, absorption, metabolism, and excretion

Medications can affect nutritional status by altering appetite, nutrient absorption, metabolism, or excretion (Table 13.4). For example, more than 250 drugs, including blood pressure medications, antidepressants, decongestants, and the pain reliever ibuprofen (found in Advil, Motrin, and Nuprin), can cause mouth dryness, which can decrease interest in eating by interfering with taste, chewing, and swallowing. Mineral oil laxatives and cholestyramine (Questran), which is used to reduce blood cholesterol, can decrease the absorption of fat-soluble vitamins and some types of diuretics can increase the excretion of potassium from the body. These effects have the greatest nutritional impact on individuals who must take medications for extended periods, those who take multiple medications, and those who already have marginal nutritional status.

Food and nutritional status affect how well medications work

Food components can either enhance or retard the absorption and metabolism of drugs. Some medications are absorbed better or faster if taken with food whereas others are absorbed faster if taken with just water. Some, such as aspirin and ibuprofen, should be taken with food because they are irritating to the gastrointestinal tract. Drugs may also interact with specific nutrients. For instance, the antibiotic tetracycline should not be taken with milk because it binds with calcium, making both unavailable.

Nutritional status can also affect drug metabolism. If nutritional status is poor, the body's ability to detoxify drugs may be altered. For example, in a malnourished individual, theophylline, used to treat asthma, is metabolized slowly, resulting in high blood levels of the drug, which can cause loss of appetite, nausea, and vomiting.

Specific nutrients can also affect the metabolism of drugs. High-protein diets enhance drug metabolism in general, and low-protein diets slow it. Vitamin K hinders the action of anticoagulants, taken to reduce the risk of blood clots. On the other hand, omega-3 fatty acids, such as those in fish oils, inhibit blood clotting and may intensify the effect of an anticoagulant drug and cause bleeding. It is safe to eat fish while taking anticoagulant drugs; however, the use of fish oil supplements is not recommended. Drugs can also interact with each other. For example, ibuprofen interferes

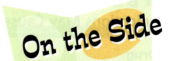

On the Side

When high aluminum levels were discovered in the brains of Alzheimer's patients, many people tried to reduce exposure by throwing out their aluminum pans and not using aluminum-containing deodorants. Unfortunately, there is little evidence that this is beneficial because Alzheimer's has not been linked to high dietary or environmental aluminum.

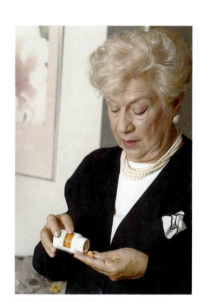

FIGURE 13.23

Most older adults take one or more medications every day. (Michael Newman/PhotoEdit)

19. CDC. Surveillance for Elevated Blood Lead Levels Among Children—United States, 1997–2001. *MMWR* 52:1–21, 2003. Available online at www.cdc.gov/mmwr/preview/mmwrhtml/ss5210a1.htm#top/Accessed September 2, 2004.

20. Fackelmann, K. Hypertension's lead connection: Does low-level exposure to lead cause high blood pressure? *Sci. News* 149:382–383, 1996.

21. Update: Blood lead levels—United States, 1991–1994. *MMWR*, 46:141–146, 1997.

22. Hindin, T. J., Contento, I. R., and Gussow, J. D. A media literacy nutrition education curriculum for Head Start parents about the effects of television advertising on their children's food requests. *J. Am. Diet. Assoc.* 104: 192–198, 2004.

23. Andersen, R. E., Crespo, C. J., Bartlett, S. J., et al. Relationship of physical activity and television watching with body weight and level of fatness among children: Results from the third National Health and Nutrition Examination Survey. *JAMA* 279:938–942, 1998.

24. Food and Nutrition Board, Institute of Medicine. *Dietary Reference Intakes for Calcium, Phosphorus, Magnesium, Vitamin D, and Fluoride.* Washington, DC: National Academy Press, 1997.

25. USDA Agriculture Research Service. 1997 Results from USDA's 1994–1996 CSFII and 1994–1996 Diet and Health Knowledge Survey. ARS Food Surveys Research Group. Available online at www.barc.usda.gov/bhnrc/foodsurvey/pdf/dhks9496.pdf Accessed September 16, 2004.

26. Food and Nutrition Board, Institute of Medicine. *Dietary Reference Intakes for Vitamin A, Vitamin K, Arsenic, Boron, Chromium, Copper, Iodine, Iron, Manganese, Molybdenum, Nickel, Silicon, Vanadium, and Zinc.* Washington, DC: National Academy Press, 2001.

27. Iron Deficiency—United States, 1999–2000. *MMWR* 51:897–899, 2002. Available online at www.cdc.gov/mmwr/preview/mmwrhtml/mm5140a1.htm/Accessed September 2, 2004.

28. American Dietetic Association. Timely statement of the American Dietetic Association: Nutrition guidance for adolescent athletes in organized sports. *J. Am. Diet. Assoc.* 96:611–612, 1996.

29. Terjung, R. L., Clarkson, P., Eichner, E. R., et al. American College of Sports Medicine Roundtable: The physiological and health effects of oral creatine supplementation. *Med. Sci. Sports Exerc.* 32:706–717, 2000.

30. Beals, K. A., and Manore, M. M. Nutritional status of female athletes with subclinical eating disorders. *J. Am. Diet. Assoc.* 98:419–425, 1998.

31. Bazzarre, T. L. Nutrition and strength. In *Nutrition in Exercise and Sport,* 3rd ed. Wolinski, I., ed. Boca Raton, FL: CRC Press, 1998, 369–419.

32. CDC. Deaths: Preliminary data for 2001, *National Vital Statistics Reports.* Vol 55, March 14, 2003. Available online at www.cdc.gov/nchs/data/nvsr/nvsr51/nvsr51_05.pdf/ Accessed September 2, 2004.

33. WHO. The World Health Report, 2001. Healthy life expectancy. Available online at www.who.int/whosis/hale/hale.cfm?path=whosis,hale&language=english/Accessed September 16, 2004.

34. CDC. Public health and aging: Trends in aging—United States and worldwide. *MMWR* 52;101–106, 2003. Available online

at http://www.cdc.gov/mmwr/preview/mmwrhtml/mm5206a2.htm/Accessed September 2, 2004.

35. U.S. Department of Health and Human Services. Administration on Aging. 1997 Census Estimates of the Older Population. Available online at www.aoa.dhhs.gov/aoa/stats/99pop/default.htm/Accessed February 17, 2001.

36. Stevens, J., Cai, J., Pamuk, E. R., et al. The effect of age on the association between body-mass index and mortality. *N. Engl. J. Med.* 338:1–7, 1998.

37. Masoro, E. J. Caloric restriction and aging: An update. *Exp. Gerontol.* 35:299–305, 2000.

38. Institute of Medicine, Food and Nutrition Board. *Dietary Reference Intakes for Thiamin, Riboflavin, Niacin, Vitamin B$_6$, Folate, Vitamin B$_{12}$, Pantothenic Acid, Biotin, and Choline.* Washington, DC: National Academy Press, 1998.

39. Russell, R. M. New views on the RDAs for older adults. *J. Am. Diet. Assoc.* 97:515–518, 1997.

40. Christen, W. G. Antioxidant vitamins and age-related eye disease. *Proc. Assoc. Am. Physicians* 111:16–21, 1999.

41. Blumberg, J. Nutritional needs of seniors. *J. Am. Coll. Nutr.* 16: 517–523, 1997.

42. Proctor, D. N., Balagopal, P., and Nair, K. S. Age-related sarcopenia in humans is associated with reduced synthetic rates of specific muscle proteins. *J. Nutr.* 128:351S–355S, 1998.

43. National Center for Health Statistics. Fast stats A to Z, arthritis. Available online at www.cdc.gov/nchs/fastats/arthrits.htm/ Accessed September 16, 2004.

44. Brief, A. A., Maurer, S. G., and Di Cesare, P. E. Use of glucosamine and chondroitin sulfate in the management of osteoarthritis. *J. Am. Acad. Orthop. Surg.* 9:71–78, 2001.

45. American Academy of Family Physicians. The nutrition checklist. Available online at www.aafp.org/nsi/Accessed September 2, 2002.

46. American Academy of Family Physicians. Nutrition Screening Initiative. Available online at www.aafp.org/nsi/index.hxml/ Accessed September 2, 2004.

47. Russell, R. M., Rasmussen, H., and Lichtenstein, A. H. Modified food guide pyramid for people over seventy years of age. *J. Nutr.* 129: 751–753, 1999.

48. Administration on Aging. A Profile of Older Americans: 2002. Available online at www.aoa.gov/prof/Statistics/profile/8.asp/ Accessed September 2, 2004.

49. U.S. Department of Health and Human Services. Administration on Aging. Fact Sheets. The Elderly Nutrition Program. Available online at www.aoa. gov/press/fact/alpha/fact_elderly nutrition.asp/Accessed September 16, 2004.

50. Roe, D. A. Development and current status of home-delivered meals programs in the United States: Are the right elderly served? *Nutr. Rev.* 52:29–33, 1994.

51. American Dietetic Association. Nutrition, aging and the continuum of care. *J. Am. Diet. Assoc.* 100:580–595, 2000.

52. American Medical Association. Harmful Consequences of Alcohol Use on the Brains of Children, Adolescents and College Students, 2002. Fact Sheet. Available online at www.ama-assn.org/ama/pub/category/9416.html/ Accessed September 2, 2004.

53. MMWR Surveillance Summaries, August 22, 2003. Vol 52, No SS-8. Available online at www.cdc.gov/mmwr/PDF/ss/ss5208.pdf/Accessed September 2, 2004.

54. National Institute on Alcohol Abuse and Alcoholism. Alcohol Alert No. 16 PH 315 Available online at www.niaaa.nih.gov/publications/aa16.htm/Accessed September 2, 2004.

55. Chick, J. Alcohol, health and the heart. *Alcohol* 33: 576–591, 1999.

56. Cleophas, T. J. Wine, beer and spirits and the risk of myocardial infarction: A systematic review. *Biomed. Pharmacother.* 53:417–423, 1999.

57. Ruh, J. C. Wine and polyphenols related to platelet aggregation and atherosclerosis. *Drugs Exp. Clin. Res.* 25:125–131, 1999.

58. Diebolt, M., Bucher, B., and Andriantsitohaina, R. Wine polyphenols decrease blood pressure, improve NO vasodilatation, and induce gene expression. *Hypertension* 38:159–65, 2001.

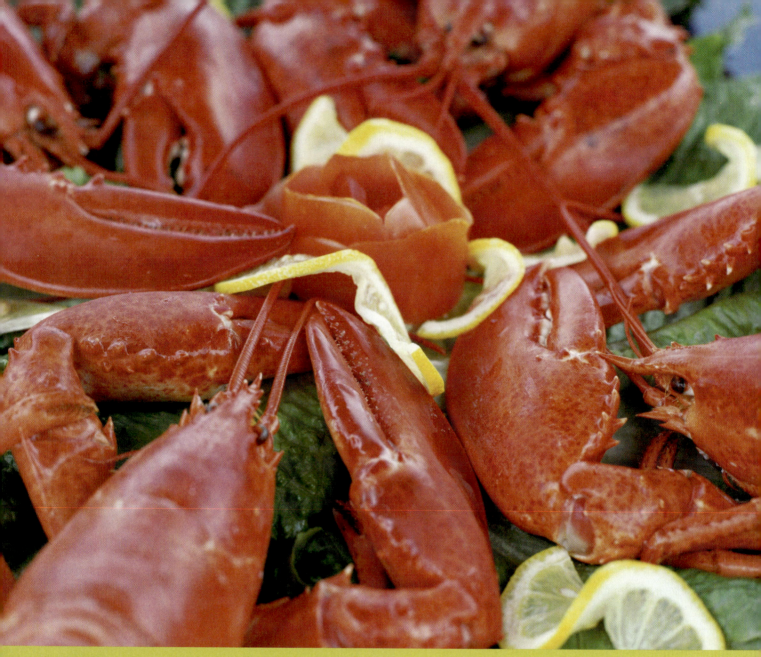

(Erik Rank/Foodpix/PictureArts Corp.)

CHAPTER 14 CONCEPTS

- Any illness related to the consumption of food is called food-borne illness.

- The safety of our food supply is the responsibility of federal, state, and local government organizations as well as individual consumers.

- Bacteria, viruses, molds, and parasites all have the potential to cause food-borne illness.

- Care in choosing, preparing, cooking, handling, and storing food can reduce the risk of food-borne illness.

- Chemicals used in agriculture and industry can make their way into the food supply.

- Technologies such as heating and cooling food, adding preservatives, and packaging are used to protect the food supply.

- Biotechnology is the newest tool used to enhance food safety but some are concerned that it may introduce new risks.

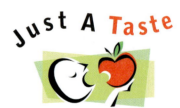

Just A Taste

Who is responsible for the safety of the food you eat?

Can you tell by looking at a food if it is contaminated?

Is it safe to eat hamburgers cooked medium rare?

Do food additives make the food supply safer?

How Safe Is Our Food Supply?

14

INTRODUCTION

USA Today

Common Food-Borne Illnesses Decline, but Not All

By *Elizabeth Weise*

April 29, 2004—The bad news: The Centers for Disease Control and Prevention estimates that 76 million people in the USA get a food-borne or diarrheal illness each year, and children are particularly at risk. The good news: Cases of at least five of the most common pathogens have significantly declined.

Common symptoms of such illnesses include diarrhea, abdominal pain and cramping. Of those who get sick, 323,000 are hospitalized, and 5,000 die. There was a dramatic decline last year in cases of deadly E. coli O157:H7 infection—36% fewer than in the previous year, according to food-borne surveillance data released Thursday by the CDC in collaboration with the Food and Drug Administration and the Department of Agriculture.

To read the entire article, go to www.usatoday.com/news/health/2004-04-29-food-usat_x.htm

If given a choice, we would only consume food that is completely safe. Unfortunately, this is almost impossible. Throughout history food has always carried risks, whether from toxins naturally found in the food or substances that contaminate it. Despite advances in science and technology these risks still exist today. The American food supply is the most carefully monitored in the world, but it is not risk-free or beyond improvement. Government agencies and food manufacturers work to ensure that the food you eat is healthy and safe, but you as a consumer also need to consider the risks and benefits when you decide which foods to buy, which to eat, and how to handle, store, and cook them.

Food-Borne Illness Is Caused by Consuming Contaminated Food

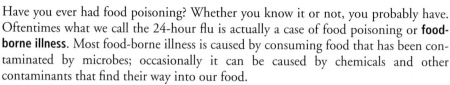

Food-borne illness An illness caused by consumption of food containing a toxin or disease-causing microorganism.

Have you ever had food poisoning? Whether you know it or not, you probably have. Oftentimes what we call the 24-hour flu is actually a case of food poisoning or **food-borne illness**. Most food-borne illness is caused by consuming food that has been contaminated by microbes; occasionally it can be caused by chemicals and other contaminants that find their way into our food.

How does this happen? Often food is contaminated where it is grown or harvested. For example, bacteria may contaminate strawberries and cantaloupes while they are still in the field (Figure 14.1), fish and seafood may be contaminated by chemicals in agricultural runoff or viruses in sewage that pollute the waters where they feed. Food can also be contaminated during processing at manufacturing plants or storage at retail facilities. You have probably heard about the recall of hamburger due to contamination with *E. coli* bacteria. *E. coli* contamination usually occurs in the processing plant when beef from one infected cow comes in contact with processing equipment, which then transfers the bacteria to all of the meat that is processed in that batch. This is referred to as **cross-contamination**. Contamination can also occur at home if food is not handled properly. Careful selection, sanitation, and handling can control most of these sources of food-borne illness.

Cross-contamination The transfer of contaminants from one food to another.

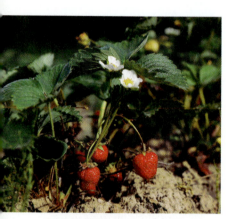

FIGURE 14.1

Strawberries and other fruits and vegetables can be contaminated with bacteria before they are even harvested. (© Bohemian Nomad Picturemakers/Corbis Images)

Contaminants in food don't always make us sick

Just because you eat a food that contains microbes or other potentially harmful substances doesn't mean you will get sick. Whether or not a contaminated food makes you sick depends on how potent the contaminant is, how much of it you consume, how often you consume it, and how big, how old, and how healthy you are. Some food contaminants cause harm even when minute amounts are consumed, and almost any substance can be toxic if a large enough amount is consumed. Small doses are more dangerous in children and small adults because the amount of toxin per unit of body weight is greater. Poor nutritional or health status may decrease the body's natural ability to detoxify harmful substances. How substances are metabolized and whether they are stored in your body also affect risk. Those that are stored are more likely to be toxic because they accumulate over time. Substances that are easily excreted are less likely to make you sick. The interaction of toxins with one another and with other dietary factors also affects toxicity. For example, mercury, which is extremely toxic, is not absorbed well if the diet is high in selenium, and the absorption of lead is decreased by the presence of iron and calcium in the diet.

Government agencies monitor the safety of the food supply

The safety of the food supply is monitored by agencies at the international, federal, and state levels. Different agencies have different responsibilities. At the international level, approximately 40 different nations work with the United States on setting food inspection and regulatory standards that help to ensure the safety of imported foods. At the federal level, the United States Department of Agriculture (USDA) and the U. S. Food and Drug Administration (FDA) along with a number of other agencies set standards and regulations for the safe and sanitary handling of food and water (Table 14.1). They also set standards for safe-handling information included on food labels. They regulate the use of agricultural chemicals, additives, and packaging materials; inspect food-processing and storage facilities; monitor both domestic and imported foods for contamination; and investigate outbreaks of food-borne illness. State agencies have the primary responsibility for milk safety and the inspection of restaurants, retail food stores, dairies, grain mills, and other food-related establishments within their borders (Figure 14.2). As a result, regulations vary from state to state.

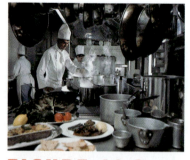

FIGURE 14.2

State and local governments are responsible for regulating the safety of food sold at restaurants. (John Miller/Stone/Getty Images)

TABLE 14.1
Who Regulates Food Safety?

Agency	What It Does
World Health Organization (WHO)	Develops international food safety policies, food inspection programs, and standards for hygienic food preparation; promotes technologies that improve food safety and consumer education about safe food practices.
Food and Drug Administration (FDA)	Ensures the safety and wholesomeness of all foods sold across state lines with the exception of red meat (beef, veal, pork, and lamb), poultry, and egg products; inspects food-processing plants; inspects imported foods with the exception of red meat, poultry, and egg products; sets standards for food composition; oversees use of drugs and feed in food-producing animals; and enforces regulations for food labeling, food and color additives, and food sanitation.
USDA Food Safety and Inspection Service (FSIS)	Enforces standards for the wholesomeness and quality of red meat, poultry, and egg products, including that imported from other countries. If a food is suspect, it can be tested for contamination, and entry into the country can be denied.
Environmental Protection Agency (EPA)	Regulates pesticide levels and must approve all pesticides before they can be sold in the United States; establishes water quality standards.
National Marine Fisheries Service	Oversees the management of fisheries and fish harvesting. Operates a voluntary program of inspection and grading of fish products.
USDA Animal and Plant Health Inspection Service (APHIS)	Monitors disease in food-producing animals.
Centers for Disease Control and Prevention (CDC)	Monitors and investigates the incidence and causes of food-borne diseases.
Bureau of Alcohol, Tobacco, and Firearms (ATF)	Enforces laws regulating the production, distribution, and labeling of alcoholic beverages.
State and local governments	Inspect food-processing plants, grocery stores, restaurants, and institutions such as schools and hospitals.

The National Food Safety Initiative coordinates food safety efforts

Media coverage of outbreaks of food-borne illness on cruise ships, the deaths of children from *E. coli* infection, and the headlines about mad cow disease have heightened our concerns about food safety. These concerns led to the development of the National Food Safety Initiative. This program was designed to coordinate all aspects of food safety from the farm to the table. It established a national computer network that allows public health agencies to quickly respond to serious and widespread food contamination problems.[1] Using this system, public health officials can track the source of outbreaks of food-borne illness. This information is used to make decisions about the recall of specific batches of food products from particular stores. Food distributors can then remove contaminated products from the shelves and stop the spread of the outbreak.

Controlling contamination is more effective than screening for it

Traditional methods of protecting the food supply use visual spot checks and random testing of food samples to screen for contamination. The National Food Safety Initiative has improved on this by promoting the use of a system that helps prevent food contamination rather than catch it after it occurs. This newer **Hazard Analysis Critical Control Point (HACCP)** approach involves developing procedures to prevent or control contamination. To accomplish this, food production, processing, and transport systems are analyzed to identify points where contamination can occur. Then, by monitoring these critical control points, contamination can be limited or prevented. For example, contamination with the bacteria *Salmonella* has been identified as a risk in the production of shelled frozen eggs. To produce this product, eggs are mixed

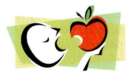

Federal, state, and local governments are all involved in keeping the food supply safe, but it is also the responsibility of the consumer. You control the handling and safety of foods once they enter your home. Safe food handling, storage, and cooking can reduce the risk of food-borne illness.

Hazard Analysis Critical Control Point (HACCP) A food safety system that focuses on identifying and preventing hazards that could cause food-borne illness.

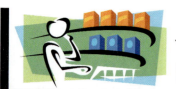

Your Choice: Should You Give Up Beef to Avoid Mad Cow Disease?

Two days before Christmas 2003 it was announced that a case of mad cow disease had been identified in the United States. The announcement created an uproar in the cattle industry and prompted federal officials to inform us that they were still eating prime rib for Christmas dinner. Why should be we care about a cattle disease? What does this mean in terms of human health?

Mad cow disease, or bovine spongiform encephalopathy (BSE), is a degenerative neurological disease that affects cattle. Symptoms begin with weight loss and changes in temperament. Within weeks or months, the animal is dead. It was first diagnosed in England in 1986 and later spread to other parts of Europe. Within 10 years of its appearance in cattle, a human form of this untreatable, incurable, and always fatal disease was identified. The human form of this disease is called variant Creutzfeldt-Jakob Disease (vCJD). People are believed to "catch it" by eating tissue from a cow infected with BSE. Symptoms of vCJD begin as mood swings and numbness and within about 14 months, progress to dementia and death.[1]

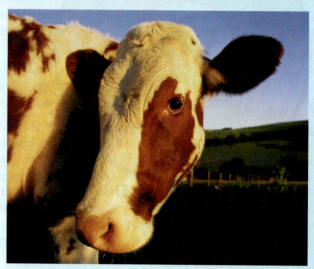

(Peter Cade/Stone/Getty Images)

So, why don't we just get rid of the infected cattle so we don't have to worry about whether it's in our hamburgers? The problem is that the only way to diagnose the disease is to kill the cow and analyze its brain tissue. By the time the results are in, the meat is on the shelf. Once it is in our meat there is no way to destroy the infectious agent. Most diseases we get from food can be prevented by cooking the food thoroughly; high temperatures kill the microbes that cause the illness. The problem with BSE is that it is caused by a protein; it can't be killed because it isn't alive. The mysterious agent that causes BSE in cows, as well as vCJD in humans and similar diseases in sheep, deer, and elk, is a protein called a prion, short for proteinaceous infectious particle. It differs from the normal brain protein in the way it is folded—its three-dimensional structure. This rouge protein reproduces itself by corrupting neighboring proteins, essentially changing their shape so they too become prions. The abnormal prion proteins are not degraded normally, so they accumulate, forming clumps called plaques. These plaques cause the deadly nervous tissue damage.

Where did these prions come from? We now know that they can be passed from an infected animal to an uninfected host, most likely from consumption of a food product containing central nervous system tissue from an infected animal.[2] BSE is believed to have originated from sheep that carried a similar disease called scrapie, which has been present in British sheep for over 200 years. It moved into cattle when the remains of slaughtered diseased sheep

began to be included in protein supplements that were fed to cattle. It was then passed to people when they ate products from infected cows.

To prevent people from getting vCJD, we need to prevent cows from getting BSE and prevent humans from eating products from infected cows. Safeguards that have been in place for some time have helped keep U.S. cows BSE-free until now. Restrictions on the import of all ruminants from countries where BSE was known to exist have been in place since 1989. In 1997, the USDA took further steps by restricting the import of ruminants and most ruminant products from all of Europe.[3] To prevent BSE from emerging in the United States, mammalian proteins cannot be used in protein supplements for ruminant animal feeds.

When the first case of mad cow disease was diagnosed in the United States authorities took immediate and long-term action. The origin of the cow was traced and the meat was recalled. Other parts of the cow were retrieved to make sure they did not get into animal feed or other products. More long-term precautions that are being put in place include increasing the number of cows tested for BSE at slaughter and holding products from cattle being tested until the results of tests are in. In addition, material from cows that can't walk will be banned from entering the food supply; high-risk tissues such as brain, spinal cord, eyes, and intestines will be kept out of the human food supply; and only slaughter methods that do not cause brain tissue to contaminate other parts of the cow will be used.[4]

So, should we all become vegetarians? Or at least have a grilled chicken sandwich instead of a hamburger for lunch? Because not all cows in the United States are tested, it is possible that a few infected animals could enter the food supply. Even if this happens and you eat meat from such a cow the risk of acquiring vCJD is extremely small. BSE is believed to be transmitted from brain and nervous tissue, intestines, eyes, and tonsils, but thus far, meat and milk have not been demonstrated to transmit BSE or vCJD. Even in Britain where over 180,000 cows were infected with BSE only about 146 cases of vCJD have been reported. It is likely that the precautions taken by U.S agencies will continue to prevent U.S. cows from getting BSE and infected meat from reaching the shelves. Because of these precautions, the risk

of animals being exposed to BSE and humans contracting vCJD in the United States remains extremely low.

References
1. U.S. Department of Agriculture. Animal and Plant Health Inspection Service. Bovine spongiform encephalopathy. Available online at www.aphis.usda.gov/lpa/issues/bse/bse.html/Accessed September 3, 2004.
2. Mad cow and human prion disease. *Neuro News*, May 18, 1998. Available online at neuroscience.about.com/science/neuroscience/library/weekly/aa051898.htm/Accessed March 5, 2001.
3. Bren, L. Trying to keep mad cow disease out of U.S. herds. *FDA Consumer*, March/April 2001. Available online at www.fda.gov/fdac/features/2001/201_cow.html/Accessed September 3, 2004.
4. Bren, L. Agencies work to corral mad cow disease. *FDA Consumer*, pp. 29–35, May/June, 2004.

improper handling. *Salmonella* outbreaks have been caused by contaminated meat, meat products, dairy products, seafood, fresh vegetables, and cereal, but poultry and eggs are the most common food sources. Poultry products are often contaminated because poultry farms house large numbers of chickens in close proximity, allowing one infected chicken to infect thousands of others. The *Salmonella* from an infected hen can enter eggs before they are laid so it is present inside the shell. Even if a food such as eggs that is contaminated with *Salmonella* is brought into the kitchen, careful handling and cooking of the food can prevent the organisms from causing illness. Washing hands, cutting boards, and utensils can prevent cross-contamination and thorough cooking can kill the bacteria.

E. coli is another bacterium that comes in contact with food through fecal contamination of water or unsanitary handling of food. Some strains of *E. coli* are harmless, but others can cause serious food-borne illness. One strain, found in water contaminated by human or animal feces, is the cause of "travelers' diarrhea." Another strain, *E. coli O157:H7*, produces a toxin that causes abdominal pain, bloody diarrhea, and, in severe cases, kidney failure and even death. This strain was responsible for the deaths of several children who consumed undercooked, contaminated hamburgers from a fast-food chain in 1993.

Although *E. coli* on food can multiply slowly even at refrigerator temperatures, if a contaminated food is thoroughly cooked to 160° F, both the bacteria and the toxin are destroyed. Ground beef contaminated with *E. coli O157:H7* is a particular risk because, unlike steaks and chops that are only contaminated on the surface, the grinding mixes the bacteria throughout the beef and other ground meats. The *E. coli* on the outside of the meat are quickly killed during cooking, but those in the interior survive if the meat is not cooked thoroughly. Transmission of *E. coli* is a risk at day-care centers from cross-contamination if caregivers do not carefully wash their hands after diaper changes.

Campylobacter is the most frequent cause of acute infectious diarrhea in developed countries. Common sources are undercooked chicken, unpasteurized milk, and untreated water. This organism grows slowly in the cold and is killed by heat, so, as with *Salmonella*, thorough cooking and careful storage help prevent infection.

Another cause of bacterial infection is *Listeria monocytogenes*. Although most cases of *Listeria* infection result in flulike symptoms, in high-risk groups such as pregnant women, children, the elderly, and the ill, it can cause meningitis and serious blood infections. It has one of the highest fatality rates of all food-borne illnesses. *Listeria* survives at higher and lower temperatures than most bacteria; it can survive and grow at refrigerator temperatures. *Listeria* frequently contaminates dairy products, but it is destroyed by pasteurization. It can contaminate processed ready-to-eat foods such as hot dogs and lunchmeats. Because consumers consider ready-to-eat foods safe, they often do not handle them as carefully as raw foods. To prevent infection, ready-to-eat meats should be heated to steaming and unpasteurized dairy products should be avoided.

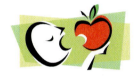

If a food looks spoiled don't eat it. But, just looking at a food, or even smelling or tasting it can't always detect contamination.

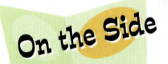

On the Side

A new way to reduce *Salmonella* infection in chickens is to spray chicks with a shower of beneficial bacteria. The chicks eat the bacteria as they preen themselves. These harmless bacteria grow in the chickens inhibiting the growth of pathogenic strains.

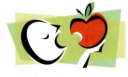

A medium-rare hamburger is not the safest choice because the center of the burger is not heated to a high enough temperature to kill bacteria that are in the middle.

TABLE 14.3
Which Bug Has You Down

Microbe	Where Do You Get It?	What Are the Symptoms?	When Do They Start?	How Long Does It Last?
Bacteria				
Salmonella	Fecal contamination, raw or undercooked eggs and meat, especially poultry	Nausea, abdominal pain, diarrhea, headache, fever	6–48 hrs	1–2 days
Campylobacter jejuni	Unpasteurized milk, under-cooked meat and poultry	Fever, headache, diarrhea, abdominal pain	2–5 days	1–2 wks
Listeria monocytogenes	Raw milk products, raw and undercooked poultry and meats, raw and smoked fish, produce	Fever, headache, stiff neck, chills, nausea, vomiting	Days to weeks	6 wks
Vibrio vulnificus	Raw seafood from contaminated water	Cramps, abdominal pain, weakness, watery diarrhea, fever, chills	15–24 hrs	2–4 days
Staphylococcus aureus	Human contamination from coughs and sneezes; eggs, meat, potato and macaroni salads	Severe nausea, vomiting, diarrhea	2–8 hrs	24–48 hrs
Escherichia coli O157:H7	Fecal contamination, undercooked ground beef	Abdominal pain, bloody diarrhea, kidney failure	5–48 hrs	3 days to 2 wks or longer
Clostridium perfringens	Fecal contamination, deep-dish casseroles	Fever, nausea, diarrhea, abdominal pain	8–22 hrs	6–24 hrs
Clostridium botulinum	Canned foods, deep casseroles, honey	Lassitude, weakness, vertigo, dizziness, respiratory failure, paralysis	18–36 hrs	10 days or longer (must administer antitoxin)
Shigella	Fecal contamination of water or foods, especially salads such as chicken, tuna, shrimp, and potato salad	Diarrhea, abdominal pain, fever, vomiting	12–50 hrs	5–6 days
Yersinia enterocolitica	Pork, dairy products, and produce	Diarrhea, vomiting, fever, abdominal pain; often mistaken for appendicitis	24–48 hrs	Weeks
Viruses				
Norovirus	Fecal contamination of seafood	Diarrhea, nausea, vomiting	1–2 days	2–6 days
Hepatitis A virus	Human fecal contamination of food or water, raw shellfish	Jaundice, liver inflammation, fatigue, fever, nausea, anorexia, abdominal discomfort	10–50 days	1–2 wks to several months
Parasites				
Giardia lamblia	Fecal contamination of water and uncooked foods	Diarrhea, abdominal pain, gas, anorexia, nausea, vomiting	5–25 days	1–2 wks but may become chronic
Cryptosporidium parvum	Fecal contamination of food or water	Severe watery diarrhea	Hours	2–4 days but sometimes weeks
Trichinella spiralis	Undercooked pork, game meat	Muscle weakness, flu symptoms	Weeks	Months
Anisakis simplex	Raw fish	Severe abdominal pain	1 hr to 2 wks	3 wks
Toxoplasma gondii	Meat, primarily pork	Toxoplasmosis (can cause central nervous system disorders, flu-like symptoms, and birth defects in women exposed during pregnancy)	10–23 days	May become chronic carrier

Source: U.S. Food and Drug Administration, Center for Food Safety and Nutrition. Foodborne Pathogenic Microorganisms and Natural Toxins Handbook: The "Bad Bug Book." Available online at vm.cfsan.fda.gov/~mow/intro.html/Accessed August 1, 2004.

Vibrio vulnificus infection usually causes gastrointestinal upset but can be deadly in vulnerable populations. Foods that pose a risk include raw and undercooked seafood. The bacteria are most common in mollusks such as oysters, clams, and mussels harvested from the Gulf of Mexico in the summer when the water is most likely to be contaminated with human fecal matter.

Food-borne intoxication is caused by consuming toxins in food

Food-borne intoxication is caused by consuming food containing toxins produced by microbes; the symptoms are caused by the toxin, not the organism itself. Unlike food-borne infections, which are caused by ingesting large numbers of bacteria, intoxication can be caused by only a few microorganisms that have produced a toxin. Although the bacteria are fairly easy to kill, some food toxins may be difficult to destroy.

Staphylococcus aureus is a common cause of microbial food-borne intoxication. These bacteria live in human nasal passages and can be transferred to food through coughing or sneezing. They can grow on the food, producing a toxin that causes vomiting soon after ingestion. Foods that are common sources include cooked ham, salads, bakery products, and dairy products.

The bacterium *Clostridium perfringens* may cause illness by both infection and intoxication. It thrives in conditions with little oxygen and is difficult to kill because it forms heat-resistant **spores**, which are a stage of bacterial life that remains dormant until environmental conditions favor growth. *Clostridium perfringens* is often called the "cafeteria germ" because foods stored in large containers like those used in cafeteria lines have little oxygen at the center, thus providing an excellent growth environment. Sources include improperly prepared roast beef, turkey, pork, chicken, and ground beef.

Another strain of *Clostridium, Clostridium botulinum*, produces the deadliest of all bacterial food toxins. Although the bacteria themselves are not harmful, consuming the toxin, produced as the spores begin to grow and develop, blocks nerve function, resulting in vomiting, abdominal pain, double vision, dizziness, and paralysis that leads to respiratory failure. If untreated, botulism poisoning is often fatal, but today modern detection methods and rapid administration of antitoxin have reduced mortality. *Clostridium botulinum* grows in low-oxygen, low-acid conditions, so foods such as potatoes or stew that are held in large containers provide optimal conditions for botulism spores to germinate. Canned foods, particularly improperly home-canned foods, can also be a source of botulism. Bulging cans should be discarded because this indicates the presence of gas produced by bacteria as they grow. Once formed, botulism toxin can be destroyed by boiling, but if the safety of a food is in question, it should be discarded; even a taste of botulism toxin can be deadly.

The most common form of botulism is infant botulism.[4] It occurs when the botulism spores are ingested. The spores germinate in the infant's body, producing toxin, some of which is absorbed into the bloodstream causing weakness, paralysis, and respiratory problems. Only infants are affected because in adults competing intestinal microflora prevent spores from germinating. Because honey can be contaminated with botulism spores, it should never be fed to infants under 1 year of age (Figure 14.5).

Viral infections can be contracted from food

Viruses make us sick by turning our cells into virus-making factories. The viruses that cause human disease cannot grow and reproduce in foods, but the virus particles can contaminate food and then infect consumers when they eat the food. Shellfish are notorious carriers of viral infections. Norovirus causes what is commonly known as the stomach flu. It is one of the leading causes of vomiting and diarrhea in the United States. Norovirus is found in water polluted with human or animal feces and infection is spread by contaminated food or water as well as person to person contact. Because norovirus is destroyed by cooking, water and uncooked foods such as raw shellfish and salads are the most common cause of food-borne illness from this virus.

Food-borne intoxication Illness caused by consuming a food containing a toxin.

Spore A dormant state of some bacteria that is resistant to heat but can germinate and produce a new organism when environmental conditions are favorable.

On the Side

Botulism toxin, the most poisonous substance known, is now used to get rid of wrinkles. When injected into tiny muscles around a wrinkle, the toxin, known as botox, causes the muscles to relax and the wrinkles smooth out. This treatment is not permanent so the injections need to be repeated to keep the wrinkles at bay. Botox has also been used to treat people who suffer from migraines, muscle spasms, and an overactive bladder.

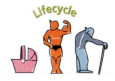

Lifecycle

On the Side

Over half of the gastroenteritis outbreaks reported aboard cruise ships in 2002 were associated with noroviruses. Because health officials track illnesses on cruise ships they are found and reported more quickly than outbreaks that occur on land.

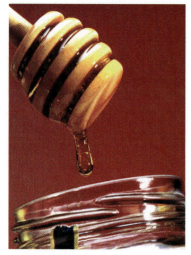

FIGURE 14.5

Spores from the bacterium *Clostridium botulinium* often contaminate honey. These spores can germinate in the intestinal tracts of infants so honey should never be fed to babies under 1 year of age. (Corbis Digital Stock)

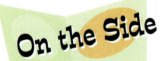

▲ **Parasites** Organisms that live at the expense of the host without contributing to its survival.

On the Side

In 1993 an outbreak of diarrhea in Milwaukee, Wisconsin affected about 403,000 people. The outbreak was traced to the parasite *Cryptosporidium* in the city water supply. The contamination is believed to have come from runoff from cattle farms.

Hepatitis A is a highly contagious viral disorder that can be contracted from food contaminated by unsanitary handling or from eating raw or undercooked shellfish caught in sewage-contaminated waters. Hepatitis A can require a long recovery period and, in some cases, results in permanent liver damage. Individuals who have contracted the hepatitis A virus may remain carriers for years. Hepatitis in drinking water is destroyed by chlorination. Cooking destroys the virus in food, and good sanitation can prevent its spread (Figure 14.6).

Molds produce toxins that can lead to food-borne intoxication

Many types of molds grow on foods such as bread, cheese, and fruit. Under certain conditions molds produce toxins. More than 250 different mold toxins have been identified. Aflatoxin is a mold toxin that is among the most potent mutagens and carcinogens known. It is commonly found in corn, cotton seed, peanuts, and tree nuts. The level of aflatoxin that may be present in foods is regulated to prevent toxicity. Another mold toxin that contaminates grain, particularly rye, is ergot. It causes hallucinations and is a natural source of the hallucinogenic drug LSD. Today, modern milling removes the part of the grain that harbors the mold, so the disease ergotism is rare. Cooking and freezing stops mold growth but does not destroy the mold toxins that have already been produced. If a food is moldy, it should be discarded, the area where it was stored should be cleaned, and neighboring foods should be checked to see if they have also become contaminated.

Parasites we eat in food can then live in us

Some **parasites** are microscopic single-celled animals, while others are worms that can be seen with the naked eye. Parasites are killed by thorough cooking. Most infections occur when food is exposed to contaminated water. *Giardia lamblia* is a single-celled parasite that is the most frequent cause of diarrhea not due to bacteria.[3] *Giardia* is sometimes contracted by hikers who drink untreated water from streams contaminated with animal feces, and it is becoming a problem from cross-contamination in day-care centers. *Cryptosporidium parvum* is another parasite that is commonly spread by contaminated water, but cases have also been reported from consuming raw fruits and vegetables that have been contaminated.[5]

Trichinella spiralis is a parasite found in raw and undercooked pork, pork products, and game meats, particularly bear. Once ingested, these small, wormlike organisms

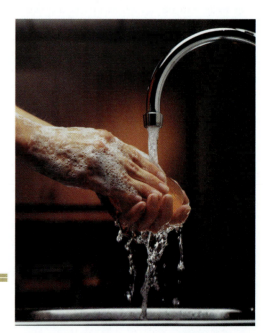

FIGURE 14.6

Good sanitation, especially hand washing, when preparing food is important for preventing food-borne illness. (Dick Clintsman/Corbis Images)

find their way to the muscles, where they grow, causing flulike symptoms, muscle weakness, fever, and fluid retention. Trichinosis, the disease caused by *Trichinella* infection, can be prevented by thoroughly cooking meat to kill the parasite before it is ingested. The parasites are also destroyed by curing, smoking, canning, or freezing.

Fish are a common source of parasitic infections. Fish can carry the larvae (a wormlike stage of an organism's life cycle) of parasites such as roundworms, flatworms, flukes, and tapeworms. One such infection, anisakis disease, is caused by the larval form of the small roundworm *Anisakis simplex*, or herring worm, found in raw fish.[3] Once consumed, these parasites invade the stomach and intestinal tract, causing severe abdominal pain. As the popularity of eating raw fish has increased, so has the incidence of parasitic infections from fish. The fresher the fish is when it is eviscerated, the less likely it is to cause this disease because the larvae move from the fish's stomach to its flesh only after the fish dies. Parasitic infections from fish can be avoided by consuming cooked fish or freezing fish for 72 hours before consumption. If raw fish is consumed, it should be very fresh (Figure 14.7).

Careful handling can prevent most microbial food-borne illness

Consumers can reduce their risk of food-borne illness by making wise choices (Table 14.4). Food should be fresh when purchased and consumed. Frozen foods should not contain frost or ice crystals, and food packaging should be secure.

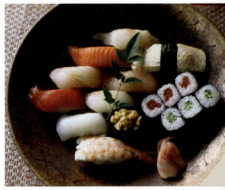

FIGURE 14.7

The incidence of parasitic infections has increased with the popularity of raw fish, such as this sushi. (Glenn Beanland/Lonely Planet Images)

On the Side

In North America, anisakis disease is often diagnosed when the affected individual feels a tingling or tickling sensation in their throat and coughs up a worm.

On the Side

There is no standard system for dating food products in the United States and it is not required by federal regulation. However, manufacturers often voluntarily include dates on some products: A "sell by" date indicates when the grocery store should take the product off the shelf. A "use by" date indicates the last date that is recommended for using the product at peak quality. "Best if used by" tells you how long the product will retain its best flavor or quality.

TABLE 14.4
What Can You Do?

To Keep Your Food Safe...

Choose wisely

Jars should be closed and seals unbroken. Cans should not be rusted, dented, or bulging. Check product expiration dates. Select frozen foods from below the frost line in the freezer.

Store foods properly

Fresh or frozen foods brought from the store should be refrigerated or frozen immediately. Food that has been in your refrigerator for longer than is safe should be discarded.

Wash

Hands, cooking utensils, and surfaces should be washed with warm soapy water before each food preparation step. This will prevent cross-contamination.

Thaw

Frozen foods should be thawed in the refrigerator or microwave.

Cook thoroughly

Foods should be cooked thoroughly to destroy most bacteria, toxins, viruses, and parasites. Use a meat thermometer.

Refrigerate promptly

Cooked food can be recontaminated, so it should be refrigerated as soon as possible after it is served.

Reheat thoroughly

Cooked foods should be thoroughly reheated to 165° F to destroy microorganisms that have recontaminated them and toxins that have been produced.

When in doubt, throw it out.

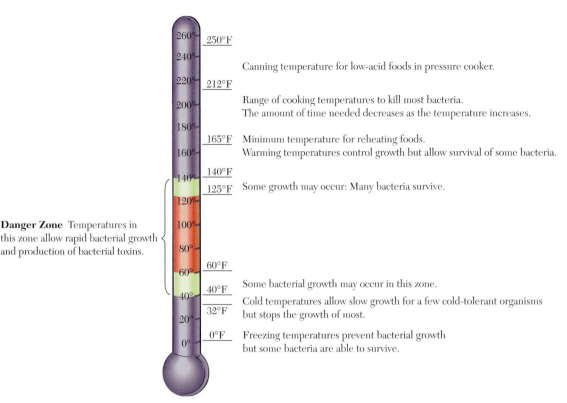

Danger Zone Temperatures in this zone allow rapid bacterial growth and production of bacterial toxins.

250°F
Canning temperature for low-acid foods in pressure cooker.

212°F

Range of cooking temperatures to kill most bacteria.
The amount of time needed decreases as the temperature increases.

165°F Minimum temperature for reheating foods.
Warming temperatures control growth but allow survival of some bacteria.

140°F
125°F Some growth may occur: Many bacteria survive.

60°F
40°F Some bacterial growth may occur in this zone.
Cold temperatures allow slow growth for a few cold-tolerant organisms
32°F but stops the growth of most.

0°F Freezing temperatures prevent bacterial growth
but some bacteria are able to survive.

FIGURE 14.8

Bacteria grow slowly at cold temperatures and are killed by very high temperatures. Avoid storing food in the danger zone—temperatures that favor microbial growth.

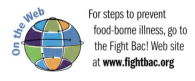

For steps to prevent food-borne illness, go to the Fight Bac! Web site at **www.fightbac.org**

Once purchased, food should be stored safely. The optimal temperature for microbial growth is between 40° and 140° F, so foods should only be allowed to remain in this temperature range for minimal amounts of time (Figure 14.8). This requires that cold foods be kept cold, frozen foods frozen, and that cooked foods be cooked thoroughly and kept hot until served.

Freezers should be set to 0° F, refrigerators to less than 40° F. Cold foods should be refrigerated as soon as possible after purchase. Fresh meat, poultry, and fish should be frozen immediately if they will not be used within a day or two. Processed meats such as hot dogs and bologna should also be refrigerated but can be kept longer than fresh meat.

Cooking food thoroughly destroys most harmful microorganisms. Meats should be cooked until they reach an internal temperature that will ensure that microorganisms have been killed. A meat thermometer should be used because color is not a good indicator of safety. Red meat and fish should be cooked to an internal temperature of 160° F and poultry to 180° F. Shellfish should be cooked to an internal temperature of 145° F. Eggs should not be eaten raw, because *Salmonella* can contaminate the inside of the shell; they should be boiled for 7 minutes, poached for 5 minutes, or fried for 3 minutes on a side (Table 14.5).

Cooked food should be refrigerated as soon as possible after serving. The best temperatures for bacterial growth are the temperatures at which food usually sets between service and storage. Large portions of food should be divided before refrigeration so they will cool quickly. Most leftovers should only be kept for a few days (Table 14.6) and when reheated, they should be heated thoroughly to destroy any bacteria that may have grown in them.

A clean kitchen is essential for food safety. Hands, countertops, cutting boards, and utensils should be washed with warm soapy water before each food preparation step. Food should be thawed in the refrigerator, in the microwave oven, or under running water—not at room temperature. In order to prevent cross-contamination foods that

TABLE 14.5

What Cooking Temperatures Are Safe?

Food Item	Internal Temperature (°F)
Beef, veal, lamb	
Ground products	160
Nonground products	
Medium-rare	145
Medium	160
Well-done	170
Poultry	
Ground products	165
Whole bird	180
Breasts and boneless roasts	170
Thighs, wings, drumsticks	180
Duck	180
Stuffing	165
Pork	
Noncured products	
Medium	160
Well done	170
Ham	160
Eggs	160
Leftovers	165

Source: American Dietetic Association. Available online at www.eatright.org/Accessed September 3, 2004.

TABLE 14.6

How Long Can You Refrigerate Leftovers?

Food Item	Keep Up To
Cooked vegetables	3–4 days
Cooked pasta	3–5 days
Cooked rice	1 week
Deli meats	5 days
Greens	1–2 days
Soups and stews	3–4 days
Stuffing	1–2 days
Meat	
Ham	3–4 days
Cooked beef, poultry, pork, and fish	3–4 days
Cooked seafood	2 days
Meat in gravy	1–2 days

Source: American Dietetic Association. Available online at www.eatright.org/Accessed September 3, 2004.

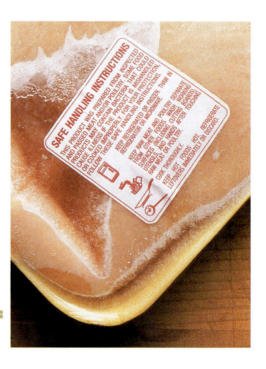

FIGURE 14.9

Meat carries labels offering safe-handling guidelines. (Dennis Drenner)

are going to be cooked should not be prepared on the same surfaces as foods that are eaten raw. For example, if a chicken contaminated with *Salmonella* is cut up on a cutting board and the unwashed cutting board is then used to chop vegetables for a salad, the vegetables will become contaminated with *Salmonella*. When the chicken is cooked, the bacteria will be killed, but the contaminated vegetables are not cooked, so the bacteria can grow and cause food-borne illness when the vegetables are eaten. Cross-contamination can also occur when uncooked foods containing live microbes come in contact with foods that have already been cooked. Therefore, cooked meat should never be returned to the same dish that held the raw meat, and sauces used to marinate uncooked foods should never be used as a sauce on cooked food. To remind consumers how to handle meat, the packaging is labeled with safe handling guidelines (Figure 14.9).

Consumers have less control over the safety of food eaten away from home

Although most of the food-borne illness in the United States is caused by food prepared in homes, an outbreak in a commercial or institutional establishment usually involves more people and is more likely to be reported. Food in retail establishments has many opportunities to be contaminated because of the large volume of food that is handled and the large number of people involved in food preparation.

Even when a restaurant uses extreme care in food preparation, customers can be a source of contamination. Because customers serve themselves at salad bars, cross-contamination from one customer to another is a risk. Salad and dessert bars in restaurants are usually equipped with "sneeze guards"—clear plastic shields placed above the food to prevent contamination from coughs and sneezes (Figure 14.10). Customers are also asked to use a clean plate if they go back for second helpings.

Picnics and other large events where food is served provide a prime opportunity for microbes to flourish because food is often left at room temperature or in the sun for hours before it is consumed. Foods that last well without refrigeration, such as fresh fruits and vegetables, breads, and crackers, should be selected for these occasions.

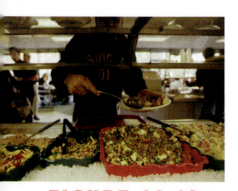

FIGURE 14.10

Clear plastic shields, or "sneeze guards," above salad bars prevent customers from contaminating food with microorganisms transmitted by coughs and sneezes. (Catherine Karnow/Corbis Images)

PIECE IT TOGETHER

Using HAACP at Home

Jennifer is organizing the annual class picnic. In order to help reduce the chances of causing food-borne illness, she decides to try to apply the principles of HAACP (Hazard Analysis Critical Control Point) she learned in her food science class. HAACP is designed to prevent or eliminate potential food hazards before they can make anyone sick. The first step in HAACP is to analyze the points in food preparation and storage where food contamination can occur.

WHAT ARE THE POINTS WHERE CONTAMINATION CAN OCCUR?

The picnic is a potluck so the food will be made in many people's homes; most contamination occurs in home-prepared foods. Another point where food can become unsafe is during storage. It is summer and the food will be outside in the temperature danger zone for several hours so pathogenic bacteria present on food will have the opportunity to multiply and produce toxins.

HOW CAN JENNIFER PREVENT FOOD FROM BEING CONTAMINATED DURING PREPARATION?

Jennifer can analyze the steps where contamination can occur during the preparation of food in her own kitchen, but it is not possible to check every step in the preparation of each food that others are making for the picnic. She can however find out what people are bringing and perhaps suggest some different choices if the foods seem to present a significant risk. She collects the following list of food items that her friends intend to bring:

Chicken salad   Cheese and crackers
Tamales   Apple pie
Fruit salad   Cookies
Raw vegetables   Mushrooms stuffed
   and onion dip   with crab meat
Chips and salsa   Fried chicken

WHICH FOODS ARE THE LEAST RISKY?

The safest foods are those that involve no home preparation and are intended to be served at room temperature such as the chips, cookies, and cheese and crackers. Store-bought dips are a good choice because they can remain unopened until the party begins. Acidic dips such as tomato-based salsa are safe because the acid inhibits bacterial growth. The apple pie is also probably safe during the picnic as long as it has been refrigerated beforehand. The raw fruits and vegetables are safe as long as they are washed before serving.

HOW MIGHT RAW VEGETABLES AND FRUIT SALAD BECOME CONTAMINATED?

Your answer:

WHICH FOODS CARRY THE HIGHEST RISKS?

The more food is handled, the more likely it is to be contaminated. The chicken salad, tamales, and mushrooms pose a risk because they are handled extensively in preparation. The fried chicken, stuffed mushrooms, and tamales are cooked, but when left at room temperature, the inside may stay warm enough to provide a good environment for microbial growth.

WHAT CAN JENNIFER DO TO REDUCE THE RISK OF FOOD SPOILAGE DURING THE PICNIC?

Your answer:

AFTER THE PICNIC IS OVER, WHAT FOODS WOULD YOU CONSIDER SAFE TO KEEP AS LEFTOVERS AND WHAT WOULD YOU THROW OUT?

Your answer:

Chemical Contaminants Can Enter the Food Supply

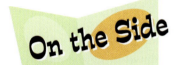

Many toxic substances can find their way into the food supply from the environment. These environmental pollutants are taken up by plants and consumed by small animals that are then eaten by larger animals that are in turn eaten by still larger animals, thus passing the contaminants up through the food chain to all levels of the food supply. Contaminants are found in the greatest concentration in foods of animal origin because animals are at the top of the food chain (Figure 14.11). If consumed in large enough amounts some of these compounds can make you ill.

The toxins that occur naturally in plants help protect the plant from bacterial and viral infections, molds, insect pests, and animal predators. For example, the toxins found in various poisonous mushrooms ensure they stay on the forest floor, rather than end up on your dinner plate. As with manmade toxins, natural toxins move through the food supply and can cause illness if consumed in large enough amounts. For example, a cow that has foraged on toxic plants can pass the toxin into her milk. Abraham Lincoln's mother died from drinking milk from a cow than had eaten poisonous snakeroot plants. The potential for toxicity depends on the dose of the toxin consumed and the health of the consumer. Most natural toxins in the food supply are consumed in doses that pose little risk to the consumer.

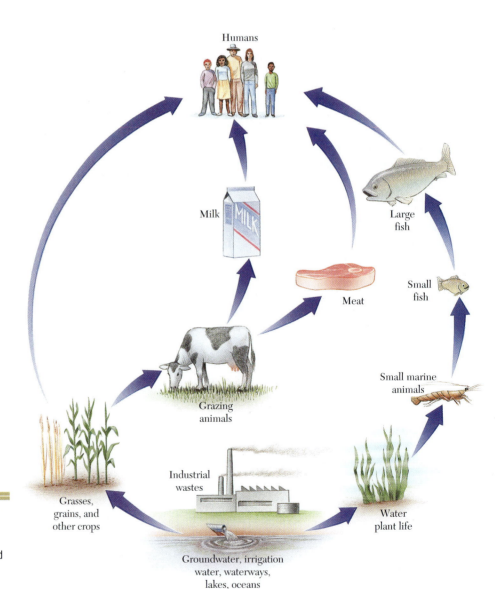

FIGURE 14.11

Industrial pollutants that contaminate the water supply become more and more concentrated as they are passed up the food chain. Large organisms like cattle and large fish may have high levels of these contaminants in their adipose tissue.

Pesticides have many benefits and some risks

Crops grown using pesticides generally produce higher yields and look more appealing because they have less insect damage. However, residues of these chemicals can remain on the fruits and vegetables that reach your plate, and they can pollute water supplies and soil. Because pesticides enter the environment, residues of these chemicals are found not only on produce, but also in meat, poultry, fish, and dairy products. The potential risks of pesticides to consumers depend on the type and amount consumed as well as who consumes them.

Pesticide use is regulated The types of pesticides that can be used on food crops and the amounts of residues that can remain when foods reach consumers are regulated. The Environmental Protection Agency (EPA) must approve and register pesticides that are used in food production and establish allowable limits, or **tolerances**. The FDA and USDA then monitor pesticide levels in foods. To establish tolerances for pesticides, the risk of toxicity is weighed against the benefit that the pesticide provides. The risks are based on the known incidence of toxicity and the predicted exposure that consumers will have to the toxin. Tolerance levels are then set at the minimum amount of the pesticide needed to be effective; these levels are often several hundred times lower than the level found to cause reactions in test animals. Because the same amount of pesticide provides a larger dose per unit of body weight for a child, the EPA is required to set tolerances that are safe for children as well as adults.

⚠ **Tolerances** The maximum amounts of pesticide residues that may legally remain in food, set by the EPA.

   In general, the amounts of pesticides to which people are exposed through foods are small. A report by the National Research Council concluded that the majority of synthetic chemicals, including pesticides, in the diet are present at levels below which any significant adverse biological effect is likely and that they are unlikely to pose a cancer risk.[6] Although special-interest groups concerned with overuse of pesticides disagree with this conclusion, the fact remains that repeated consumption of large doses of any one pesticide is unlikely because most people consume a variety of foods produced in many different locations.

Better pesticides and agricultural methods help reduce pesticide risk To reduce the risks of pesticide contamination more effective, less toxic chemical pesticides are being developed, and the use of older, more toxic products is decreasing in the United States. In addition to developing safer pesticides, safer production methods are being implemented to make low-pesticide and pesticide-free produce available to the consumer.

Integrated pest management minimizes pesticide use
Integrated pest management (IPM) is a method of agricultural pest control that combines chemical and nonchemical methods and emphasizes the use of natural toxins and more effective pesticide application. For example, increasing the use of naturally pest-resistant crop varieties that thrive without the use of added pesticides can reduce costs and do less environmental damage. Integrated pest management programs use information about the life cycle of pests and their interaction with the environment to manage pest damage economically, and with the least possible hazard to people, property, and the environment.

⚠ **Integrated pest management (IPM)** A method of agricultural pest control that integrates nonchemical and chemical techniques.

Organic farming does not use synthetic pesticides **Organic food** production is based on biological methods that avoid the use of synthetic pesticides, herbicides, or fertilizers. It applies many of the same concepts as IPM but restricts the use of pesticides to those that are produced from natural sources. Consumer demand for these products has been increasing due in part to the belief that organic foods are safer or superior in quality, taste, or nutrient content to conventionally grown foods; however, this is not necessarily the case. In addition, organic foods are usually more expensive and available in less variety than conventionally grown foods.

⚠ **Organic food** Food produced without the use of synthetic fertilizers or pesticides, sewage sludge, irradiation, or genetically modified ingredients according to the standards of the USDA's National Organic Program.

TABLE 14.8
What Do Additives Do?

Additive	What It Does	Where It Is Used
Acetic acid	Provides acidity	Gives tartness to dressings and sauces.
Ascorbic acid	Preservative, nutrient	Keeps fruit from darkening, inhibits rancidity in fatty foods, enhances nutritional value of beverages.
Baking soda (sodium bicarbonate)	Leavening agent	Generates gas so ensures baked goods rise.
Beet extract	Natural color	Gives deep red color to foods.
BHA (butylated hydroxyanisole)	Preservative	Acts as an antioxidant to prevent rancidity of fats, oils, and dried meats; keeps baked goods fresh.
BHT (butylated hydroxytoluene)	Preservative	Acts as an antioxidant to prevent rancidity in potato flakes, enriched rice and shortenings.
Calcium silicate	Anticaking agent	Absorbs moisture to keep powdered foods like baking powder free-flowing.
Carrageenan	Stabilizer, texturizer	Improves consistency and texture of chocolate milk, frozen desserts, puddings, and syrup.
Citric acid	Preservative, provides acidity	Provides acidity in beverages and dessert products.
FD&C colors	Color	Adds color to foods, drugs, and cosmetics.
Gelatin	Thickener	Provides texture to desserts, confectionery products, and canned meat products.
Glycerides (monoglycerides and diglycerides)	Emulsifier	Prevents ice cream from separating while melting, keeps oil in peanut butter from separating.
Glycerine (glycerol)	Humectant	Binds water to prevent moisture losses in flaked coconut, marshmallows, and toaster foods.
Guar gum	Thickener	Thickens liquids such as gravies and sauces.
Gum arabic	Stabilizer, emulsifier	Keeps butter mixed in buttered syrups and stabilizes flavors in dry-mix food products.
Lactic acid	Preservative	Controls molds in pickles, sauerkraut, cheese, buttermilk, and yogurt.
Lecithin	Emulsifier	Prevents separation of oil and vinegar in mayonnaise.
Magnesium stearate	Anticaking agent	Prevents clumping in flour.
Pectin	Thickener	Gels jams, jellies, and preserves.
Potassium sorbate	Preservative	Controls surface molds on cheese, syrups, margarine, and mayonnaise.
Propylene glycol	Humectant	Improves texture of foods by holding moisture.
Sodium benzoate	Preservative	Controls molds in syrup, margarine, soft drinks, and fruit products.
Sodium chloride	Preservative, flavor agent	Prevents microbial growth in cured meats, adds flavor to soups.
Sodium nitrite	Preservative	Prevents botulism growth in cured meats, fish, and poultry.
Sorbitol	Sweetener, humectant	Keeps fruit snacks and gummy candies soft.
Sulfites (sulfur dioxide, sodium sulfide, sodium and potassium bisulfite, and sodium and potassium metabisulfite)	Preservative	Acts as an antioxidant to prevent discoloration in fruits and vegetables like dried apples and dehydrated potatoes.
Tartaric acid	Increases acidity	Adds tartness to carbonated fruit-flavored drinks.

Additives can maintain or improve the nutritional value of a food Nutrients that are added to foods are considered additives. As discussed in Chapter 8, refined grains have iron and some of the B vitamins added in enrichment; these are considered additives. Although the addition of these to foods benefits the population by increasing the nutrient content of the diet, it can also increase the risk of nutrient toxicities. For example, high intakes of foods fortified with folic acid can mask the symptoms of a vitamin B_{12} deficiency.

Additives improve and maintain texture Many different types of additives are used in product processing and preparation. Emulsifiers such as lecithin and mono- and diglycerides improve the homogeneity, stability, and consistency of products like ice cream and peanut butter. Stabilizers, thickeners, and texturizers, such as pectins and gums, are used to improve consistency or texture in pudding and to stabilize emulsions in foods such as salad dressing. Leavening agents are added to incorporate gas into breads and cakes, causing them to rise. Acids are added as flavor enhancers, preservatives, and antioxidants. Humectants, such as propylene glycol, cause moisture to be retained so products stay fresh. Anticaking agents prevent crystalline products such as powdered sugar from absorbing moisture and caking or lumping.

Additives affect color and flavor Additives are also used to enhance the flavor and color of foods. Both natural and artificial sweeteners are added to sweeten foods such as yogurt and fruit drinks. Color additives enhance the appearance of foods. They are used in foods for many reasons, including to balance color loss due to storage or processing, to even out natural variations in food color, and to make foods appear more appetizing. However, they cannot be used as deception to conceal inferiority. Colors permitted for use in foods are classified as certified or exempt from certification. Certified food colors are synthetic dyes that have been tested to ensure safety, quality, consistency, and strength of color. Colors derived from plant, animal, and certain mineral sources are exempt from certification. Examples include beet juice, caramel, and paprika extract.

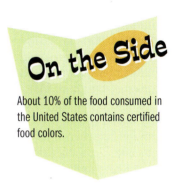

Food additives are regulated by the FDA
Food additives improve food quality and help protect us from disease, but if the wrong additive is used or if the wrong amount is added, it could do more harm than good. To prevent this, the Federal Food, Drug, and Cosmetic (FD&C) Act of 1938, gave the Food and Drug Administration (FDA) authority over food and food ingredients and defined requirements for truthful labeling of ingredients. This act provided exemptions and safe tolerance levels for additives that were necessary or unavoidable in production and established what are called **standards of identity** for certain foods. Standards of identity define exactly the ingredients that can be contained in certain foods such as mayonnaise, jelly, and orange juice. The Food, Drug, and Cosmetic Act also gave the FDA the responsibility of testing food additives for safety. Because the FDA could not possibly test all additives, the 1958 Food Additives Amendment transferred the responsibility for testing from the FDA to the manufacturer. Today, when a manufacturer wants to use a new food additive, they must submit a petition to the FDA. The petition must describe the chemical composition of the additive, how it is manufactured, and how it is detected and measured in food. The manufacturer must prove that the additive will be effective for its intended purpose at the proposed levels, that it is safe for its intended use, and that its use is necessary. Additives may not be used to disguise inferior products or deceive consumers. They cannot be used if they significantly destroy nutrients or where the same effect can be achieved by sound manufacturing processes.

Standards of identity Regulations that define the allowable ingredients, composition, and other characteristics of foods.

Some additives used before 1958 are regulated differently
The Food Additives Amendment of 1958 exempted two groups of substances from the food additive regulation process. One group included substances that the FDA or the USDA had determined were safe; these were designated as prior-sanctioned substances. The nitrates and nitrites used to retard the growth of *Clostridium botulinum* in cured meats such as ham and hot dogs are on the prior-sanctioned list. However, the use

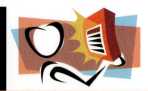

Off the Label: What's Been Added to Your Food?

For many of us, the ingredients listed on food labels sound like a chemical soup. Calcium propionate is added to bread, disodium EDTA is added to canned kidney beans, and BHA is in potato chips. Are these chemical additives safe?

For most individuals, concerns about food additives are unfounded. The FDA does not approve food additives unless they are safe for most consumers. Understanding what these chemicals are used for can help make the ingredient list a source of information rather than a cause for concern (see Table 14.6).

For individuals who are sensitive or allergic to certain additives the ingredient list provides lifesaving information about what additives are present. For example, in sensitive individuals, sulfites can cause symptoms that range from stomachaches and hives to severe asthmatic reactions. Sulfites are preservatives used in foods such as baked goods, canned vegetables, dried fruits, condiments, and maraschino cherries. Sulfites that may appear in the ingredient list of packaged foods include sulfur dioxide, sodium sulfite, sodium and potassium bisulfite, and sodium and potassium metabisulfite.[1] Individuals sensitive to sulfites should read food labels to identify foods that contain them, and should be aware that foods served in restaurants could contain sulfites. For example, a potato dish served in a restaurant may be prepared using potatoes that were peeled and soaked in a sulfite solution before cooking.

Food colors can also cause reactions in sensitive individuals. For instance, the color additive FD&C Yellow No. 5, which is listed as tartrazine on medicine labels, may cause itching and hives in sensitive people. It is found in beverages, desserts, and processed vegetables. The ingredient list of the food label can be used to identify the presence of color additives. All foods that contain FDA-certified color additives must list them by name in the ingredient list. Colors that are exempt from certification, such as dehydrated beets and carotenoids, do not have to be specifically identified and may be listed on the label collectively as "artificial color."[2]

Reactions to food ingredients are relatively rare. The FDA estimates that 1 in 100 people are sulfite-sensitive and that sensitivity to FD&C Yellow No. 5 occurs in fewer than 1 in 10,000 people. The FDA monitors problems related to food additives using the Center for Food Safety and Applied Nutrition's Adverse Event Reporting System. Adverse reactions can be reported by contacting the FDA district office listed in your phone directory or in an emergency by calling the FDA's main emergency number, 301-443-1240.

References
1. Papazian, R. Sulfites: Safe for most, dangerous for some. *FDA Consumer* 30:11–14, December 1996. Available online at www.cfsan.fda.gov/~dms/fdsulfit.html/Accessed September 20, 2004.
2. U.S. Food and Drug Administration. Food Color Facts. January 1993. Available online at vm.cfsan.fda.gov/~lrd/colorfac.html/Accessed August 1, 2004.

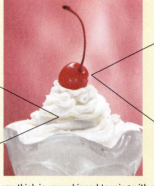

INGREDIENTS: Cream, milk, sugar, dextrose, sorbitan monostearate, artificial flavor, carrageenan, mixed tocopherols (vitamin E) to protect flavor, beta carotene (color), propellant: Nitrous oxide

INGREDIENTS: CHERRIES, WATER, CORN SYRUP, SUGAR, CITRIC ACID, NATURAL AND ARTIFICIAL FLAVOR, POTASSIUM SORBATE AND SODIUM BENZOATE ADDED AS PRESERVATIVE, FD&C RED #40 (ARTIFICIAL COLOR), AND SULFUR DIOXIDE (PRESERVATIVE).

There are more additives than you think in your whipped topping with a cherry on top. (Comstock Images/Getty Images)

of these has been controversial because they form carcinogenic **nitrosamines** in the digestive tract. They are still allowed in foods because there is little evidence that they pose a serious risk in the amounts consumed in the human diet.[15] To minimize any risk posed by nitrosamines without increasing the risk of bacterial illness, the FDA has limited the amount of nitrites that can be added to food and has required the addition of antioxidants, which reduce nitrosamine formation, to foods containing nitrites. Consumers can reduce the risk of nitrites by limiting cured meat consumption to 3 to 4 ounces per week and maintaining adequate intakes of the antioxidant vitamins C and E.

A second category excluded from the food additive regulation process is substances **generally recognized as safe (GRAS)**. GRAS substances are those whose use is generally recognized as safe, based on their extensive history of use in food before 1958 or based on published scientific evidence.

Just because a substance is on the GRAS or prior-sanctioned list doesn't mean it is safe or that it will stay on these lists. If new evidence emerges that suggests that a substance in either of these categories is unsafe the FDA may take action to remove the substance from food products.

The Delaney Clause prevents carcinogens from being added to foods
The 1958 Food Additives Amendment also included the **Delaney Clause**, which was designed to protect the public from additives found to be carcinogenic. The Delaney Clause states that a substance that induces cancer in either an animal species or humans at any dosage, no matter how large, may not be added to food. Currently, support is growing to amend the Delaney Clause to allow the use of substances that are added at a level so low that they would not represent a significant health risk.

Packaging helps protect food

How long does it take an open package of cheddar cheese to grow mold in your refrigerator? How about an unopened package? The open package will be moldy in a few days but the unopened package will stay fresh for weeks. Packaging plays an important role in food preservation; it keeps molds and bacteria out, keeps moisture in, and protects food from physical damage. Food packaging is continuously being improved.

Consumer demand for fresh foods has led to the packaging of fresh refrigerated foods such as pasta, vegetables, fish, chicken, and beef. To make fresh refrigerated foods—for example, beef teriyaki—the raw ingredients are sealed in plastic pouches, the air is vacuumed out, and the pouch and its contents are partially precooked and immediately refrigerated. This type of processing eliminates the need for the extreme cold of freezing or the extreme heat of canning, so flavor and nutrients are better preserved. Unlike canned foods, fresh refrigerated products are not heated to sufficient temperatures to kill all bacteria, and unlike frozen foods, they are not kept at temperatures low enough to prevent all bacteria from growing. In some products, the oxygen in the package is replaced with a gas such as carbon dioxide or nitrogen, in which microbes are unlikely to grow. This is called **modified atmosphere packaging (MAP)**. These foods should be purchased only from reputable vendors, used by the expiration date printed on the package, refrigerated constantly until use, and heated according to the time and temperature on the package directions.

Packaging can protect food from spoilage, but even the best packaging can introduce risk if it becomes a part of the food. A variety of substances leach into foods from plastics, paper, and even dishes. Substances that are known to contaminate foods are indirect food additives and the amounts and types are regulated by the EPA and the FDA. However, these regulations apply only to the intended use of the product. When used improperly, substances from packaging can migrate into food. These are accidental contaminants, which are not regulated by the FDA. It is the consumer's responsibility to prevent these substances from entering food. For instance, some plastics migrate into food when heated in a microwave oven. Thus, only packages designed for microwave cooking should be used.

Nitrosamines Carcinogenic compounds produced by reactions between nitrites and amino acids.

Generally recognized as safe (GRAS) A group of chemical additives defined by the FDA as safe based on their long-standing presence in the food supply without obvious harmful effects.

Delaney Clause A clause added to the 1958 Food Additives Amendment of the Pure Food and Drug Act that prohibits the intentional addition to foods of any compound that has been shown to induce cancer in animals or humans at any dose.

Modified atmosphere packaging (MAP) A type of food packaging in which the gases inside the package control or retard chemical, physical, and microbiological changes.

Biotechnology could introduce toxins or allergens to food Safety concerns related to bioengineered foods include the possibility that an allergen or toxin may have inadvertently been introduced into a previously safe food, or that the nutrient content of a food may have been negatively affected. For example, if DNA from fish or peanuts—foods that commonly cause allergic reactions—is introduced into tomatoes or corn, these foods that were previously safe could cause allergic reactions. Or, if tomatoes, which are a good source of vitamin C, were modified to have no vitamin C, people who rely on tomatoes for the vitamin would no longer meet their needs.

Another potential health concern is that the antibiotic resistance genes used in biotechnology may promote the development of antibiotic-resistant strains of bacteria. If bacteria that cause human disease acquire the antibiotic-resistant traits, then the effectiveness of antibiotic treatments will be reduced.

Biotechnology could harm the environment One of the arguments against the use of genetically modified crops is that they will harm the environment by reducing diversity, promoting the evolution of pesticide-resistant insects, and creating "superweeds" that will overgrow our agricultural and forest lands. Diversity is a concern because the ability of populations of organisms to adapt to new conditions, diseases, or other hazards depends on the presence of many different species that provide a diversity of genes. If farmers only plant new insect-resistant high-yielding varieties of crops other varieties may eventually become extinct. This is a concern with genetically engineered crops, but no more so than with crops developed by traditional plant breeding.

The evolution of pesticide-resistant insects is also a concern. An illustration of this problem is insects that feed on plants that have been modified to produce the Bt toxin. As more and more of the insect's food supply is made up of plants that produce this pesticide, only insects that carry genes making them resistant to Bt can survive and reproduce. This increases the number of Bt-resistant insects and therefore reduces the effectiveness of Bt as a method of pest control. Although an important concern, the risk of this occurring is no greater for genetically modified crops than for pesticides that are sprayed on crops.

Concern about the development of super weeds has arisen because it is hypothesized that traits introduced into domesticated plant species might be passed on to wild relatives, causing them to become fast-growing weeds. Although this is unlikely to occur, as a safeguard plant developers are avoiding introducing traits that could increase plant competitiveness or other undesirable properties of weedy relatives.

The use of biotechnology is regulated

Experts estimate that 70% to 75% of all processed foods on U.S. grocery shelves contain genetically modified ingredients.[19] The most common genetically modified foods are soybeans, corn, cotton, and rapeseed (canola) oil. Therefore foods produced in the U.S. that contain field corn or high-fructose corn syrup, such as many breakfast cereals, snack foods, and soft drinks; foods made with soybeans; and foods made with cottonseed and canola oils could contain genetically modified ingredients. The reason you didn't know these foods were genetically modified is they appear no different from other foods and special labeling of these foods is only required if they pose a potential risk.

To prevent harm to the consumer and to the environment three U.S. government agencies, the FDA, the USDA, and the EPA, are involved in regulating genetically modified plants and foods. Guidelines established by these agencies help researchers address safety and environmental issues at all stages of the process, from the early development of genetically engineered plants through field-testing and, eventually, commercialization. Companies that develop new plant varieties must provide data to support the safety and wholesomeness of their products. Crops created by both traditional breeding and biotechnology methods must be field-tested for several seasons to make sure only desirable changes have been made. Plants are examined to ensure that

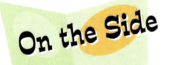

On the Side

The United States accounts for over two-thirds of all GM crops planted globally. GM food crops grown by U.S. farmers include corn, cotton, soybeans, canola, squash, and papaya.

they look right, grow right, and produce food that is safe, not nutritionally altered, and tastes right.[18]

The FDA regulates the safety of GM foods The FDA policy is that the safety of a food product should be determined based on the characteristics of the food or food product, not the method used to produce it. Foods developed using biotechnology are therefore evaluated to determine their equivalence to foods produced by traditional plant breeding. Labeling of foods containing GM ingredients is only required if the nutritional composition of the food has been altered; if it contains potentially harmful allergens, toxins, pesticides, or herbicides; if it contains ingredients that are new to the food supply; or if it has been changed significantly enough that its traditional name no longer applies. For example, if DNA from a Brazil nut—a food that commonly causes allergic reactions—were introduced into wheat, it would have to be labeled unless the manufacturer could prove the food does not cause allergies. To keep a regulatory eye on GM foods manufacturers must notify the FDA before putting GM foods on the market.

The USDA regulates GM crops The USDA regulates agricultural products and research concerning the development of new plant varieties. The Animal and Plant Health Inspection Service (APHIS) of the USDA helps to ensure that the cultivation of a new plant variety poses no risk to agricultural production or to the environment. For example, if there is a high probability that a new plant variety will crossbreed with a weed and that the transfer of the new trait could allow the weed plant to survive better, APHIS may not allow further development of this plant. If a plant has been studied and tested and does not pose environmental risks, field-testing is allowed. APHIS continues to oversee the testing until it is determined that the plant is safe.

The EPA regulates GM pesticides The EPA regulates any pesticides that may be present in foods and sets tolerance levels for these pesticides. This includes genetically modified plants containing proteins that protect them from insects or disease. The EPA assesses the safety of these proteins for human consumption, for other organisms, and for the environment.

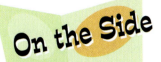

On the Side

Genetically modified foods look the same as other foods. The difficulty of tracking all genetically modified ingredients was brought to the public's attention in 2000 when genetically modified corn that had not been approved for human consumption was used to make taco shells. The product had to be recalled from grocery shelves. The taco shells caused no health problems but this incident served to highlight the fact that it is difficult to identify the presence of genetically modified ingredients and to segregate crops at all phases of food production.

THINKING FOR YOURSELF

1. How could contamination from one food spread throughout a picnic? After 67 people became ill from consuming food at a company picnic, investigators determined that the tossed salad, the egg salad, and the turkey slices were all contaminated with *Salmonella*. Invent a scenario that would explain how all three became contaminated.

2. Can your kitchen pass the food safety test? To find out go to www.foodsafety.gov/~fsg/kitchen.html. After you complete the exercise answer the following questions.
   a. Based on how you answered these questions, what changes should you make in the way you store and handle foods in your kitchen?
   b. Based on how you answered these questions, are there foods that you will eliminate from your diet? Why?

3. What are the risks and benefits for each scenario described below?
   a. A restaurant decides not to replace their old dishwasher even though it no longer heats the water to above 140° F.
   b. A town decides that they can improve the health of their citizens and the environment by banning the production and sale of all but organically produced foods.
   c. A new wheat variety that provides readily absorbable iron has been produced by genetic engineering. It is used to make bread and other bakery products that are consumed by almost everyone in the population.

SUMMARY

1. Most food-borne illness is caused by consuming food that has been contaminated by disease-causing microbes called pathogens; occasionally it can be caused by chemicals that find their way into our food. The harm caused by contaminants in the food supply depends on the type of toxin, the dose, the length of time over which it is consumed, and the size and health status of the consumer.

2. The food supply is monitored for safety by food manufacturers and regulatory agencies at the international, federal, state, and local levels. The National Food Safety Initiative was designed to coordinate all aspects of food safety from the farm to the table. It promotes the use of the HACCP system to prevent and eliminate food contamination rather than catching it after it occurs. Consumers can prevent most cases of food-borne illness by using safe food-handling procedures.

3. Most cases of food-borne illness involve a short bout of abdominal pain, nausea, diarrhea, and vomiting. Some bacteria cause food-borne infection because they are able to grow in the gastrointestinal tract when ingested. Others produce toxins in food and consumption of the toxin causes food-borne intoxication. Viruses consumed in food can also cause food-borne illness, as can toxins produced by molds that grow on foods, and parasites consumed in contaminated water or food.

4. The risk of food-borne illness can be decreased by proper food selection, preparation, and storage. Consumers should choose the freshest meats and produce, select frozen foods that do not contain frost or ice crystals, and avoid packages with broken seals or contents that appear spoiled. Foods prepared at home should be cooked thoroughly and leftovers stored properly. Kitchen surfaces, hands, and cooking utensils should be cleaned between preparation steps.

5. Contaminants such as pesticides applied to crops, drugs given to animals, and industrial wastes that leach into water may find their way into the food supply. Industrial pollutants such as PCBs, radioactive substances, and toxic metals have contaminated some waterways and the fish that live in them. Contaminants are found in the greatest concentration in foods of animal origin because animals are at the top of the food chain.

6. Pesticides help increase crop yields and the quality of produce. To decrease the potential risk of pesticides, safer ones are being developed and U.S. farmers are reducing the amounts applied by using integrated pest management and organic methods.

7. Consumers can reduce the amounts of pesticides and other environmental contaminants in food by careful selection and handling of produce; selection of low-fat saltwater varieties of fish caught well offshore in unpolluted waters; and trimming fat from meat, poultry, and fish before cooking.

8. Technology is used to prevent food spoilage and lengthen shelf life. Cold temperatures slow or prevent microbial growth. High temperatures used in canning, pasteurization, sterilization, and cooking kill microorganisms.

9. Irradiation preserves food by exposing it to radiation. This kills microorganisms, destroys insects, and slows the germination and ripening of fruits and vegetables.

10. Food additives include all substances that can reasonably be expected to find their way into a food during processing. This includes direct food additives, which are used to preserve or enhance the appeal of food, and indirect food additives, which are substances known to find their way into food during cooking, processing, and packaging. Direct and indirect food additives are regulated by the FDA. Accidental contaminants that enter food when it is used or prepared incorrectly are not regulated by the FDA.

11. Packaging also preserves foods. Aseptic processing sterilizes the food and the package; modified atmosphere packaging reduces the oxygen available for microbial growth.

12. Biotechnology produces genetically engineered plants, animals, and microorganisms that have the potential to improve the amount, safety, and quality of the food supply. However, there are some concerns with this new technology. Health concerns include the potential to introduce allergens or toxins into foods or to negatively affect nutrient content. Environmental concerns include the reduction of biologic diversity, the evolution of pesticide-resistant insects, and the creation of super weeds.

REVIEW QUESTIONS

1. What is the major cause of food-borne illness in the United States today?
2. List three factors that determine the likelihood that a contaminant will cause food-borne illness in an individual.
3. How is the federal government involved in providing a safe food supply?
4. How does HACCP differ from traditional methods of monitoring food safety?
5. List three common bacterial food contaminants. What can be done to avoid the food-borne illnesses caused by them?
6. What temperature range allows the most rapid bacterial growth?
7. Explain how cross-contamination can occur in home kitchens.
8. How do pesticides applied to crops find their way into animal products?

9. List some food-processing techniques that reduce food-borne illnesses.
10. What is the GRAS list?
11. What is food irradiation? Is it safe?

12. How does genetic engineering introduce new traits into plants?
13. List three benefits of food biotechnology and three potential risks.

REFERENCES

1. U.S. Department of Health and Human Services. National computer network in place to combat foodborne illness (press release). May 22, 1998. Available online at www.cdc.gov/od/oc/media/pressrel/r980522.htm/Accessed September 3, 2004.

2. Knabel, S. J. Institute of Food Technologists Scientific Status Summary: Foodborne illness: Role of home food handling practices. *Food Technol.* 49:119–131, 1995.

3. U.S. Food and Drug Administration, Center for Food Safety and Nutrition. Foodborne Pathogenic Microorganisms and Natural Toxins Handbook: The "Bad Bug Book." Available online at vm.cfsan.fda.gov/~mow/intro.html/Accessed August 1, 2004.

4. Infant Botulism—New York City 2001–2002. *MMWR* 52:21–24, January 17, 2003.

5. Centers for Disease Control and Prevention. Cryptospiridium fact sheet. Available online at www.cdc.gov/ncidod/dpd/parasites/cryptosporidiosis/factsht_cryptosporidiosis.htm/Accessed August 1, 2004.

6. National Research Council, Committee on Comparative Toxicology of Naturally Occurring Carcinogens. Individual chemicals in the diet generally pose no risk to Americans, NRC concludes. *Food Chem. News* 37:32–33, 1996.

7. U.S. Department of Agriculture. Agricultural Marketing Service. National Organic Program: Final Rule. Available online at www.ams.usda.gov/nop/nop2000/nop/finalrulepages/finalrulemap.htm/Accessed March 1, 2004.

8. U.S. Food and Drug Administration. Center for Veterinary Medicine, Communications and Education Branch. Monitoring for residues in food animals. Revised March 1994. Available online at www.fda.gov/cvm/index/memos/cvmm19.html/Accessed September 3, 2004.

9. Bren, L. Battle of the bugs: Fighting antibiotic resistance *FDA Consumer* 52:24–27, July 2003. Available online at www.fda.gov/fdac/features/2002/402_bugs.html/Accessed August 1, 2004.

10. Ropp, K. L. New animal drug increases milk production. *FDA Consumer* 28:24–27, May 1994. Available online at www.cfsan.fda.gov/~ear/BSTQUEST.html/Accessed August 1, 2004.

11. U.S. Department of Health and Human Services. Questions and answers about dioxin. Available online at www.cfsan.fda.gov/%7Elrd/dioxinqa.html/Accessed July 31, 2004.

12. U.S. Department of Health and Human Services and U.S. Environmental Protection Agency. What you need to know about mercury in fish and shellfish. EPA-823-R-04-005, March 2004. Available online at www.cfsan.fda.gov/~dms/admehg3.html/Accessed August 1, 2004.

13. U.S. General Accounting Office. Food irradiation: Available research indicates that benefits outweigh risks. Washington DC, August 2000. Available online at www.foodsafety.gov/~fsg/irradiat.html/Accessed September 3, 2004.

14. U.S. Food and Drug Administration. Food irradiation: A safe measure. January 2000. Available online at www.fda.gov/opacom/catalog/irradbro.html/Accessed August 1, 2004.

15. Eichholzer, M., and Gutzwiller, F. Dietary nitrates, nitrites, and N-nitroso compounds and cancer risk: A review of the epidemiologic evidence. *Nutr. Rev.* 56:95–105, 1998.

16. Smith, N. Seeds of opportunity: An assessment of the benefits, safety and oversight of plant genomics and agricultural biotechnology. U.S. House of Representatives Report. April 13, 2000. Available online at www.house.gov/science/documents.htm/Accessed September 3, 2004.

17. National Academy of Sciences, National Research Council. *Genetically Modified Pest-Protected Plants: Science and Regulation.* Washington, DC: National Academy Press, 2000.

18. Thompson, L. Are bioengineered foods safe? *FDA Consumer* 18–23, January/February 2000.

19. Bren, L. Genetic engineering: The future of foods? *FDA Consumer* November/December 2003. Available online at www.fda.gov/fdac/features/2003/603_food.html/Accessed September 17, 2004.

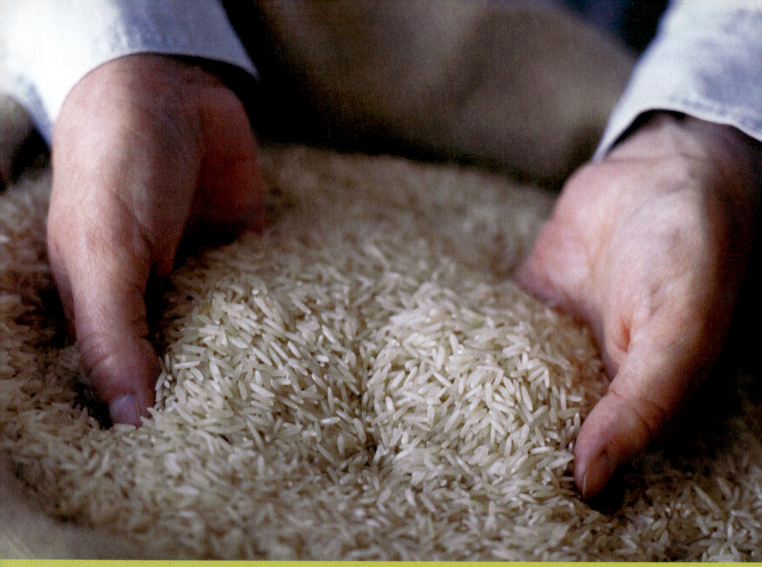

(Joann Frederick/Age Fotostock America, Inc.)

CHAPTER 15 CONCEPTS

- There are two faces of malnutrition in the world today—overnutrition from too much of the wrong foods and undernutrition from too little of the right foods.
- Undernutrition is primarily a problem in developing countries where a cycle of malnutrition produces poorly nourished children who grow into unhealthy adults.
- Undernutrition can be caused by food shortages, which are due to an imbalance between the number of people and the resources available to feed them.
- Undernutrition can be caused by poor-quality diets, especially in people with high nutrient needs.
- Preventing undernutrition involves short-term relief to feed the hungry and long-term policies that work to balance the number of people with available resources.
- In the United States, the majority of the population is at risk for overnutrition, but some segments also suffer from undernutrition.
- Solutions to hunger at home involve providing access to affordable food, education, and medical care.

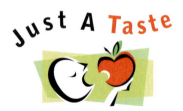

Just A Taste

Is obesity a problem in developing countries?

Is there enough food to feed the world?

Do environmental issues affect nutrition?

Is hunger a problem in the United States?

Feeding the World

15

INTRODUCTION

Times News Network

Diabetes, Obesity Haunt Slum-Dwellers: Study

Saturday, Apr. 10, 2004—There was a time when diabetes mellitus and obesity were regarded as lifestyle diseases of the rich. But a study among slum-dwellers by AIIMS has shattered that myth.

The three-year-long study is a part of a larger study on migrant Indian populations the world over. It deals with inter- and intra-country migration and nearly 550 slum-dwellers who had migrated to Delhi from Haryana, UP and Rajasthan . . . [who] were surveyed for signs of diabetes mellitus, obesity and high blood cholesterol levels. Ten percent of the surveyed population had diabetes, 11% was suffering from hypertension, more than 25% had excess body fat and 27% had high levels of cholesterol. Dr. Anoop Misra, professor of medicine, AIIMS, said: "The findings were startling because all of them had migrated to the city from villages where the incidence of all these diseases has been found to be less than 1%."

To read the entire article, go to www.timesofindia.indiatimes.com/cms. dll/html/uncomp/articleshow?msid=609154

The image we have of slum dwellers—especially from third world countries, is that they are under-nourished and underweight. Diabetes and hypertension are problems for overweight Westerners, not the poor of the developing world. Yet, the rising incidence of these diseases of overconsumption in slum dwellers in India is not an isolated phenomenon. More and more, as diets in developing countries shift toward more Western-style meal patterns that are higher in meat and fat and lower in plant foods, people are beginning to suffer from diabetes, high blood pressure, obesity, and high blood cholesterol. The focus of feeding the world's hungry has shifted from simply providing food to providing the right foods to keep people healthy today and in the future.

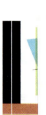

One c
concerr
animal
destroy
water. 7
produce
argume
animals
on how
thousar
grazed
efficien
family f
impact

On a
kitchen
turn the
contribu
agribusi
scraps. 7
animals
have go
plant m
cow and
1 pound
and cost
the tota
In the U
to anim
gallons
The wor
land to
America

Mana
environr
local fiel
a small a
pollute r
overgrov
pollutioi
gases tha
to acid r

The s
to the er
grazing
continue
Amazon
cattle. Fc
deforesta
atmosph

SUMMARY

1. Overnutrition coexists with undernutrition in both developed and developing nations around the world. The underlying cause of world hunger is that the food available in the world is not distributed equitably. The reason for the growing problem of overnutrition is the change in diet and lifestyle to a more Western pattern that occurs in developing nations as economic conditions improve.

2. In poorly nourished populations, a cycle of malnutrition exists in which malnourished women give birth to low-birth-weight infants at risk of disease and early death. If these children survive, they grow into adults who are physically unable to fully contribute to society. In populations where malnutrition is prevalent low-birth-weight, infant mortality, stunting, and infections are more common.

3. Hunger and undernutrition occur when there is a shortage of food. Famine is an example of a short-term food shortage that occurs when food production and distribution are disrupted. Chronic food shortage occurs when economic inequities result in lack of money, health care, and education for individuals or populations; when overpopulation and limited natural resources create a situation in which there are more people than food; when environmental resources are misused, limiting the ability to continue to produce food; and when cultural practices limit food choices.

4. Malnutrition also occurs when the available diet does not contain adequate nutrients. High-risk groups with special nutrient needs, such as pregnant women, children, the elderly, and the ill, may not be able to meet their nutrient

needs by consuming this diet. Deficiencies of protein, iron, iodine, and vitamin A are common worldwide.

5. Short-term solutions to undernutrition provide food through relief at the local, national, and international levels. Long-term solutions include control of population growth, economic and agricultural policies that promote self-sufficiency and alleviate poverty, improvements in the quality of the food supply, and the development of sustainable systems that will provide food without damaging the environment.

6. Food fortification and dietary supplementation can be used to increase protein quality, alleviate micronutrient deficiencies, and improve the overall quality of the diet.

7. New crops and food products can be produced using biotechnology. These genetically engineered products increase crop yields, improve insect resistance, and enhance the nutrient content of foods.

8. Both undernutrition and overnutrition are problems in the United States. As in developing nations, undernutrition and food insecurity are associated with poverty. The homeless, women, children, the elderly, and minority groups are most often food-insecure.

9. Nutrition programs in the United States focus on maintaining a nutrition safety net that will provide access to affordable food and promote healthy eating in the United States. Some programs designed to help feed the hungry address the general population, whereas others focus on specific high-risk groups. Most programs provide access to food and some provide nutrition education.

REVIEW QUESTIONS

1. Why is overnutrition a concern around the world?
2. What is the cycle of malnutrition?
3. How does poverty contribute to world hunger?
4. What happens to birth rates when education and income level increase?
5. How does overpopulation contribute to food shortage?
6. What segments of the world population are at greatest risk for undernutrition?
7. List three micronutrient deficiencies that are world health problems.

8. Why are environmental issues important in maintaining the world's food supply?
9. How does sustainable agriculture reduce environmental damage?
10. How can food fortification be used to help eliminate malnutrition?
11. List four population subgroups in the United States that are at risk for undernutrition.
12. List three federal programs that address malnutrition in the United States.

REFERENCES

1. Bread for the World Institute. Hunger Basics: International Facts on Hunger and Poverty. Available online at www.bread.org/hungerbasics/international.html/Accessed May 6, 2004.
2. Vorster, H. H., Bourne, L. T., Venter, C. S., and Oosthuizen, W. Contribution of nutrition to the health transition in developing countries: A framework for research and intervention. *Nutr. Rev.* 57:341–349, 1999.
3. American Dietetic Association. Addressing world hunger and malnutrition and food insecurity. *J. Am. Diet. Assoc.* 103:1046–1057, 2003.

4. Infant Mortality Rates. Available online at www.geographyiq.com/ranking/ranking_Infant_Mortality_Rate_aall.htm/ Accessed April 28, 2004.
5. UNICEF End Decade Report on Malnutrition. Available online at www.childinfo.org/eddb/malnutrition/Accessed April 28, 2004.
6. Are We on Track to End Hunger? Hunger Report 2004. Bread for the World Institute. Available online at www.bread.org/institute/hunger_report/index.html/ Accessed May 7, 2004.

7. World Health Organization. Micronutrient deficiencies. Battling iron deficiency anaemia. Available online at www.who.int/nut/ida.htm/Accessed April 28, 2004.

8. World Health Organization. Micronutrient deficiencies. Eliminating iodine deficiency disorders: The challenge. Available online at www.who.int/nut/idd.htm/Accessed May 7, 2004.

9. World Health Organization. Micronutrient deficiencies. Combating vitamin A deficiency: The challenge. Available online at www.who.int/nut/vad.htm/Accessed May 7, 2004.

10. Raven, P. H., Berg, L. R., and Aliff, J. *Environment*, 4th ed. Hoboken: John Wiley & Sons, 2003.

11. Matson, P. A., Parton, W. J., Power, A. G., and Swift, M. J. Agricultural intensification and ecosystem properties. *Science* 277:504–509, 1997.

12. Ye, X., Al-Babili, S., Kloti, A., et al. Engineering the provitamin A (beta-carotene) biosynthetic pathway into (carotenoid-free) rice endosperm. *Science* 287:303–305, 2000.

13. Shintani, D., and DellaPenna, D. Elevating the vitamin E content of plants through metabolic engineering. *Science* 282:2098–2100, 1998.

14. Obesity and Overweight: A Public Health Epidemic. Centers for Disease Control and Prevention. Available online at www.cdc.gov/nccdphp/dnpa/obesity/index.htm/Accessed March 20, 2004.

15. American Dietetic Association. Domestic food and nutrition security. *J. Am. Diet. Assoc.* 102:1840–1847, 2002.

16. America's Second Harvest, Current Hunger and Poverty Statistics. Available online at www.secondharvest.org/site_content.asp?s=59#1/Accessed May 17, 2004.

17. Centers for Disease Control and Prevention. Deaths: Final data for 2001. National Vital Statistics Report Vol. 52, No. 3, September 18, 2003. Available online at www.cdc.gov/nchs/data/nvsr/nvsr52/nvsr52_03.pdf/Accessed September 22, 2004.

18. Native Economic Development Guidance and Empowerment. Available online at www.occ.treas.gov/cdd/edge.pdf/Accessed May 18, 2004.

19. Variyam, J. N., Blaylock, J., and Smallwood, D. U.S. Department of Agriculture. USDA's Healthy Eating Index and Nutrition Information. Economic Research Service. No. 1866, May 1998. Available online at www.ers.usda.gov/publications/TB1866/Accessed September 22, 2004.

ADDITIONAL DRI TABLES
All other DRI tables are included in the front and back covers of this text

Dietary Reference Intakes: Recommended Intakes for Individuals: Essential Amino Acids

Life Stage Group	Histidine (mg/kg/day)	Isoleucine (mg/kg/day)	Leucine (mg/kg/day)	Lysine (mg/kg/day)	Methionine + Cysteine (mg/kg/day)	Phenylalanine + Tyrosine (mg/kg/day)	Threonine (mg/kg/day)	Tryptophan (mg/kg/day)	Valine (mg/kg/day)
Infants									
0–6 mo*	23	88	156	107	59	135	73	28	87
7–12 mo	32	43	93	89	43	84	49	13	58
Children									
1–3 y	21	28	63	58	28	54	32	8	37
4–8 y	16	22	49	46	22	41	24	6	28
Males									
9–13 y	17	22	49	46	22	41	24	6	28
14–18 y	15	21	47	43	21	38	22	6	27
19–30 y	14	19	42	38	19	33	20	5	24
31–50 y	14	19	42	38	19	33	20	5	24
51–70 y	14	19	42	38	19	33	20	5	24
> 70 y	14	19	42	38	19	33	20	5	24
Females									
9–13 y	15	21	47	43	21	38	22	6	27
14–18 y	14	19	44	40	19	35	21	5	24
19–30 y	14	19	42	38	19	33	20	5	24
31–50 y	14	19	42	38	19	33	20	5	24
51–70 y	14	19	42	38	19	33	20	5	24
> 70 y	14	19	42	38	19	33	20	5	24
Pregnancy	18	25	56	51	25	44	26	7	31
Lactation	19	30	62	52	26	51	30	9	35

*Values for this age group are AI (Adequate Intakes).

Source: Institute of Medicine, Food and Nutrition Board "Dietary Reference Intakes for Energy, Carbohydrates, Fiber, Fat, Protein and Amino Acids." Washington, DC: National Academy Press, 2002.

1983 Metropolitan Life Insurance Co. Height and Weight Tables

Height	Small Frame	Medium Frame	Large Frame
		lb	
Men*			
5'2"	128–134	131–141	138–150
5'3"	130–136	133–143	140–153
5'4"	132–138	135–145	142–156
5'5"	134–140	137–148	144–160
5'6"	136–142	139–151	146–164
5'7"	138–145	142–154	149–168
5'8"	140–148	145–157	152–172
5'9"	142–151	148–160	155–176
5'10"	144–154	151–163	158–180
5'11"	146–157	154–166	161–184
6'0"	149–160	157–170	164–188
6'1"	152–164	160–174	168–192
6'2"	155–168	164–178	172–197
6'3"	158–172	167–182	176–202
6'4"	162–176	171–187	181–207
Women†			
4'10"	102–111	109–121	118–131
4'11"	103–113	111–123	120–134
5'0"	104–115	113–126	122–137
5'1"	106–118	115–129	125–140
5'2"	108–121	118–132	128–143
5'3"	111–124	121–135	131–147
5'4"	114–127	124–138	134–151
5'5"	117–130	127–141	137–155
5'6"	120–133	130–144	140–159
5'7"	123–136	133–147	143–163
5'8"	126–139	136–150	146–167
5'9"	129–142	139–153	149–170
5'10"	132–145	142–156	152–173
5'11"	135–148	145–159	155–176
6'0"	138–151	148–162	158–179

*Weights at ages 25 to 59 based on lowest mortality. Weight in pounds according to frame (in indoor clothing weighing 5 lb, shoes with 1" heels).

†Weights at ages 25 to 59 based on lowest mortality. Weight in pounds according to frame (in indoor clothing weighing 3 lb, shoes with 1" heels).

Source: Courtesy of Metropolitan Life Insurance Company.

Birth to 36 months: Girls
Length-for-age and Weight-for-age percentiles

NAME ———————————————

RECORD # ——————————

AGE (MONTHS)

Birth   3   6   9   12   15   18   21   24   27   30   33   36

LENGTH

WEIGHT

95
90
75
50
25
10
5

Mother's Stature ——————————
Father's Stature ——————————
Gestational Age: ———— Weeks

Date	Age	Weight	Length	Head Circ.	Comment
	Birth				

Published May 30, 2000 (modified 4/20/01).

Source: Developed by the National Center for Health Statistics in collaboration with the National Center for Chronic Disease Prevention and Health Promotion (2000). www.cdc.gov/growthcharts

SAFER · HEALTHIER · PEOPLE™

Birth to 36 months: Boys
Length-for-age and Weight-for-age percentiles

NAME _____

RECORD # _____

AGE (MONTHS)

Birth   3   6   9   12   15   18   21   24   27   30   33   36

LENGTH

95
90
75
50
25
10
5

WEIGHT

95
90
75
50
25
10
5

AGE (MONTHS)

12   15   18   21   24   27   30   33   36

Mother's Stature _____			Gestational		
Father's Stature _____			Age: _____ Weeks		Comment
Date	Age	Weight	Length	Head Circ.	
	Birth				

Birth   3   6   9

Published May 30, 2000 (modified 4/20/01).

Source: Developed by the National Center for Health Statistics in collaboration with the National Center for Chronic Disease Prevention and Health Promotion (2000). www.cdc.gov/growthcharts

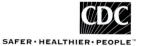

CDC

SAFER · HEALTHIER · PEOPLE™